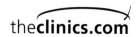

OTOLARYNGOLOGIC CLINICS OF NORTH AMERICA

Phonosurgery

GUEST EDITOR
Gregory A. Grillone, MD, FACS

February 2006 • Volume 39 • Number 1

SAUNDERS

An Imprint of Elsevier, Inc.
PHILADELPHIA   LONDON   TORONTO   MONTREAL   SYDNEY   TOKYO

W.B. SAUNDERS COMPANY
A Division of Elsevier Inc.

1600 John F. Kennedy Boulevard, Suite 1800, Philadelphia, PA 19103–2899

http://www.theclinics.com

THE OTOLARYNGOLOGIC CLINICS	Volume 39, Number 1
OF NORTH AMERICA	ISSN 0030–6665
February 2006	ISBN 1-4160-3376-9
Editor: Molly Jay	

The ideas and opinions expressed in *The Otolaryngologic Clinics of North America* do not necessarily reflect those of the Publisher. The Publisher does not assume any responsibility for any injury and/or damage to persons or property arising out of or related to any use of the material contained in this periodical. The reader is advised to check the appropriate medical literature and the product information currently provided by the manufacturer of each drug to be administered to verify the dosage, the method and duration of administration, or contraindications. It is the responsibility of the treating physician or other health care professional, relying on independent experience and knowledge of the patient, to determine drug dosages and the best treatment for the patient. Mention of any product in this issue should not be construed as endorsement by the contributors, editors, or the Publisher of the product or manufacturers' claims.

The Otolaryngologic Clinics of North America (ISSN 0030–6665) is published bimonthly by W.B. Saunders, 360 Park Avenue South, New York, NY 10010-1710. Months of publication are February, April, June, August, October, and December. Business and Editorial Offices: 1600 John F. Kennedy Blvd., Suite 1800, Philadelphia, PA 19103-2899. Accounting and Circulation Offices: 6277 Sea Harbor Drive, Orlando, FL 32887-4800. Periodicals postage paid at New York, NY and additional mailing offices. Subscription price is $205.00 per year (US individuals), $370.00 per year (US institutions), $100.00 per year (US student/resident), $270.00 per year (Canadian individuals), $455.00 per year (Canadian institutions), $285.00 per year (international individuals), $455.00 per year (international institutions), $145.00 per year (international & Canadian student/resident). Foreign air speed delivery is included in all *Clinics'* subscription prices. All prices are subject to change without notice. **POSTMASTER:** Send address changes to *The Otolaryngologic Clinics of North America*, Elsevier Periodicals Customer Service, 6277 Sea Harbor Drive, Orlando, FL 32887-4800. **Customer Service: 1-800-654-2452 (US). From outside the US, call 407-345-4000.**

The Otolaryngologic Clinics of North America is also published in Spanish by McGraw-Hill Interamericana Editores S.A., P.O. Box 5-237, 06500 Mexico D.F., Mexico.

The Otolaryngologic Clinics of North America is covered in *Index Medicus, Current Contents/Clinical Medicine, Excerpta Medica, BIOSIS, Science Citation Index,* and *ISI/BIOMED.*

Printed in the United States of America.

GUEST EDITOR

GREGORY A. GRILLONE, MD, FACS, Associate Professor and Vice Chairman; Director, Center for Voice and Swallowing Disorders, Department of Otolaryngology-Head and Neck Surgery, Boston University Medical Center, Boston, Massachusetts

CONTRIBUTORS

JENNIFER G. ANDRUS, MD, Resident, Department of Otolaryngology-Head & Neck Surgery, Boston Medical Center, Boston, Massachusetts

AMINDRA S. ARORA, MBBChir, Assistant Professor, Department of Gastroenterology, Mayo Clinic College of Medicine, Rochester, Minnesota

GERALD S. BERKE, MD, Professor, Division of Head and Neck Surgery, University of California Los Angeles Medical Center, Los Angeles, California

ANDREA BOLZONI, MD, Department of Otolaryngology, University of Brescia, Brescia, Italy

JAMES A. BURNS, MD, FACS, Assistant Professor, Harvard Medical School; Surgeon, Center for Laryngeal Surgery and Voice Rehabilitation, Massachusetts General Hospital, Boston, Massachusetts

TERESA CHAN, MD, Resident, Department of Otolaryngology-Head and Neck Surgery, Boston University Medical Center, Boston, Massachusetts

DINESH K. CHHETRI, MD, Assistant Professor, Division of Head and Neck Surgery, University of California Los Angeles Medical Center, Los Angeles, California

SETH H. DAILEY, MD, Assistant Professor, Division of Otolaryngology-Head and Neck Surgery, Department of Surgery, University of Wisconsin School of Medicine, University of Wisconsin Hospital and Clinics, Madison, Wisconsin

EILEEN H. DAUER, MD, Staff Physician, Department of Otolaryngology-Head and Neck Surgery, Malcolm Grown Medical Center, Andrews Air Force Base, Maryland

CHARLES N. FORD, MD, Professor and Chairman, Division of Otolaryngology-Head and Neck Surgery, Department of Surgery, University of Wisconsin School of Medicine, University of Wisconsin Hospital and Clinics, Madison, Wisconsin

GREGORY A. GRILLONE, MD, FACS, Associate Professor and Vice Chairman; Director, Center for Voice and Swallowing Disorders, Department of Otolaryngology-Head and Neck Surgery, Boston University Medical Center, Boston, Massachusetts

JACQUES JAMART, MD, Center for Statistics and Scientific Documentation, University Hospital of Louvain at Mont-Godinne, Yvoir, Belgium

GEORGES LAWSON, MD, Department of ORL-Head & Neck Surgery, University Hospital of Louvain at Mont-Godinne, Yvoir, Belgium

HANS F. MAHIEU, MD, PhD, Professor of Otolaryngology, Department of Otolaryngology/Head and Neck Surgery, Vrije Universiteit Medical Center, Amsterdam, The Netherlands; Otolaryngologist, Otolaryngology Group Sonoor, Meander Medical Center, Amersfoort, The Netherlands

DOMINIQUE MORSOMME, Speech Th, Department of ORL-Head & Neck Surgery, University Hospital of Louvain at Mont-Godinne, Yvoir, Belgium

J. PIETER NOORDZIJ, MD, Clinical Instructor, Department of Otolaryngology-Head and Neck Surgery, Vanderbilt University Medical Center, Nashville, Tennessee

MIRIAM A. O'LEARY, MD, Resident, Department of Otolaryngology–Head and Neck Surgery, Boston University Medical Center, Boston, Massachusetts

ROBERT H. OSSOFF, DMD, MD, Professor and Chairman, Department of Otolaryngology, Vanderbilt University Medical Center, Nashville, Tennessee

CESARE PIAZZA, MD, Department of Otolaryngology, University of Brescia, Brescia, Italy

GIORGIO PERETTI, MD, Department of Otolaryngology, University of Brescia, Brescia, Italy

MARC REMACLE, MD, PhD, Department of ORL-Head & Neck Surgery, University Hospital of Louvain at Mont-Godinne, Yvoir, Belgium

YVONNE ROMERO, MD, Assistant Professor, Department of Gastroenterology, Mayo Clinic College of Medicine, Rochester, Minnesota

STANLEY M. SHAPSHAY, MD, FACS, Professor, Department of Otolaryngology-Head & Neck Surgery, Mount Sinai School of Medicine, New York, New York

JEFFREY H. SPIEGEL, MD, FACS, Chief, Facial Plastic and Reconstructive Surgery; Associate Professor, Department of Otolaryngology-Head and Neck Surgery, Boston University School of Medicine, Boston, Massachusetts

DANA M. THOMPSON, MD, Associate Professor, Department of Otorhinolaryngology, Mayo Clinic College of Medicine; Chair, Division of Pediatric Otolaryngology, Mayo Clinic College of Medicine, Rochester, Minnesota

PEAK WOO, MD, FACS, Professor, Department of Otolaryngology, Mount Sinai School of Medicine, The Grabscheid Voice Center, Mount Sinai Medical Center, New York, New York

STEVEN M. ZEITELS, MD, FACS, Eugene B. Casey Chair of Laryngeal Surgery, Harvard Medical School; Director, Center for Laryngeal Surgery and Voice Rehabilitation, Massachusetts General Hospital, Boston, Massachusetts

CONTENTS

and disturb the viscoelastic properties that are essential for vocal fold function. Sulcus vocalis is a specific example of vocal fold scarring, and it presents the same essential challenge in restoration of function. Vocal fold scar and sulcus vocalis share glottic insufficiency, breathy voice quality, and resistance to tissue alteration as hallmarks. Multiple surgical strategies have been devised to help improve vocal fold closure and pliability. The approaches are open and endoscopic, conceptually direct or indirect, and may or may not involve direct tissue implantation to the vocal fold cover. Specific commentary is provided regarding these different surgical techniques. Future treatment pathways are explored.

Injection laryngoplasty has developed from decades of experience by otolaryngologists, yet continues to offer exciting opportunities and breakthroughs. Indications for this treatment have expanded widely, and now including a large variety of voice disorders. Likewise, new materials are emerging continually in the field to accommodate these increasing indications. As innovative techniques are developed, more and more patients will benefit from injection laryngoplasty in the future. This article discusses available and investigational materials, indications, and techniques for injection laryngoplasty.

Laryngeal framework surgery (LFS) procedures enable functionally monitored correction of vocal-fold position as well as vocal-fold tension, without jeopardizing the delicate structure of the vocal folds, producing good results with few and usually minor complications. Modern phonosurgery requires versatile surgeons to adequately comply with the demands of dysphonic patients. The different types of LFS are rewarding but occasionally demanding procedures, which should be part of the armamentarium of the phonosurgeon.

Many procedures for pitch alteration have been developed. This chapter reviews current techniques and their possible value in adjusting vocal pitch.

Laryngeal dystonia (spasmodic dysphonia) is a focal dystonia that affects laryngeal motor control. There are four major types:

adductor, abductor, mixed type, and adductor laryngeal breathing dystonia. Over the past 20 years, major advances have been made in the diagnosis, evaluation, and treatment of spasmodic dysphonia. The genetic and neurologic origins of spasmodic dysphonia and other dystonias are being sought actively, and will lead to further advances in treatment. Botulinum toxin remains the most safe and effective treatment of symptoms of adductor and abductor spasmodic dysphonia.

Spasmodic dysphonia (SD) is a voice disorder characterized by abnormal intermittent spasms of intralaryngeal muscles, resulting in voice breaks during speech. Patients who have SD typically have no other associated chronic medical problems or handicaps and are highly functioning individuals, but they perceive their voice significantly limits them functionally, physically, and emotionally. One main hurdle toward achieving a cure for SD is that the cause and pathophysiology of SD remain unclear; there are no animal models for this disorder. What is known from laryngoscopic and electromyographic examinations is that voice breaks in SD are associated with abnormal electrical activity of the laryngeal nerves, resulting in increased muscle movements. This article focuses on the surgical management of the adductor variant of spasmodic dysphonia by selective laryngeal adductor denervation and reinnervation.

This article outlines the procedures that are amenable to being performed under local anesthesia in the general otolaryngologist's office. These procedures can be performed without a lot of expensive equipment and can be done with existing diagnostic equipment that is supplemented by a few simple instruments. This article gives details about the technique of office anesthesia, and the necessary office equipment and instruments.

Occurring in children and adults, recurrent respiratory papillomatosis (RRP) is the most common neoplasm in humans. Although benign, malignant transformation of these human papillomavirus-associated lesions is well documented, but rare. More commonly, RRP can be life threatening because of airway obstruction from growth and proliferation of the papilloma lesions. Successful long-term eradication of RRP lesions is unreliable; however, there has been some improvement in reducing the number and frequency of procedures that require general anesthesia through the use of adjuvant treatments and in-office procedures.

Laser Applications in Laryngology: Past, Present, and Future

Steven M. Zeitels and James A. Burns

Since their introduction in laryngology over 30 years ago, lasers have facilitated critically important innovations. These advances accommodated well to otolaryngology, which has led in minimally invasive surgical approaches since mirror-guided interventions in the nineteenth century. The lasers discussed in this article will provide new platform technologies that will likely lead to enhanced treatment of a number of benign and malignant laryngeal disorders. There is an expanding group of centers in which fiber-based technologies have already caused many procedures to be performed by means of local anesthesia in the clinic or office, especially for chronic diseases such as papillomatosis and dysplasia. This approach is likely to expand significantly because of the diminished patient morbidity along with socioeconomic pressures of health care delivery.

Endoscopic Treatment for Early Glottic Cancer: Indications and Oncologic Outcome

Giorgio Peretti, Cesare Piazza, and Andrea Bolzoni

The authors' treatment approach for the comprehensive management of early glottic cancer can be divided into two basic therapeutic scenarios. Tis and T1a lesions of the midcord are treated preferably by an excisional biopsy, which, after appropriate pre- and intraoperative diagnostic work-up, allows precise diagnosis and definitive treatment of these lesions. This approach is associated with minimal morbidity, short hospitalization time, and a high cost-effectiveness ratio. Moreover, the postoperative voice has been shown to be comparable to that of controls because most of the vocalis muscle is preserved. On the other hand, T1b and T2 tumors deserve special attention because comparable oncologic outcomes may be seen with other therapeutic modalities. Therefore, appropriate preoperative counseling, including other voice-sparing options (eg, radiation or chemoradiation therapy) should always be part of the informed consent discussion.

Reconstruction of Glottic Defects after Endoscopic Cordectomy: Voice Outcome

Marc Remacle, Georges Lawson, Dominique Morsomme, and Jacques Jamart

Although there is no linear correlation between the amount of tissue removed and vocal outcome, a significant glottic gap that persists after endoscopic cordectomy may lead to poor voice quality. Development of thick and sometimes partially stenosing synechia at the anterior commissure also is a major factor that leads to poor voice result after extended cordectomy. Medialization thyroplasty for correction of glottic gap, transoral placement of a keel after laser-assisted section, and topical application of mitomycin-C for anterior glottic synechiae are effective procedures for managing glottic abnormalities after endoscopic cordectomy. This article focuses on our experience with the management of glottic gaps and anterior commissure synechiae, including patient selection, surgical technique, and outcome.

Eosinophilic esophagitis (EE) is a unique clinicopathologic entity that has slowly gained attention over the past decade but has not been well recognized in the field of otolaryngology. The precise cause of the disease is not known but is likely associated with food and environmental allergic antigens. Otolaryngologists should be familiar with the presentation because many patients experience concomitant pharyngolaryngeal and airway symptoms. As the otolaryngologist's role in the evaluation and management of esophageal disease continues to expand, it will be imperative to consider EE as a potential diagnosis among young children with feeding disorders and adolescents and adults with dysphagia. Esophagoscopy, with biopsies of the proximal, mid, and distal esophagus are essential tests for diagnosing EE, and food allergy testing may be helpful in identifying possible causative agents that should be restricted or eliminated.

FORTHCOMING ISSUES

RECENT ISSUES

The Clinics are now available online!

Access your subscription at
www.theclinics.com

Otolaryngol Clin N Am
39 (2006) xi–xii

OTOLARYNGOLOGIC
CLINICS
OF NORTH AMERICA

Preface

Phonosurgery

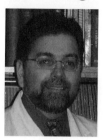

Gregory A. Grillone, MD, FACS
Guest Editor

Laryngeal and voice disorders can affect anyone regardless of age, sex, or social status. Altered or complete loss of voice can have devastating effects on an individual's ability to work, social interaction, and lifestyle. The field of laryngology began in the mid-nineteenth century after Garcia's description of mirror laryngoscopy. The term *phonosurgery* was coined in the early 1960s by Hans von Leden and refers to surgical procedures designed primarily to restore normal voice quality. Although there have been many advances in both laryngology and phonosurgery, these fields are still evolving. Many changes have occurred even since the last issue of the *Otolaryngologic Clinics of North America* devoted to this topic 5 years ago.

Although this issue cannot cover all areas of laryngology and phonosurgery, I selected topics that I believe are of significance to current practice, such as office-based laryngeal procedures and new laser applications in laryngology. I also selected topics that I believe represent the greatest challenges, such as the management of vocal fold scar and sulcus vocalis. To obtain a broader perspective, I invited some of our European colleagues to contribute articles, including Giorgio Peretti from Italy, Marc Remacle from Belgium, and Hans Mahieu from The Netherlands. It is my hope that readers will find this issue both informative and practical.

I am grateful to all of the authors for contributing their time and expertise to this issue of the *Otolaryngologic Clinics of North America*. I would also like to thank Elsevier for the opportunity to participate in the creation of this issue, particularly Molly Jay for her editorial assistance. I also wish to acknowledge my early mentors in laryngology, including Stuart Strong,

doi:10.1016/j.otc.2005.11.013

Charles Vaughan, and Stanley Shapshay, as well as several colleagues who have influenced me greatly, including Steven Zeitels and Jamie Koufman. Finally, and most importantly, I would like to dedicate this issue to my wife Diane and my children Gregory James and Deanna Rose for their constant support and patience.

Gregory A. Grillone, MD, FACS
Center for Voice and Swallowing Disorders
Department of Otolaryngology–Head and Neck Surgery
Boston University Medical Center
88 East Newton Street, D-616
Boston, MA 02118, USA

E-mail address: gregory.grillone@bmc.org

ELSEVIER
SAUNDERS

Otolaryngol Clin N Am
39 (2006) 1–10

OTOLARYNGOLOGIC
CLINICS
OF NORTH AMERICA

Anatomy and Physiology of the Larynx

J. Pieter Noordzij, MD*, Robert H. Ossoff, DMD, MD

*Vanderbilt Voice Center, Department of Otolaryngology, 7302 Medical Center East,
South Tower 1215, 21st Avenue South, Nashville, TN 37232-8783, USA*

Assessing the function of vocal folds begins with a thorough understanding of vocal fold anatomy (histologic and gross) and physiology. This knowledge is important not only in understanding normal vibratory behavior, but it is also critical in appreciating how alterations in normal structure will adversely affect vibratory behavior and thereby voice. This article covers the latest understanding in vocal fold anatomy and physiology that would be relevant to the practicing otolaryngologist.

Histologic anatomy

One key to understanding the vocal fold anatomy is to focus on vocal fold histology. The covering of the free edge of the vocal fold is especially adapted for phonatory vibration. This vocal fold epithelium is squamous rather than respiratory and contains no mucous glands [1]. The arrangement of connective tissue within the vocal fold allows the mucous membrane to undulate with minimal restriction from the underlying vocalis muscle.

Histologically, the vocal fold consists of five layers (Fig. 1):

1. The squamous epithelium layer of the mucosa is very thin and helps to hold the shape of the vocal fold. There are no mucous glands located within this epithelium; therefore, mucoserous secretions covering the vocal fold must travel from glands located superiorly, inferiorly, anteriorly, and posteriorly to the edge of the membranous vocal fold.
2. The superficial layer of the lamina propria consists primarily of loose fibers and matrix. Clinically, it is referred to as Reinke's space. This layer has the lowest concentration of both elastic and collagenous fibers. It offers the least resistance to vibration and can be thought of as a soft

* Corresponding author.
E-mail address: jpnoordzij@pol.net (J.P. Noordzij).

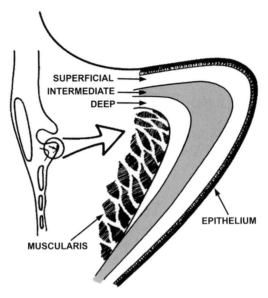

Fig. 1. The three layers of the lamina propria of the vocal fold. (*From* Gray SD, Dove H, Bie-lamowicz SA, et al. Experimental approaches to vocal fold alteration introduction to the mini-thyrotomy. Ann Otol Rhinol Laryngol 1999;108:2; with permission.)

    gelatinous mass. This layer, in particular, is vital for proper phonatory function.

3. The intermediate layer of the lamina propria also consists of elastic and collagenous fibers but at a higher concentration than the superficial layer of the lamina propria.

4. The deep layer of the lamina propria consists primarily of a high concentration of collagen bundles. This deep layer is dense and fibrous and together with the intermediate layer forms the vocal ligament. The vocal ligament is the uppermost portion of the conus elasticus. Some collagenous fibers of the deep layer of the lamina propria insert into the muscle fibers of the vocalis muscle. The intermediate and deep layers are not easily separated.

5. The vocalis (also known as thyroarytenoid) muscle provides the main mass of the vocal fold. The muscle fibers run parallel to the free edge of the vocal fold.

    The vocal fold histologic characteristics described above are fairly consistent along the length of the vocal fold with the following exceptions: at the anterior-most portion of the vocal fold there is a mass of collagenous fibers known as the anterior commisure tendon or Broyle's tendon. These fibers are attached to the inner thyroid perichondrium. The intermediate layer of the lamina propria is thickened at the anterior and posterior ends of the membranous vocal fold. These regions are known as the anterior and posterior macula flava. These structures serve as a transition zone between the stiff thyroid and arytenoid cartilage and the pliable membranous vocal fold. These structures may cushion the vocal folds and provide protection from mechanical damage caused by vibration [2].

The vocal fold epidermis is secured to the superficial lamina propria through the basement membrane zone [3]. The basement membrane zone is a collection of protein and nonprotein structures that, together, help the basal cells of the epidermis secure themselves to the rather amorphous mass of proteins present in the lamina propria. The basal cells have anchoring filaments and fibers that attach themselves to laminar proteins in the lamina propria (Fig. 2). This delicate and flexible anchoring system allows the primarily cellular epidermis to adhere to the amorphous and gelatinous lamina propria.

Any disruption in this anchoring system can have serious consequences in voice production. For example, the number of anchoring fibers per unit area appears to be genetically determined [4]. A person with fewer anchoring fibers might be predisposed to the development of vocal fold nodules [3].

The lamina propria of the vocal fold can be categorized by its cellular and noncellular (or extracellular) components [3]. The lamina propria contains a variety of important cells including fibroblasts, myofibroblasts, and macrophages. Macrophages are found in higher concentrations just below the basement membrane zone and in the superficial layer of the lamina propria. Their location suggests that these cells are present to combat inflammatory agents crossing the epithelial layer. Fibroblasts are cells that replace damaged proteins of the lamina propria. They are present in similar concentrations throughout all layers of the vocal fold. Myofibroblasts are fibroblasts

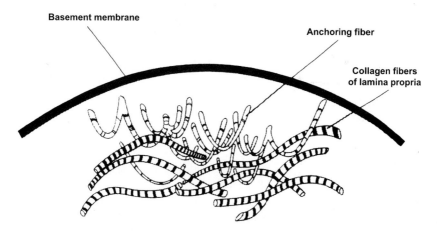

Fig. 2. The basement membrane zone of the vocal fold. (*From* Gray SD, Pignatari SN, Harding P. Morphologic ultrastructure of anchoring fibers in the normal vocal fold basement membrane zone. J Voice 1994;8:48–52; with permission.)

that have differentiated into cells of repair [5], which are present when injury has occurred and repair is needed. Myofibroblasts are found in most human vocal folds and are found in a higher density in the superficial layer of the lamina propria. It is speculated that their presence indicates that the human vocal fold is constantly going through a cycle of minor injury and repair. It is believed that the extent of this tissue injury is likely greatest in the superficial lamina propria. By maintaining this constant presence of myofibroblasts, the vocal folds appear very capable of repairing minor injuries efficiently, without significant compromise in vocal fold tissue or function. However, the myofibroblasts must be given time to perform this repair. If a patient develops a minor injury because of overuse, the voice must be rested to allow the myofibroblasts the chance to perform needed repairs. This typically happens in 2 to 3 days. Obviously, larger, more macroscopic injuries would overwhelm the myofibroblasts and result in the degradation of voice production.

The noncellular or extracellular component of the lamina propria is also known as the extracellular matrix and refers essentially to the molecules found between the cells [3]. The extracellular matrix contains a variety of molecules, including fibrous and interstitial proteins and other interstitial molecules such as carbohydrates and lipids [6,7]. The two most important fibrous proteins are collagen and elastin. Collagen provides strength and structure to the vocal fold. Elastin, on the other hand, is elastic in nature and allows the vocal fold to be deformed and then return to its original shape [3]. Interstitial proteins, also known as proteoglycans, include hyaluronic acid, decorin, fibromodulin, versican, heparin sulfate proteoglycan, and aggregan biglycan [8]. Interstitial proteins affect tissue viscosity and bestow a dampening or shock-absorbing property [9].

The extracellular matrix of the lamina propria is regulated by fibroblasts and is influenced by age and gender. Older or damaged proteins in this matrix are constantly being replaced by fibroblasts. With aging, the extracellular matrix turnover slows, that is, the collagen turnover decreases with age. With age, collagen is older before being replaced or destroyed. In addition, older proteins also undergo a process known as cross-linking. Cross-linking results in less elastic elastin [10] and stiffer collagen [11]. As a result, the vocal folds become less elastic and stiffer as the human body ages [3].

Gross anatomy

We now shift away from histologic anatomy to focus on the macroscopic or gross anatomic features of the larynx. Vocal fold shape and movement are primarily the result of intrinsic laryngeal muscle activity (Fig. 3). To a lesser degree, extrinsic laryngeal muscles also affect vocal fold shape and movement. The muscles that act to adduct or close the vocal folds are the lateral cricoarytenoid, thyroarytenoid, and interarytenoid muscles. The lateral cricoarytenoid muscle originates on the lateral aspect of the cricoid

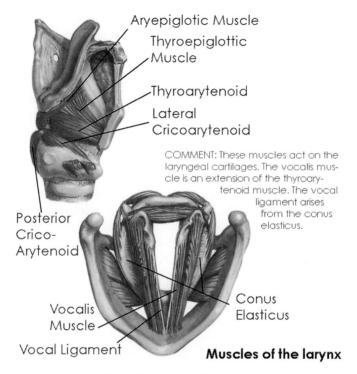

Aryepiglotic Muscle

Thyroepiglottic Muscle

Thyroarytenoid

Lateral Cricoarytenoid

COMMENT: These muscles act on the laryngeal cartilages. The vocalis muscle is an extension of the thyroarytenoid muscle. The vocal ligament arises from the conus elasticus.

Posterior Crico-Arytenoid

Vocalis Muscle

Vocal Ligament

Conus Elasticus

Muscles of the larynx

Fig. 3. The muscles of the larynx.

cartilage and inserts onto the muscular process of the arytenoid cartilage. The thyroarytenoid muscle arises from the inner thyroid cartilage and inserts on the vocal process of the arytenoid cartilage.

The posterior cricoarytenoid muscle is the only muscle that abducts or opens the vocal folds. It originates from the posterior surface of the cricoid cartilage and inserts onto the muscular process of the arytenoid. When both posterior cricoarytenoid muscles become denervated (eg, in bilateral recurrent laryngeal nerve injury from thyroidectomy surgery), serious airway obstruction can ensue. The cricothyroid muscle narrows the gap between the thyroid and cricoid cartilages, thereby stretching of the vocal folds. Professional singers rely particularly on proper cricothyroid muscle control to reach higher pitches while singing.

Compartmentalization of the intrinsic laryngeal muscles allows for ultrafine control of the vocal fold position. The posterior cricoarytenoid, cricothyroid, and thyroarytenoid muscles all have subdivisions, each with separate nerve branches [12–14]. The division of the thyroarytenoid muscle into superior and inferior subcompartments, which appear to contract independently, allows the human larynx to produce sounds with a variety of intensities, registers, and qualities that would not otherwise be possible [15].

The vagus nerve provides motor and sensory innervation to the larynx through two branches, the superior and recurrent laryngeal nerves. The superior laryngeal nerve has two branches, the external branch of the superior laryngeal nerve, which provides motor innervation to the cricothyroid muscle, and the internal branch of the superior laryngeal nerve, which provides sensory innervation of the supraglottis and the glottis. The internal branch of the superior laryngeal nerve enters the laryngopharynx through an opening in the thyrohyoid membrane.

The recurrent laryngeal nerves provide motor innervation for the remaining intrinsic laryngeal muscles (thyroarytenoid, lateral cricoarytenoid, posterior cricoarytenoid, and interarytenoid) and sensory innervation to the upper trachea and subglottis. The recurrent laryngeal nerves usually travel from the skull base downward into the upper thorax before heading back superiorly into the lower neck. The left recurrent laryngeal nerve travels around the aortic arch before turning superiorly, whereas the right recurrent laryngeal travels around the right subclavian artery. The left recurrent laryngeal nerve travels more medially in the tracheoesophageal groove as it heads toward the larynx compared with the right recurrent laryngeal nerve. Both left and right recurrent laryngeal nerves may be nonrecurrent, meaning the nerve does not travel into the thorax but rather directly from the skull base through the neck into the larynx. This occurs on the right side in approximately 0.5% of cases [16] and much less commonly on the left side. A nonrecurrent laryngeal nerve has important surgical implications when operating along the external larynx (eg, as in thyroidectomy).

Phonation

Physiologically, the human larynx is required for airway protection, respiration, swallowing, and phonation. This article focuses on phonation. During phonation, the vocal folds act as an energy transducer that converts aerodynamic power generated by the chest, diaphragm, and abdominal musculature into acoustic power that is heard as the voice [17]. This energy transformation occurs primarily in the space between the vocal folds; however, it is also influenced by subglottic and supraglottic parameters. For normal phonation, adequate respiratory support, appropriate glottal closure, a normal vocal fold cover, and control of vocal fold length and tension are required.

The vibratory motion of vocal folds is a complex cycle that results in voice production (Fig. 4). The modulation (ie, glottal opening and closing) of the air stream during phonation is what results in voice production. As the subglottic pressure increases against closed vocal folds, this pressure eventually opens the glottis. At its maximum opening, the upper lip of the vocal fold continues to move laterally, while the lower lip begins to move medially. Eventually the upper lip also begins to move medially. The medial movement of the vocal folds results from a passive recoiling force (because of an innate elasticity of the vocal folds), a drop in subglottic pressure, and

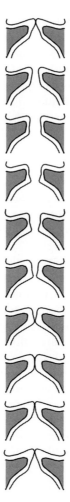

Fig. 4. Vocal fold vibration showing a coronal view of a complete glottal cycle.

the negative pressure caused by the Bernoulli effect. This negative pressure pulls the vocal folds toward each other. The initial recontact occurs at the lower lip of the vocal folds. The contact area of the vocal folds increases until the subglottic pressure becomes high enough to push the vocal folds apart. This aeromechanical cycle is repeated over and over and results in phonation.

This glottal cycle results in the occurrence of a traveling wave of mucosa from the inferior to superior surface of the vocal folds, known as the mucosal wave. This mucosal wave is present only if there is a pliable mucous membrane covering the vocal fold. The speed at which the mucosal wave travels is increased with the vocal fold lengthening [18,19], greater airflow [18], greater subglottic pressure [20], and laryngeal muscle contraction, which is associated with increased fundamental frequency [20].

Normal vocal folds can produce three typical vibratory patterns: falsetto, modal voice, and glottal fry. In the falsetto or light voice, no complete glottal closure takes place. During this high-pitched voice, only the upper edge of the vocal fold vibrates. In the modal voice, complete glottal closure occurs and results in the majority of the midfrequency range voice. During the modal phonation, the vocal fold mucosa vibrates independently of the underlying vocalis muscle. Glottal fry, or very low-frequency phonation, is characterized by a closed phase, which is relatively long compared with the open phase. During glottal fry, the mucosal cover and underlying muscle vibrate as a unit.

Knowledge of videostroboscopic vibratory parameters is important for the clinician when assessing videostroboscopic images of the larynx. The first such parameter is fundamental frequency, which describes the modal or basic frequency at which a person phonates. The fundamental frequency for an adult male is approximately 120 Hz (number of vibratory cycles per second), whereas for an adult female, the frequency is approximately 200 Hz. Another major parameter is the horizontal (or lateral) excursion of the vocal fold edge. The vocal fold edge is the medial-most part of the vocal fold, and this is not a fixed point on the vocal fold. Rather, the medial-most portion of the vocal fold is at varying vertical points along the vocal fold, depending on where the vocal fold is in its glottal cycle (see Fig. 4). The horizontal displacement of the vocal folds is called amplitude. The distance between the vocal folds is known as the glottal width. The area between the two vocal fold edges (when viewed from above) is called the glottal area.

The vibratory cycle is divided into the open and closed phases [21]. The open phase denotes the time at which the vocal folds are at least partially open. The closed phase denotes the time at which the membranous vocal folds are fully closed. The open phase is further divided into the opening and closing phases. The opening phase is defined as the time when the vocal folds are moving away from each other, whereas the closing phase is defined as the time when the vocal folds are moving together.

There are several other important vocal fold physiologic parameters that should be assessed when visually examining the vocal folds. One parameter is the mucosal wave of the vocal fold, which represents an undulation of the mucous membrane during the glottal cycle. During normal phonation, the mucosal wave travels in an inferior-to-superior direction. The speed of the mucosal wave ranges from 0.5 to 1 m per second [21]. The symmetry of vocal fold vibratory behavior is another important parameter to assess. Any asymmetry of vocal fold excursion (one vocal fold compared with the other) represents a pathologic process. Finally, the periodicity of the glottal cycles also should be assessed. Periodicity denotes a regular repetition of vibratory cycles such that each cycle is the same in amplitude and duration. Any deviation from periodic vibratory cycles is known as aperiodicity.

Summary

A sound understanding of laryngeal anatomy and physiology is crucial when managing patients with vocal complaints. This article covers the basics in vocal fold anatomy (histologic and gross) and vocal fold physiology. A better understanding of the lamina propria and the basement membrane zone and of the fine neuromuscular control of laryngeal muscles may result in improved treatments of dysphonia in the future.

References

[1] Nassar VH, Bridger P. Topography of the laryngeal mucous glands. Arch Otolaryngol 1971; 94:490–8.
[2] Hirano M, Sato K, Nakashima T. Fibroblasts in human vocal fold mucosa. Acta Otolaryngol 1999;119(2):271–6.
[3] Gray SD. Cellular physiology of the vocal folds. Otolaryngol Clin North Am 2000;33(4): 679–97.
[4] Gray SD, Pignatari SN, Harding P. Morphologic ultrastructure of anchoring fibers in the normal vocal fold basement membrane zone. J Voice 1994;8:48–52.
[5] Darby I, Skalli O, Gabbiani G. Alpha-smooth muscle action is transiently expressed by myo-fibroblasts during experimental wound healing. Lab Invest 1990;63:21–9.
[6] Gray SD, Titze IR, Chan R, et al. Vocal fold proteoglycans and their influence on biome-chanics. Laryngoscope 1999;109:845–54.
[7] Labat-Robert J, Bihari-Varga M, Robert L. Extracellular matrix. FEBS Lett 1990;268: 386–93.
[8] Pawlak A, Hammond T, Hammond E, et al. Immunocytochemical study of proteoglycans in vocal folds. Ann Otol Rhinol Laryngol 1996;105:6–11.
[9] Balazs EA, Gibbs DA. The rheological properties and biological function of hyaluronic acid. In: Balazs EA, editor. Chemistry and molecular biology of the intercellular matrix. volume 3. New York: Academic Press; 1970. p. 1241–53.
[10] Niewwoeher DE, Kleinerman J, Liotta L. Elastic behavior of postmortem human lungs: effects of aging and mild emphysema. J Appl Physiol 1975;39:943.
[11] Schneider SL, Kohn RR. Effects of age and diabetes mellitus on the solubility of collagen from human skin, tracheal cartilage and dura mater. Exp Gerontol 1982;17:185.
[12] Bryant NJ, Woodson GE, Kaufman K, et al. Human posterior cricothyroid muscle compart-ments: anatomy and mechanics. Arch Otolaryngol Head Neck Surg 1996:1331–6.
[13] Sanders I, Jacobs I, Wu BL, et al. The three bellies of the canine posterior cricoaryte-noid muscle: implications for understanding laryngeal function. Laryngoscope 1993;103: 171–7.
[14] Sanders I, Han Y, Wang J, et al. Muscle spindles are concentrated in the superior vocalis subcompartment of the human thyroarytenoid muscle. J Voice 1998;12:7–16.
[15] Sanders I, Rai S, Han Y, Biller HF. Human vocalis contains distinct superior and inferior subcompartments: possible candidates for the two masses of vocal fold vibration. Ann Otol Rhinol Laryngol 1998;107(10 Pt 1):826–33.
[16] Henry JF, Audiffret J, Denizot A, Plan M. The nonrecurrent inferior laryngeal nerve: review of 33 cases, including two on the left side. Surgery 1988;104:977–84.
[17] Titze IR. Regulation of vocal power and efficiency by subglottal pressure and glottal width. In: Fujimura O, editor. Vocal physiology: voice production, mechanisms and functions. New York: Raven Press; 1988. p. 227–37.
[18] Jiang J, Yomoto E, Lin S, et al. Quantitative measurement of mucosal wave by high-speed photography in excised larynges. Ann Otol Rhinol Laryngol 1998;107:98–103.

[19] Titze IR, Jiang JJ, Hsiao T-Y. Measurement of mucosal wave propagation and vertical phase difference in vocal fold vibration. Ann Otol Rhinol Laryngol 1993;102:58–63.
[20] Nasri S, Sercarz JA, Berke GS. Noninvasive measurement of traveling wave velocity in the canine larynx. Ann Otol Rhinol Laryngol 1994;103:758–66.
[21] Hirano M, Bless DM, editors. Videostroboscopic examination of the larynx. San Diego (CA): Singular; 1993. p. 23–34.

ELSEVIER
SAUNDERS

Otolaryngol Clin N Am
39 (2006) 11–22

OTOLARYNGOLOGIC
CLINICS
OF NORTH AMERICA

Diagnostic and Therapeutic Pitfalls in Phonosurgery

Seth Dailey, MD

*Division of Otolaryngology-Head and Neck Surgery, Department of Surgery,
University of Wisconsin School of Medicine, University of Wisconsin Hospital and Clinics,
K4/720, 600 Highland Avenue, Madison, WI 53792-7375, USA*

"Good judgment is the product of experience. Experience is the product of bad judgment." This frequently quoted statement is wholly applicable to phonomicrosurgery. Learning from our collective mistakes is the privilege and obligation of all care providers. As such, it is crucial to examine both diagnostic and therapeutic pitfalls carefully to highlight areas of common error and to propose clear solutions. These solutions may come in the form of awareness of pitfalls or the use of technology to enhance our abilities to find and resolve a given problem. For phonomicrosurgery, the importance of a thorough diagnosis, patient preparation and selection, surgical set-up, and tissue handling in the context of anatomic and physiologic principles of the glottis are the foundations of good outcomes.

A few words are required about the current understanding of vocal-fold anatomy and physiology because this understanding has an impact on surgical decision making. The vocal fold is a multilayered structure composed of muscle, vocal ligaments, superficial lamina propia (SLP), and overlying epithelium. When the vocal folds are brought together by the intrinsic laryngeal muscles acting on the arytenoid cartilages, they can be set into motion by air emanating from the trachea. Although still controversial, the SLP and epithelium (cover) move independently over the ligament and muscle (body). Closure of the vocal folds on a cycle-to-cycle basis provides the basis for regular oscillation and a stable sound source for the supraglottis to modulate. When closure is reduced by a mass lesion or by the loss of pliability of the cover, the glottal valve becomes inefficient, producing a breathy quality. More effort is required for the patient to phonate. Also, when asymmetry of tension and viscoelasticity between the vocal folds are introduced, an irregular oscillatory pattern starts, yielding the psychoacoustic phenomenon of

---

E-mail address: dailey@surgery.wisc.edu

0030-6665/06/$ - see front matter © 2005 Elsevier Inc. All rights reserved.
doi:10.1016/j.otc.2005.10.006

hoarseness. Thus, alterations of vocal-fold closure, pliability, and symmetry will yield abnormal voices. The surgical reestablishment of the microlayered structure to achieve proper closure, pliability, and symmetry is the goal of phonomicrosurgery.

Diagnostics

History

The first part of any proper evaluation is to take a complete patient history. Elements must include standard components of medical problems, previous surgery, medications, and gynecologic history when appropriate. A complete laryngeal history would be insufficient without noting whether the patient has swallowing or airway complaints. Specific to voice, issues such as previous intubations, laryngeal or head and neck trauma, previous voice surgery, and vocal history, including training, are mandatory. Cigarette smoking, alcohol consumption, allergies, and symptoms of laryngopharyngeal reflux must be explored. Furthermore, because hoarseness is a general term, an understanding of the specific voice complaint is essential. For example, a patient who has vocal cord paralysis will often be exhausted by glottal insufficiency and desire a reduction in vocal effort, whereas a jazz singer may want the return of his or her top octave. This initial probing is critical for a discussion of postoperative expectations. Importantly, the treating physician must also have the grounding to recognize when treatment may not be able to satisfy a patient's expectations and to request another opinion from colleagues.

Office examination

Relying only on mirror examination for surgical decision making may introduce errors that affect vocal outcomes. Although a mirror examination is performed rapidly and has excellent color resolution, the examination is often short, uncomfortable for the patient, cannot be reviewed by the patient or physician afterward, and most importantly, cannot evaluate the pliability of the vocal folds during vocalization. It is well recognized that the addition of videostroboscopy to the armamentarium of office procedures has enhanced the ability to accurately identify vocal-fold lesions [1,2]. Videostroboscopy is also helpful in the identification of lesions not seen by mirror or flexible fiber-optic transnasal examination. Sataloff and colleagues [1] have noted that 18% of lesions were incorrectly identified by mirror or flexible examination and that 29% of patients had other lesions when videostroboscopy was performed. Woo [2] has also found that the specific addition of the stroboscope to rigid telescopic transoral endoscopy yields information that alters therapy in 10% of cases. Furthermore, Woo found that postoperative scarring was a common finding in postoperative dysphonia, making clear the need to assess vocal-fold pliability.

Telescopic rigid videostroboscopy allows digital recording of the examination and slow-motion review by the clinician for maximal diagnostic certainty and patient teaching. Also, stroboscopy is the only commonly available tool to assess the pre- and postoperative pliability of the vocal-fold cover. Focal stiffness can help to distinguish a polyp from a cyst, for example, or may reveal stiffness of the contralateral vocal fold, which, if unidentified, could lead to an unexpectedly poor voice result in the face of excellent ipsilateral surgery [3]. A careful examination of arytenoid mobility may also help to uncover vocal-fold paresis, which is believed to promote the development of phonotraumatic lesions, specifically the paresis "podule" (Fig. 1). Koufman and Belafsky [4] point out that vocal-fold paresis, if unrecognized, may lead to lesion recurrence after surgery because the irregular shear stresses on the vocal folds during phonation will remain. Probe tasks such as serial "ee"-sniffs, whistling, or running speech may exaggerate any arytenoid dysmobility, which help to secure the diagnosis. Also, given that the identification of vocal-fold paresis can be elusive, electromyography is critical in these cases. Heman-Ackah and Batory [5] recently report that a comprehensive work-up for vocal-fold hypomobility in 49 patients yielded a potential cause in 41 patients (84%). Direct or indirect injury to the recurrent laryngeal nerve was the principal source. Furthermore, the advent of high-speed digital imaging and new software to quantify arytenoid motion may be of clinical use in the future [6,7].

Operative examination

To be a complete phonosurgeon, it is imperative to perform a gentle inspection under high magnification and palpation of the inferior, medial, and superior surfaces of both vocal folds, once they are exposed. Sweeping slowly from inferior to superior in the anterior, middle, and posterior thirds of the musculomembranous segments of the vocal folds with a right-angle blunt probe is

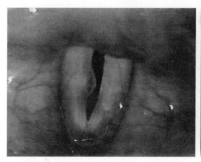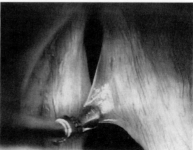

Fig. 1. (*left*) Stroboscopic image of a right vocal-fold "podule," a benign subepithelial nonhemorrhagic lesion. (*right*) Microlaryngoscopic image of a right vocal-fold "podule" being examined with a microinstrument. (*From* Koufman JA, Belafsky PC. Unilateral or localized Reinke's edema (pseudocyst) as a manifestation of vocal-fold paresis: the paresis podule. Laryngoscope 2001;111(4 Pt 1):576–80; with permission.)

the recommended practice. This examination allows for tactile feedback regarding the nonpathologic segments of the vocal fold and will help to evaluate the native pliability, contour, and vascularity of both the pathologic and normal segments. Palpation will also help to distinguish mucus from keratinous cysts as well as how scarred and firm a mass lesion may be.

Concordant with previous studies by Bouchayer and Poels, Dailey and colleagues recently identified sulcal deformities as the most commonly missed benign vocal-fold disorder before surgical exploration (Fig. 2) [8–10]. Indeed, the authors found that even a retrospective review of the preoperative stroboscopic examinations did not reveal the sulcal deformities. Mucosal bridges were also noted to be a commonly unrecognized entity by stroboscopy alone. These observations have a bearing on surgical planning and medicolegal aspects of care. In cases of uncertain pathology, the surgeon and patient must decide before surgery whether additional findings such as sulcus vocalis, discovered at surgery, can be acted on immediately or whether additional procedures should be used to address the new findings.

Timing

Responses to medical regimens and to voice therapy play an important role in the accuracy of office endoscopy. For example, in the face of glottic

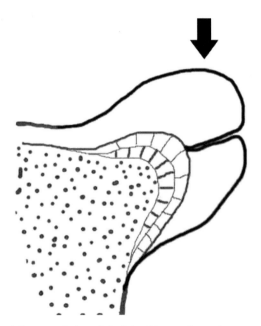

Fig. 2. Rendition of the coronal view of the left mid-musculomembranous vocal fold in a patient who had Reinke's edema and a concomitant sulcal deformity. The arrow notes the optical vector during stroboscopy. Note that the sulcus is hidden from view by overlying SLP and epithelium.

edema caused by allergies or laryngopharyngeal reflux, lesions such as cysts within the SLP may be masked, but as the edema resolves, the lesion often becomes more prominent and thus recognized more confidently. Also, with a trial of aggressive voice therapy, vocal-fold nodules often resolve so significantly that surgery is no longer required [11]. One would certainly not rush to operate on vocal-fold nodules when faced with a patient who has limited self-monitoring and who has limited tools to prevent recurrence. On the other hand, there is a strong argument to be made for proceeding expediently in patients with large vocal-fold polyps, poorly defined lesions, or masses that may induce worsening ipsilateral or contralateral stiffness and scar.

Preparatory considerations

Adjusting to factors that influence the readiness of the patient for surgery should be considered carefully. For example, excessive cigarette and alcohol use in the perioperative period should be discouraged strongly because healing of the vocal-fold epithelium and SLP is believed to occur best without undue inflammatory sources [12–15]. Similarly, medical management of allergies and laryngopharyngeal reflux will help to provide a more neutral environment after surgery. For women of the appropriate age, vocal-fold surgery is best performed before or after the premenstrual time because excessive secretions, glottic edema, and vessel and epithelial fragility create a suboptimal atmosphere for healing and may induce postoperative bleeding (Fig. 3) [16]. For each of these medical conditions, there is a tendency toward increased throat clearing as well, which is to be discouraged because

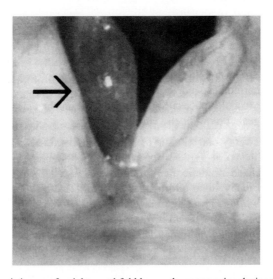

Fig. 3. Stroboscopic image of a right vocal-fold hemorrhage occurring during the premenstrual time secondary to bleeding into the superficial lamina propria. (*From* Abitbol J, Abitbol P, Abitbol B. Sex hormones and the female voice. J Voice 1999;13(3):424–46; with permission.)

of additional aerodynamic glottic trauma after surgery. The alteration of vocal use, perhaps permanently, may also be of value in the patient who clearly is overtaxed; for example, the person who is a singer by night but works at a call center by day should understand that a change of day job may have a significant long-term benefit.

Expectations

The limitations of an existing pathology and surgical technique dictate that it is unrealistic to have perfect restoration of glottic function. Thus, for the patient and the surgeon to be satisfied, specific discussion about vocal outcomes must take place. Johns and colleagues [17] have recently reported statistically significant improvements in Vocal Handicap Index (VHI) measures in patients who presented with cysts and polyps. Acoustic improvements were noted in female patients, with respect to jitter, shimmer, and range. Importantly, the difference between pre- and postoperative VHI measures in patients with scarring did not reach statistical significance, indicating that this group will likely experience more a modest benefit from surgery and should be counseled accordingly. Also Zeitels and colleagues [18] have reported on vocal results after phonomicrosurgery in 185 singers and performing artists. They found statistically significant improvement in 8 of 24 objective measures centered on the efficiency of voice production, indicating a positive outlook for this surgical population with the conditions of careful diagnosis, precise surgery, and active voice rehabilitation. Behrman and colleagues [19] call into question how patients' perception of dysphonia correlates with standard evaluations of voice, namely the VHI, auditory-perceptual evaluation of dysphonia severity, and other factors. They found that patient perception did not correlate with these commonly used measures, which raises more questions than it answers. Until some of these issues are resolved better, open-ended questions to the patient about what specifically (eg, fatigue, projection, range, loss of high notes, and other qualities) bothers them about their voice are of the greatest value and help the surgeon to determine realistically the chances of resolving their complaints. As in all surgical consultations, a well-informed patient and a realistic, honest, and caring physician form the best combination.

Surgical considerations

Special attention to anesthesia, exposure, instrumentation, hemostasis, and ergonomics will optimize the procedure itself. For the intubation, it is essential to discuss with the anesthesia team the potential difficulties in ventilating and intubating the patient. Factors such as obesity, a short thyromental distance, a short and thick neck, retrognathia, and a history of difficult intubation will raise red flags about extra consideration [20]. Given that the masses to be excised might be easily stripped from the vocal folds with an endotracheal tube, it is important to decide who should place the endotracheal tube. If there is any doubt, the most experienced person is usually the best choice. This clarity may help reduce the chance of a rushed and traumatic intubation that could jeopardize the integrity of the glottis. When jet ventilation techniques are selected to eliminate the need for endotracheal tubes, the surgeon and anesthesia staff must be familiar and comfortable with the technique [21,22]. The preoperative identification of patients with challenging laryngoscopic exposure will warrant the selection of laryngoscopes with smaller examining specula [23,24]. An increased thyroid-mandibular angle in both men and women has been identified recently as a reliable measure of difficult laryngoscopic exposure [25]. Patients with large tongues and those who are obese may also present challenges.

The adage "you can't cut what you can't see" is highly relevant in this setting. The basic technique for direct laryngoscopic exposure has been addressed previously by Zeitels and colleagues [26] and others and includes several key points: the neck of the supine patient should be flexed with extension at the atlanto-occipital joint; external counterpressure should be applied posteriorly to the proximal trachea for enhanced exposure; conformation of the laryngoscope to the triangular glottis is optimal; distention of the false vocal folds away from the glottis enhances exposure; mechanical suspension of the laryngoscope leaves both of the surgeon's hands free to operate.

Magnification and adequate lighting provide the surgeon with the best opportunity for assessment of color, tissue pliability, vasculature of the cover, and assurance of proper tissue contouring. Distinguishing between normal and abnormal tissue can be quite difficult, and sacrificing this opportunity can lead to poor tissue plane definition and the sacrifice of normal SLP [27]. The advent of xenon light sources and higher resolution microscopes is helpful in this regard. Angled telescopes are also useful in the examination of the inferior vocal-fold edge and the ventricle. Exposure also comes in the form of hemostasis. When bleeding from small vessels in the cover is encountered, reduction of the bleeding can be controlled with different modalities, each having relative benefits. Tiny cotton balls soaked in epinephrine (1:10,000 dilution) can be applied gently to the area. Care must be taken not to wipe away normal SLP and not to tear the epithelial flap. Microbipolar forceps (no. MCL34, Microfrance, Montreal, Quebec, Canada) have been produced for controlling vessels and are effective when used conservatively. Thermal injury, especially to the cover, can induce an exuberant inflammatory reaction and lead to scar formation. Larger unipolar devices are to be avoided for this reason.

A full set of microlaryngeal instruments is helpful for manipulating both the epithelium and the lesion. For example, gentle grasping of the epithelial flap along a broad base with a heart-shaped forceps rather than an alligator forceps will reduce the risk of tearing the flap (the pressure on the tissue is reduced because the surface area used is larger [pressure = force/area]). Also, when the lesion is densely adherent to the undersurface of the epithelium, only sharp dissection will be effective in establishing a tissue plane between the two; if the scissors are too dull or if blunt dissection is selected because of a lack of instruments, undue epithelial loss is likely to occur. Furthermore, given the small size of benign vocal-fold lesions (often 2–3 mm in size), instruments with working ends that are twice the size of the lesion are awkward and usually ineffective; therefore, having instruments with small distal tips allows greater precision. For example, in the excision of ectasias and varices, without the proper instruments, such as fine picks, a frustrated surgeon might resort to the use of CO_2 laser, which has been reported to induce more scarring than cold instrument dissection [28].

Surgical instruments, however, are only as stable as the surgeon who is using them. Stability in turn is enhanced by physical comfort. Mayo stands, rolling chairs with adjustable arms supports, and other devices will help to assure the resting of major arm and back muscle groups so that fine muscle groups of the forearms and hands are not unduly fatigued. In otolaryngology-head and neck surgery, the surgeon often too willingly sacrifices physical comfort for speed. For microlaryngoscopy, this sacrifice is a liability because physical discomfort will lead to excessive muscle tension, hand tremor, and possibly suboptimal results [29]. Therefore the surgeon must pay attention to the position of neck, back, arms and hands relative to the patient, especially as the length of the case increases. Removing the instruments and relaxing for a moment now and then is helpful. Hockstein and colleagues [30,31] have demonstrated the use of robotics for microlaryngeal surgery in animal and cadaveric models for the elimination of hand tremor. The high cost and further development of the robotic system limit its immediate application.

Surgical training experience certainly plays a role in outcomes. For laparoscopic splenectomies at one institution, operative time dropped from 195 to 97 minutes, whereas success rates (not converted to an open procedure) increased from 60% to 95% [32]. Similarly, for laparoscopic colorectal resection performed at a single institution, 30 cases were necessary to achieve a steady state in optimal operative time [33]. In the otologic literature, patients operated on by residents were more prone to emetic sequelae than those operated on by specialists, and the healing rate of tympanic membranes in patients operated on by residents versus specialists was 78% and 95%, respectively [34]. A recent study of experience level in stapedectomy has demonstrated that less experienced surgeons are more likely to displace the stapes prosthesis during insertion [35]. These studies reinforce the fact that real operative experiences increase efficiency and results. To achieve this end, Dailey and colleagues [36] and others have designed laryngeal training stations that will help the surgeon to work out ergonomic and technical details outside the operating room [37].

Tissue handling

Consideration given to the vocal-fold epithelium and the underlying SLP is of paramount importance in the pursuit of the reestablishment of the native glottic architecture. The epithelium and SLP cannot be replaced once they have been removed, so careful planning and respect for tissue are critical.

An excision of a benign lesion is achieved best when four tissue conditions are met. First, there should be neither too much nor too little epithelium present once the lesion is excised. Too little epithelium, which leaves the SLP exposed, mandates healing by secondary intention, which is inherently more inflammatory than primary healing. This situation may happen when resecting the fibrous tissue of a nodule away from its overlying epithelium; the nodule, being adherent to the epithelium is difficult to dissect away, leading to epithelial loss. Too much epithelium may leave an irregular edge once the excess epithelium has regressed, or it may lead to a granuloma at the healing site. This might happen after removing abnormal SLP from Reinke's space in cases of Reinke's edema; the edema, which is really altered SLP, acts as a tissue expander, leaving extra overlying epithelium that must be tailored for primary healing.

Second, no normal SLP should be resected unless it will aid in the production of a smoothly contoured straight vocal-fold edge. The SLP defect is not replaced by new SLP and will reduce local pliability and create a small volume loss, both of which lead to glottic insufficiency. This situation is noted all too often in patients who have undergone repeated surgical biopsies of premalignant epithelium that have removed some underlying SLP each time. Indeed, the reestablishment of a pliable and volumetrically correct vocal fold is a source of much interest in laryngology today [38–42].

Third, excessive undermining of the epithelium away from the SLP should be avoided because anchoring basement membrane proteins, as identified by Gray and colleagues [43] help to maintain the integrity of the cover; additional dissection mandates an inflammatory process for reintegrating these structures. Fourth, smooth straight vocal-fold edges with minimal volume loss will likely produce the best vocal result because there is restoration of closure, pliability, and symmetry.

To these ends, epithelial incisions and dissection within the cover are considered. The position, direction, length, and the epithelial incision (cordotomy) are all essential factors to be considered before performing them. All incisions may be aided by the technique of subepithelial infusion. The technique allows for hemostasis and increased space for placement of cutting instruments [44]. The lateral microflap is best used when examining pathology deeper in the vocal fold (close to the vocal ligament), such as a sulcus vocalis (Fig. 4) [45]. A lengthy longitudinal incision is made. The flap is easy to manipulate, coapts well when released, and can be sutured without risk to the medial striking surface. It is less likely to tear because it is more robust, containing both epithelium and some underlying SLP. The medial microflap, based immediately laterally to the lateral extent of a benign lesion, is more of an epithelium-only flap and is more likely to tear. Also, it is closer to the medial striking surface of the vocal fold and should be developed gently. This flap is best used for small benign lesions such as nodules and polyps [46,47].

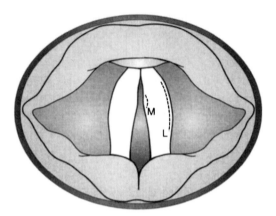

Fig. 4. Rendition of the endolarynx in the surgical position. Dotted lines mark the incisions of the medial microflap cordotomy (M) and the lateral microflap cordotomy (L). (*From* Ford CN. Advances and refinements in phonosurgery. Laryngoscope 1999;109(12):1891–900; with permission.)

All cordotomies should be performed parallel to the long axis of the vocal fold. When force from retraction is applied perpendicularly to the incision, it is thus less likely to tear. If the cordotomy is canted or is curvilinear rather than linear, then tearing is more likely. Torn flaps must be trimmed because they will not reappose spontaneously. Of note, long cordotomies based more medially are also less likely to reappose spontaneously and may lead to an area of uncovered SLP, which then heals by secondary intention.

Summary

To avoid pitfalls and to enhance results, multiple areas of consideration are essential. Thorough diagnostics, including a history and physical examination, office endoscopy with stroboscopy, and operative examination provide a high yield combination. Timing and preparation for surgery and expectation management allow for mature decision making by the surgeon and patient. Considerations specific to surgical technique must include anesthesia, intubation, exposure of the glottis, lighting, magnification, hemostasis, instrumentation, flap design, and tissue handling. These considerations are in the context of extreme respect for the superficial layer of lamina propria, which does not regenerate well and the sacrifice of which may mean potentially irreversible dysphonia.

References

[1] Sataloff RT, Spiegel JR, Hawkshaw MJ. Strobovideolaryngoscopy: results and clinical value. Ann Otol Rhinol Laryngol 1991;100(9 Pt 1):725–7.

[2] Woo P. Diagnostic value of stroboscopic examination in hoarse patients. J Voice 1991;5(3): 231–8.

[3] Shohet JA, Courey MS, Scott MA, et al. Value of videostroboscopic parameters in differentiating true vocal fold cysts from polyps. Laryngoscope 1996;106(1 Pt 1):19–26.

[4] Koufman JA, Belafsky PC. Unilateral or localized Reinke's edema (pseudocyst) as a manifestation of vocal fold paresis: the paresis podule. Laryngoscope 2001;111(4 Pt 1):576–80.

[5] Heman-Ackah YD, Batory M. Determining the etiology of mild vocal fold hypomobility. J Voice 2003;17(4):579–88.

[6] Larsson H, Hertegard S, Lindestad PA, et al. Vocal fold vibrations: high-speed imaging, kymography, and acoustic analysis: a preliminary report. Laryngoscope 2000;110(12):2117–22.

[7] Dailey SH, Kobler JB, Hillman RE, et al. Endoscopic measurement of vocal fold movement during adduction and abduction. Laryngoscope 2005;115(1):178–83.

[8] Dailey SH, Spanou K, Zeitels K. The evaluation of benign glottic lesions: rigid telescopic stroboscopy vs. suspension microlaryngoscopy. J Voice, in press.

[9] Poels PJ, de Jong FI, Schutte HK. Consistency of the preoperative and intraoperative diagnosis of benign vocal fold lesions. J Voice 2003;17(3):425–33.

[10] Bouchayer M, Cornut G, Witzig E, et al. Epidermoid cysts, sulci, and mucosal bridges of the true vocal cord: a report of 157 cases. Laryngoscope 1985;95(9 Pt 1):1087–94.

[11] McCrory E. Voice therapy outcomes in vocal fold nodules: a retrospective audit. Int J Lang Commun Disord 2001;36(Suppl):S19–24.

[12] Morrison MD. Is chronic gastroesophageal reflux a causative factor in glottic carcinoma? Otolaryngol Head Neck Surg 1988;99(4):370–3.

[13] Vecerina Volic S, Kirincic N, Markov D. Some morphological, histological, cytological and histochemical aspects of Reinke's oedema. Acta Otolaryngol 1996;116(2):322–4.

[14] Koufman JA, Aviv JE, Casiano RR, et al. Laryngopharyngeal reflux: position statement of the committee on speech, voice, and swallowing disorders of the American Academy of Otolaryngology Head and Neck Surgery. Otolaryngol Head Neck Surg 2002;127(1):32–5.

[15] Verdolini K, Min Y, Titze IR, et al. Biological mechanisms underlying voice changes due to dehydration. J Speech Lang Hear Res 2002;45(2):268–81.

[16] Abitbol J, Abitbol P, Abitbol B. Sex hormones and the female voice. J Voice 1999;13(3): 424–46.

[17] Johns MM, Garrett CG, Hwang J, et al. Quality-of-life outcomes following laryngeal endoscopic surgery for non-neoplastic vocal fold lesions. Ann Otol Rhinol Laryngol 2004;113(8): 597–601.

[18] Zeitels SM, Hillman RE, Desloge R, et al. Phonomicrosurgery in singers and performing artists: treatment outcomes, management theories, and future directions. Ann Otol Rhinol Laryngol Suppl 2002;190:21–40.

[19] Behrman A, Sulica L, He T. Factors predicting patient perception of dysphonia caused by benign vocal fold lesions. Laryngoscope 2004;114(10):1693–700.

[20] Merah NA, Wong DT, Ffoulkes-Crabbe DJ, et al. Modified Mallampati test, thyromental distance and inter-incisor gap are the best predictors of difficult laryngoscopy in West Africans. Can J Anaesth 2005;52(3):291–6.

[21] Rubin JS, Patel A, Lennox P. Subglottic jet ventilation for suspension microlaryngoscopy. J Voice 2005;19(1):146–50.

[22] Shikowitz MJ, Abramson AL, Liberatore L. Endolaryngeal jet ventilation: a 10-year review. Laryngoscope 1991;101(5):455–61.

[23] Hochman II, Zeitels SM, Heaton JT. Analysis of the forces and position required for direct laryngoscopic exposure of the anterior vocal folds. Ann Otol Rhinol Laryngol 1999;108(8): 715–24.

[24] Zeitels SM. Universal modular glottiscope system: the evolution of a century of design and technique for direct laryngoscopy. Ann Otol Rhinol Laryngol Suppl 1999;179:2–24.

[25] Hsiung MW, Pai L, Kang BH, et al. Clinical predictors of difficult laryngeal exposure. Laryngoscope 2004;114(2):358–63.

[26] Zeitels SM, Vaughan CW. "External counterpressure" and "internal distention" for optimal laryngoscopic exposure of the anterior glottal commisure. Ann Otol Rhinol Laryngol 1994; 103(9):669–75.

[27] Zeitels S. Atlas of phonomicrosurgery and other endolaryngeal procedures for benign and malignant disease. San Diego: Singular; 2001.

[28] Hochman I, Sataloff RT, Hillman RE, et al. Ectasias and varices of the vocal fold: clearing the striking zone. Ann Otol Rhinol Laryngol 1999;108(1):10–6.

[29] Hemal AK, Srinivas M, Charles AR. Ergonomic problems associated with laparoscopy. J Endourol 2001;15(5):499–503.

[30] Hockstein NG, Nolan JP, O'Malley BW Jr, et al. Robot-assisted pharyngeal and laryngeal microsurgery: results of robotic cadaver dissections. Laryngoscope 2005;115(6):1003–8.

[31] Hockstein NG, Nolan JP, O'Malley BW Jr, et al. Robotic microlaryngeal surgery: a technical feasibility study using the daVinci surgical robot and an airway mannequin. Laryngoscope 2005;115(5):780–5.

[32] Rege RV, Joehl RJ. A learning curve for laparoscopic splenectomy at an academic institution. J Surg Res 1999;81(1):27–32.

[33] Schlachta CM, Mamazza J, Seshadri PA, et al. Defining a learning curve for laparoscopic colorectal resections. Dis Colon Rectum 2001;44(2):217–22.

[34] Honkavaara PPI. Surgeon's experience as a factor for emetic sequelae after middle ear surgery. Acta Anaesthesiol Scand 1998;42:1033–7.

[35] Rothbaum DL, Roy J, Hager GD, et al. Task performance in stapedotomy: comparison between surgeons of different experience levels. Otolaryngol Head Neck Surg 2003;128(1): 71–7.

[36] Dailey SH, Kobler JB, Zeitels SM. A laryngeal dissection station: educational paradigms in phonosurgery. Laryngoscope 2004;114(5):878–82.

[37] Paczona R. A cadaver larynx holder for teaching laryngomicrosurgery. J Laryngol Otol 1997;111(1):56–7.

[38] Hertegard S, Hallen L, Laurent C, Lindstrom E, et al. Cross-linked hyaluronan versus collagen for injection treatment of glottal insufficiency: 2-year follow-up. Acta Otolaryngol 2004;124(10):1208–14.

[39] Hertegård S, Dahlqvist Å, Goodyer E, et al. Viscoelasticity in scarred rabbit vocal folds after hyaluronan injection: short term results. Paper presented at the Annual Meeting of the American Academy of Otolaryngology Head and Neck Surgery Foundation. New York, September 19–22, 2004.

[40] Hirano S, Bless DM, Nagai H, et al. Growth factor therapy for vocal fold scarring in a canine model. Ann Otol Rhinol Laryngol 2004;113(10):777–85.

[41] Chhetri DK, Head C, Revazova E, et al. Lamina propria replacement therapy with cultured autologous fibroblasts for vocal fold scars. Otolaryngol Head Neck Surg 2004;131(6): 864–70.

[42] Kanemaru S, Nakamura T, Omori K, et al. Regeneration of the vocal fold using autologous mesenchymal stem cells. Ann Otol Rhinol Laryngol 2003;112(11):915–20.

[43] Gray SD, Pignatari SS, Harding P. Morphologic ultrastructure of anchoring fibers in normal vocal fold basement membrane zone. J Voice 1994;8(1):48–52.

[44] Zeitels SM, Vaughan CW. A submucosal true vocal fold infusion needle. Otolaryngol Head Neck Surg 1991;105(3):478–9.

[45] Courey MS, Garrett CG, Ossoff RH. Medial microflap for excision of benign vocal fold lesions. Laryngoscope 1997;107(3):340–4.

[46] Hochman II, Zeitels SM. Phonomicrosurgical management of vocal fold polyps: the subepithelial microflap resection technique. J Voice 2000;14(1):112–8.

[47] Sataloff RT, Spiegel JR, Heuer RJ, et al. Laryngeal mini-microflap: a new technique and reassessment of the microflap saga. J Voice 1995;9(2):198–204.

OTOLARYNGOLOGIC
CLINICS
OF NORTH AMERICA

Otolaryngol Clin N Am
39 (2006) 23–42

Surgical Management of Sulcus Vocalis and Vocal Fold Scarring

Seth H. Dailey, MD*, Charles N. Ford, MD

*Division of Otolaryngology-Head and Neck Surgery, Department of Surgery,
University of Wisconsin School of Medicine, University of Wisconsin Hospital and Clinics,
K4/720, 600 Highland Avenue, Madison, WI 53792-7375, USA*

Sulcus vocalis and vocal fold scarring are fibroplastic anomalies of the normally pliable vocal fold cover. The two conditions share the hallmarks of refractory dysphonia, glottal insufficiency, and difficulty of repair. Consequently, except when important differences exist, they will be considered interchangeably. Difficulties in their definition, pathophysiology, clinical characteristics, identification, and treatment have proven to be barriers to adequate management. As understanding of these entities has evolved, surgeons have devised various strategies to improve glottic efficiency and restoration of more normal vocal fold microarchitecture with variable success. Current understanding of these entities and considerations for management are provided. Future treatment pathways are explored.

Background anatomy and physiology

The vocal fold is a multilayered structure that is composed of muscle, vocal ligament, superficial lamina propria (SLP), and overlying epithelium (Fig. 1). When the vocal folds are brought together by the intrinsic laryngeal muscles that act upon the arytenoid cartilages, the folds of tissue can be set into motion by air that emanates from the trachea. At normal pitch and loudness, the cover of the vocal fold (made up of the SLP and epithelium) is believed to move freely over the vocal fold body (made up of the intermediate and deep layers of lamina propria [the vocal ligament] and thyroarytenoid muscle). The vocal ligament links the cover to the muscular component of the vocal fold body. Concordant with Bernoulli's principle, the high air

---

* Corresponding author.
E-mail address: dailey@surgery.wisc.edu (S.H. Dailey).

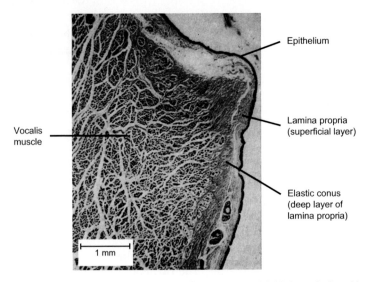

Fig. 1. Photomicrograph of a coronal section of a human vocal fold through the mid-musculomembranous section depicting the microarchitectural layers (hematoxylin-eosin). (*From* Hirano M. Morphological structure of the vocal cord as a vibrator and its variations. Folia Phoniatr (Basel) 1974;26(2):90; with permission.)

flow from the trachea upon expiration creates an area between the vocal folds of low relative pressure that leads to the entrainment of pliable (not stiff) tissues, such as the vocal fold cover. A multimass model of vocal fold oscillation that specifies the upper and lower borders of the vocal folds as individual masses helps to explain the sequential opening of the vocal folds from inferior to superior. The sequential opening creates variable aerodynamic pressures within the glottis that allow for flow-induced oscillation (continuous vibration produced by the passage of air). Ordered oscillation of the vocal folds yields efficient cycle-to-cycle closure of the vocal folds, and is a reliable sound source for voicing. When the pliability or physical volume of the vocal fold cover is reduced, higher pressures and airflows are required to drive the vocal folds, respectively. Although principally a matter of pliability loss to the cover, sulcus vocalis and scar possess a volumetrically deficient vocal fold cover, which aggravates the efficiency of cycle-to-cycle closure.

Definitions

Sulcus vocalis is a migration of the vocal fold epithelium into the normally convex SLP or deeper. Ford and colleagues [1] provided a rational schema, whereby variants of the entity are categorized as one of three types. Types II and III are represented schematically in Fig. 2. Anatomically, all are noted on the medial surface of the vocal fold. Type I is a longitudinal depression of the epithelium into the SLP, but not down to the vocal ligament (Fig. 3). The depression extends most often for the full length of the

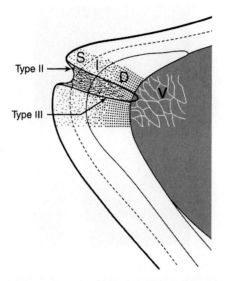

Fig. 2. Vocal fold coronally sectioned and depicting the depth of epithelial adherence in types II and III sulcus vocalis. D, deep layer of lamina propria; I, intermediate later of lamina propria; S, superficial layer of lamina propria; V, vocalis muscle. (*From* Ford CN. Advances and refinements in phonosurgery. Laryngoscope 1999;109:1894; with permission.)

musculomembranous vocal fold, from vocal process to anterior commissure. Because it is reasonably common and is associated with only mild vocal dysfunction, it has been termed "physiologic sulcus." Type II also is a full-length depression, extends down to the vocal ligament or further, and involves loss of SLP (Fig. 4). This feature produces disruption of the mucosal wave at the medial surface of the vocal fold as the wave propagates

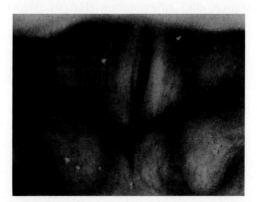

Fig. 3. Microlaryngoscopic image of a left vocal fold type I ("physiologic") sulcus vocalis deformity along the medial vocal fold edge. Note that it does not penetrate deeply into the vocal fold. (*From* Ford CN, Inagi K, Khidr A, et al. Sulcus vocalis: a rational analytical approach to diagnosis and management. Ann Otol Rhinol Laryngol 1996;105(3):193; with permission.)

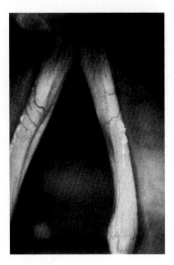

Fig. 4. Microlaryngoscopic image of bilateral type II sulcus vocalis deformities along the medial vocal fold edge. The right side may be more focal and arguably is closer to a type III ("pitlike") sulcus. (*From* Ford CN, Inagi K, Khidr A, et al. Sulcus vocalis: a rational analytical approach to diagnosis and management. Ann Otol Rhinol Laryngol 1996;105(3):195; with permission.)

from the infraglottic to the superior surface. The variation in depth corresponds to the description by Itoh and colleagues [2] of these lesions being deep, moderate, or shallow. Type III is a deep, often pitlike, focal indentation of epithelium along the medial surface of the vocal fold that does not extend for its whole length (Fig. 5). There also is loss of SLP in type III, and its focal disruption of the mucosal wave can be severe on stroboscopy. Histologic examination of excised type III deformities reveals diffuse fibrosis, neovascularization, and inflammation (Fig. 6). This tethering of the

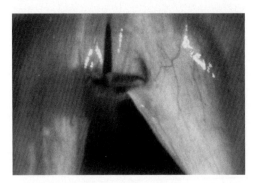

Fig. 5. Microlaryngoscopic image of right type III sulcus vocalis being demonstrated with microinstrument. (*From* Ford CN, Inagi K, Khidr A, et al. Sulcus vocalis: a rational analytical approach to diagnosis and management. Ann Otol Rhinol Laryngol 1996;105(3):195; with permission.)

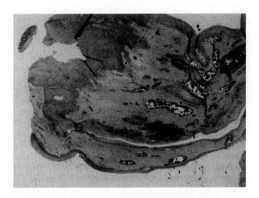

Fig. 6. Photomicrograph of a type III sulcus deformity showing massive inflammation, neovascularization, and fibrosis (hematoxylin-eosin, original magnification ×20). (*From* Ford CN, Inagi K, Khidr A, et al. Sulcus vocalis: a rational analytical approach to diagnosis and management. Ann Otol Rhinol Laryngol 1996;105(3):196; with permission.)

epithelium is similar to a scar contracture. Sato and Hirano [3] confirmed ultrastructural alterations of the collagenous and elastic fibers at the deepest extent of sulcus vocalis deformities.

Congenital and acquired theories of pathogenesis have been supported. Arnold [4] and Bouchayer and colleagues [5] supported a congenital source for these lesions. Bouchayer and colleagues [5] postulated that faulty genesis of the fourth and sixth branchial arches is responsible for the incomplete microarchitecture. Epidermoid cysts from epithelial rests within the vocal fold are believed to rupture and cause the characteristic appearance of the disorder: fibrosis, neovascularization, and inflammation, as seen in type III sulcus vocalis. Its appearance in childhood, lack of recurrence after excision, and a familial propensity buttress the congenital nature of these lesions. Conversely, the theory of acquired pathogenesis is supported by Van Caneg-ham's [6] observation of adult onset symptoms that may have been induced by trauma or mycobacterial infection. In a review of 240 patients who had vocal fold furrows, Itoh and colleagues [2] noted that 73% of the 195 patients who had sulcus vocalis reported onset of hoarseness after age 40. Furthermore, examination of whole-mount sections from the University of Wisconsin revealed a high rate (48%) of sulcus deformities on the contralateral fold of adult specimens with ipsilateral malignant lesions [7]. Itoh and colleagues [2] noted that both congenital and acquired sources of sulcus vocalis are likely, because the onset of vocal symptoms ranged from birth into the ninth decade of life in their large series.

Generically, vocal fold scar is characterized by a replacement of the native microarchitecture by disorganized collagen and loss of essential elements of the extracellular matrix. This results in contraction of the vocal fold cover and a volumetric deficiency of the affected vocal fold, as well as a loss of pliability. On office examination, vocal fold scar is noted to be a subepithelial entity that can make the normally translucent vocal fold cover appear white or opaque. On stroboscopic examination, the scarred region has a reduction of mucosal wave, loss of tissue pliability, and a loss of entrainment with the contralateral vocal folds, most often producing a spindle-shaped glottic closure pattern [2,8]. Examination under microlaryngoscopy often reveals a white medial vocal fold edge that is stiff to palpation with microinstruments (Fig. 7). Severity of scar is determined, in part, by the number of layers of the native vocal fold that have been replaced by scar. For example, a patient who has excessive phonotrauma during a bout of laryngitis might have deposition of scar only along the basement membrane in the superficial area of the SLP, whereas a patient who had a glottic cancer that was resected down to thyroarytenoid muscle by way of CO_2 laser will have replacement of the SLP and vocal ligament by scar. Given that the depth of involvement is hidden from the human eye, further definition of the three-dimensional anatomy of scar awaits the clinical availability of new tools, specifically ocular coherence tomography (OCT) and the linear skin rheometer (LSR) [9–11]. Recent reports suggest the usefulness of these dermatologically based modalities. OCT uses principles of light refraction to yield images of the most superficial 2 mm of the vocal fold, which makes it ideal to evaluate the SLP. OCT's use under microlaryngoscopy and, more recently in the clinic setting with topical anesthesia, support its proof of concept; however, images with better resolution and reliability are pending [12]. LSR uses a physical probe to displace (~ 2 mm) various sites along the surface of the vocal fold to yield force displacement curves, and thus, "pliability maps." Although they are being used in experimental models, newer production versions are in trials to yield data on patients' vocal folds while under microlaryngoscopic examination (E. Goodyer, personal communication, 2005).

Causes of vocal fold scarring have been classified by Benninger and colleagues [13] as traumatic (eg, blunt, penetrating, radiation, surgery, glottic

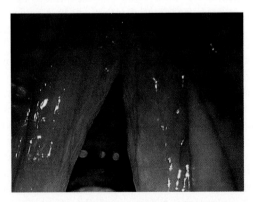

Fig. 7. Microlaryngoscopic image of bilateral scarring deformities along the medial vocal fold edges. There is incidental presence of Reinke's edema along the superior surface.

carcinoma), iatrogenic (eg, Teflon injection, injudicious vocal cord surgery, prolonged endotracheal intubation, nasogastric intubation, tracheotomy), inflammatory (eg, inhalation injury, rheumatologic diseases), and miscellaneous (eg. sulcus vocalis, congenital webs, cysts). Some of the most common causes probably are postsurgical and iatrogenic. For example, CO_2 laser treatment of glottic recurrent respiratory papillomatosis risks thermal injury to the epithelium and SLP. Despite its use as a precise laser, surrounding areas of secondary thermal trauma induce inflammation and abnormal collagen deposition [14]. Internal trauma from prolonged endotracheal intubation in ICU settings has increased the incidence of vocal fold scarring [15]. External trauma with de-epithelialization of the endolarynx and healing by secondary intention can set scar deposition into motion. Woo and colleagues [16] noted that the most common cause of dysphonia after vocal fold surgery was vocal fold scar. Serial biopsies for premalignant epithelium with keratosis also are a source of scar. Given that these biopsies have been classified as "vocal fold stripping," there is an inherent component of the procedure that pulls away underlying SLP with the overlying epithelium. Studies in feline models of serial vocal fold stripping showed increased deposition of fibrous tissue [17]. Tateya and colleagues [18] showed an increase in deposition of collagen types I and III with reduced hyaluronic acid (HA) in rats that underwent surgical biopsy similar to vocal fold stripping. That resection of the vocal fold cover yields scar is seen clearly in patients who have undergone CO_2 laser resections of the glottic larynx. Once healed, the operated vocal fold is uniformly stiff and volumetrically contracted [19,20].

Despite the differences in etiology, there is considerable overlap in clinical presentation, and ultimately, treatment options. Different investigators agree that clinical presentation is characterized by hoarseness, vocal fatigue, breathy vocal quality, and effortful voice projection [5,8,21]. Typical laryngoscopic findings in this population were described by Hirano and colleagues [8], and include bowed vocal folds with a spindle-shaped glottic closure pattern, medial furrows noted on inhalation phonation, and supraglottic hyperfunction.

Recent reports on the success of diagnosis with stroboscopic examination revealed that despite the classic findings that were noted by Hirano and colleagues [8], sulcus vocalis remains one of the most commonly missed glottic pathologies. Concordant with the observations of Poels and colleagues [22], Dailey and Zeitels noted that sulcus vocalis was the single most unidentified benign glottic entity in a population of patients who were evaluated for benign glottic pathology [23]. Given that the vector of examination is tangent to the site of pathology, there can be an "umbrella effect" that makes identification difficult (Fig. 8). This visual dilemma makes intraoperative examination that much more important, and stresses the need for other imaging modalities that permit visualization of the medial and infraglottic surfaces (eg, OCT, high-speed digital imaging) [9,12,24].

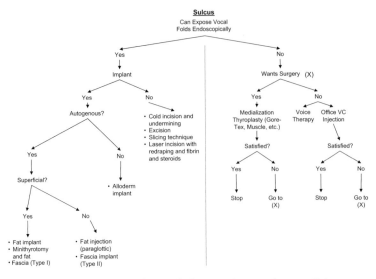

Fig. 8. Decision-making for surgical approaches to sulcus vocalis/scar.

Goals

Overall, the treatment goal is to improve glottic efficiency—reduce vocal effort and improve vocal quality. This goal is targeted by re-establishing the physical volume and microarchitecture of the vocal folds. Specifically, the goals are the elimination of restricted cover movement that is brought about by anatomic overadherence of the epithelium to deep vocal fold structures or by replacement of native SLP by less pliable scar.

Aggravating factors

Given that surgical success has been less than ideal, it is essential to maximize any benefit that is derived from control of aggravating factors. For example, suppression of laryngopharyngeal reflux (LPR) can reduce throat clearing, irregular sound production, and glottic edema. LPR may produce an environment that upregulates inflammation, which makes its control vital. Voice therapy that reduces supraglottic hyperfunction and enhances resonant characteristics can allow a pathway for improvement, and can provide the patient with different phonatory models, a certain sense of control, and access to supportive caregivers. Rosen [25] stressed the absolute requirement for 6 months of voice therapy, and noted the usefulness of "singing" therapy, in particular, for this population. Smoking, uncontrolled allergic disease, and any other inflammatory sources need to be addressed aggressively. It was noted recently that for patients who undergo surgical interventions, final outcomes should not be expected for at least 1 year [26,27]. Managing patient expectations regarding the time frame of potential improvement and the need for control of the aforementioned factors are essential. Overall, an attitude of patience and vigilance by the clinician and the patient yields the best results.

Operative considerations

Because there are multiple approaches to the repair of sulcus vocalis and vocal fold scarring, it is important to consider the various factors that may influence selection of repair by the patient and surgeon. Fig. 9 illustrates a proposed schema for clinical decision-making related to surgical approach. First, the ability of the surgeon to achieve proper direct microlaryngoscopic exposure in the operating room is an essential fork in the road of decision-making. If the surgeon cannot achieve full laryngoscopic exposure, then many techniques are eliminated. Remaining options are open medialization thyroplasty, injection thyroplasty in the office, and voice therapy. If an endoscopic approach is possible and appropriate, then the decision whether to incise and redrape the epithelium or to place an implant is the next step. If the use of an implant is selected, then the option of an autologous implant (fat, fascia) or nonautologous (Alloderm) is the last consideration.

Specific questions

The surgeon and patient must grapple with several questions as the decision-making discussion is broached (Table 1).

1. Is it an endoscopic or open approach?
2. Is there a separate harvest site?

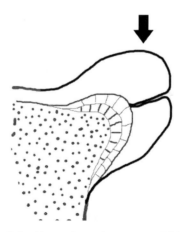

Fig. 9. Coronal view of the left midmusculomembranous vocal fold in a patient who has Reinke's edema and a concomitant sulcus deformity. The thick arrow notes the optical vector during stroboscopy. Note that the sulcus is hidden from view by overlying SLP and epithelium.

Table 1
Considerations related to surgical approach

	Endoscopic approach	Separate harvest site	Aimed at long-term solution	Appropriate for severe disease	Direct solution	Addresses gap	Adds pliability
Medialization thyroplasty	No	No	Yes	Yes	No	Yes	No
Collagen injection[a]	Yes	No	No?	Yes	Yes	Yes	Yes
Laser redrape	Yes	No	Yes	No	Yes	+/−	+/−
Cold redrape	Yes	No	Yes	No	Yes	+/−	+/−
Cold excision	Yes	No	Yes	No	Yes	+/−	+/−
Slicing technique	Yes	No	Yes	Yes	Yes	Yes	Yes
Alloderm implant	Yes	No	Yes	Yes	Yes	Yes	Yes
Fat injection	Yes	Yes	Yes	Yes	No	Yes	No
Fat implant[a]	Yes	Yes	Yes	Yes	Yes	Yes	Yes
Fascia implant – superficial	Yes	Yes	Yes	Yes	Yes	Yes	Yes
Fascia implant – deep	Yes	Yes	Yes	Yes	No	Yes	No

[a] Applies to treatment of scar also.

3. Is the approach aimed at a long-term solution?
4. Is the approach appropriate for severe cases?
5. Is the approach a direct or indirect solution?
6. Does the approach address the glottal gap, loss of pliability, or both?

Surgical approaches

Medialization thyroplasty

Medialization laryngoplasty is a well-established technique for closure of glottal gaps [28–30]. This technique has been successful for vocal fold paralysis, and uses different medializing implants (eg, Gore-Tex, silastic, hydroxylapatite) with no separate harvest site [31,32]. Koufman and Isaacson [33] affirmed the usefulness of silastic medialization for laryngeal and vocal fold scarring. Su and colleagues [34] reported on the use of strap muscle transposition if autogenous material is preferred. Gore-Tex has been used for glottal insufficiency of myriad types, including cancer defects, atrophy, and sulcus vocalis [32]. It is familiar to most surgeons and is aimed at a long-term solution because it does not resorb. With the use of Gore-Tex, it is easy to medialize selectively the healthy cover of the infraglottic edge of one or both vocal folds to narrow the glottic gap, and introduce vocal fold cover tissue of more native pliability than the stiff medial edge (S.M. Zeitels, personal communication, 2002). As a sole modality there is no objective evidence to support its use for sulcus vocalis or scar, although it can and should be considered strongly as a stand-alone or adjunctive treatment to the remaining options.

Collagen injection

Injectable collagen has a long record of safety and efficacy in the treatment of glottic insufficiency [35–38]. Results after collagen injection for glottic insufficiency have shown improvement of self-perception of voice as well as of jitter/shimmer values, signal to noise ratios, and airflow values [36]. The physical injection of the substance aids in the closure of the glottic gap, and the collagen is postulated to alter the nature of the adjacent scar and makes it more pliable by lamina propria remodeling [39]. Collagen is administered transorally in the clinic setting with no harvest site, and can offer substantial improvement for patients who cannot or will not undergo surgery. Given that collagen resorbs and that long-term data are not available, the patient should be counseled that repeat injections may be necessary, and that aggressive management of aforementioned aggravating factors is of great importance. Ford and Bless [40] noted that this modality is best applied for more modest gaps, and that large defects are not addressed well with this approach.

Cold instrument undermining of the sulcus

This microlaryngoscopic approach involves a longitudinal epithelial cordotomy with release of the depth of the sulcus from its deepest attachment, followed by simple redraping of the epithelium and SLP over the vocal fold body. Steroids may or may not be used. In a review of 20 patients who had pathologic sulcus vocalis and who underwent surgical repair, Ford and colleagues [1] noted that for three of five patients for whom postoperative voice results were available, two had notable improvement of stroboscopic parameters. This technique involves no implant and is achieved reasonably rapidly in the operating room. Its central appeal is the direct manner in which it addresses the anatomic deformity. The release of the tethered tissue may allow for better closure during oscillation, but it does not address the loss of native SLP nor the typical inflammatory and fibrotic component at the base of the sulcus. It is essential to understand that for all microlaryngoscopic approaches that address the vocal fold cover directly, a "burned bridge" phenomenon exists. After the abnormal cover has been operated upon, the healing process may induce worsening of cover pliability, such that revision surgery for sulcus must be undertaken with extreme caution.

Laser undermining with redraping, steroids, and fibrin glue application

Similar to the laryngoscopic cold instrument dissection that was described above, the CO_2 laser approach offers simultaneous hemostasis and apparent surgical precision. Steroids are injected at the time of redraping, and fibrin glue is applied to the epithelium to enhance reapproximation of the epithelial edges of the cordotomy. Remacle and colleagues [40] used this technique in 45 patients who had sulcus vocalis (type II), with a median follow-up of 5 months. They noted improvement in aerodynamic, acoustic, stroboscopic, and patient self-perception parameters. Notably, stroboscopic measures showed an improvement in symmetry, amplitude, and wave, which indicated that the release of the tethered epithelium enhanced pliability. Patients often remained "breathy and hoarse," however, which reflects the difficulty in obtaining a near normal voice, despite direct intervention upon the anatomic anomaly itself.

Cold instrument excision

For patients who have type III or pitlike sulcus deformities, formal endoscopic excision to the depth of the lesion has been performed [1]. In seven of the 10 patients for whom postoperative results were available, Ford and colleagues [1] noted variable improvement of stroboscopic parameters. The data were skewed, however, in that all patients had bilateral sulci, and those sulci often were a mix of types II and III. Intuitively, the poorer results make sense in that repair of a type III lesion often leaves a focal tissue defect or focal scarring for which correction is difficult. Relative advantages are the same as for the cold instrument redraping technique.

Slicing technique

This unique approach, which was reported by Pontes and Behlau [26], uses the principles of scar contracture repair to relieve the lines of tension in sulcus type II deformities. With the interruption of the scar band and the medial advancement of vocal fold cover, it is conceptually appealing because it can address deficits of pliability and glottic gap, respectively. Cuts of varying lengths are made in the coronal plane of the vocal fold to release the longitudinal scar band (Fig. 10). In a study of 10 patients using this technique, Pontes and Behlau [27] reported improvement of auditory–perceptual and stroboscopic parameters in 9 out of 10 patients, as well as improvement in voice spectrographic values. Ford and colleagues [1] also noted dramatic improvement of stroboscopic parameters in patients who underwent the slicing technique on one of two vocal folds for sulcus type II deformities. Because no sutures are used and the technique is unusual for most surgeons, it has had limited acceptance. It is perhaps best used in cases of severe deformity where less aggressive treatment is likely to be unsatisfactory. Aggressive year-long voice therapy is a mandatory part of this regimen, and should be made clear to any patient who is a candidate.

Alloderm implant

After the lysis of deep epithelial adhesions in type II sulcus repairs, Ford has introduced Alloderm strips longitudinally within Reinke's space to restore pliability and tissue loss within the SLP. Its placement requires epithelial suture to secure it, and thus, the repair thus been prone to granuloma

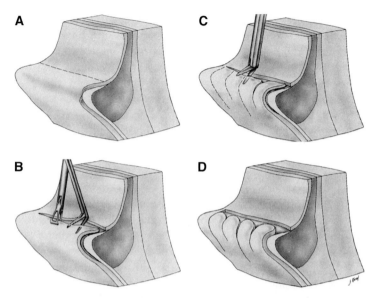

Fig. 10. Steps in the surgical management of type II sulcus vocalis, based on the technique of Pontes and Behlau. Each diagram is a simplified three-dimensional medial–sagittal construct with the vocal ligament in white. (*A*) An incision is made on the superior surface of the vocal fold parallel with the vocal fold free edge. (*B*) Microinstruments are used to grasp and incise the vocal fold cover. (*C*) Coronal incisions are made of varying lengths to perform scar release. (*D*) The vocal fold cover after incisions are made. (*From* Ford CN, Inagi K, Khidr A, Bless DM, Gilchrist KW. Sulcus vocalis: a rational analytical approach to diagnosis and management. Ann Otol Rhinol Laryngol 1996;105(3):191; with permission.)

formation and implant extrusion (unpublished data). Given these risks, it may be applied best in severe cases. Nevertheless, in eight patients who underwent fascia or Alloderm implant, there were improved acoustic, stroboscopic, and subjective perceptual values using the voice handicap index. Three of these patients underwent additional procedures (eg, thyroplasty). Three-year follow-up data suggest that vocal results continue to change over that time [41]. Work with implantation of stem cells and fascial implants suggests that the host tissues replace the implants over time, which helps to explain the vocal variability [42,43].

Fat injection (deep)

Correction of glottal insufficiency of various etiologies (including sulcus and scar) has been performed with injection techniques. Injection of fat into the paraglottic space for correction of unilateral vocal fold paralysis and glottic insufficiency has been advocated, based upon the known staying power of autologous fat (20–40% take rate) and the elimination of nonautologous materials [43–47]. Dedo [48] first reported free fat grafts into the larynx for construction of a neocord through an inconvenient laryngofissure approach. Since then, harvest with liposuction and free fat grafts injected through a Brünings gun under laryngoscopic exposure have become more popular. Hsiung and colleagues [45] demonstrated improvement of self-perceptual, acoustic, aerodynamic, and stroboscopic measures in 7 of 11 patients who had vocal fold scar patients who underwent paraglottic fat injection. Sometimes, repeated injections were necessary because of variable fat resorption. Brandenburg and colleagues [49] also reported improvement in one patient who had vocal fold scar who underwent the same approach. Issues of fat preparation to maximize viability remain unresolved.

Fat implant (superficial lamina propria)

Fat implantation into the vibratory margin and not into the paraglottic tissues was reported by Sataloff and colleagues [50] in 1997. Four patients received placement of fat into Reinke's space along with other procedures, such as medialization thyroplasty. Stroboscopic parameters were improved more reliably than were aerodynamic and acoustic measures. These data suggest improved pliability of the affected vocal folds, but a persistent gap for which more gross procedures were mandated for glottic closure. A follow-up study by the same group reported on improved stroboscopic and perceptual parameters. Eight patients underwent fat implantation often with adjunct procedures including medialization thyroplasty, fat injection into the paraglottic space, lysis of adhesions, scar excision, and steroid injection [51]. The central advantages were the ability to use autologous tissue and to improve the pliability of the vocal fold cover, which arguably is the most difficult task.

Fascia implant (superficial or deep)

Tsunoda and colleagues [52–54] reported on the use of temporalis fascia as a superficial and deep implant into the vocal fold. Six patients were treated endoscopically with a superficial implant of temporalis fascia into Reinke's space; all had improved maximum phonation time at 1 year along with a gradual improvement of maximum phonation time stroboscopic parameters. Two of three patients who underwent implantation into the paraglottic musculature experienced benefit at 1-year follow-up.

Implications of research

In general, surgical approaches do not address the presence of scar before and after sulcus repair. Biologic softening or replacement of the scar using endogenous mechanisms would be useful and represent the future of treatment options. Investigations within the last 10 years have helped to identify candidate "fillers" for the lamina propria, to characterize vocal fold scar in different animal models, and to test interventions using growth factors and stem cells for regeneration of the lamina propria.

Candidate fillers

Much of what has been learned about candidate fillers comes from animal studies and laboratory bench work. Generally, studies of humans have had small data sets and usually are not designed so that they can be considered evidence based. Consequently, much needs to be learned before we have definitive answers about the "ideal" candidate filler for correction of sulcus or scar deformities. In animal and rheologic studies, fat implants seem to be a strong candidate filler. Animal studies of fat implantation into vocal folds have demonstrated its feasibility to fill deficit areas and soften tissue [46,47]. Jiang and colleagues [55] also found that aerodynamic and acoustic parameters are near normal in injured canine vocal folds whose vibratory margins were implanted with fat. Using parallel-plate rheometry, Chan and Titze [56] found that the viscoelasticity of subcutaneous fat was closer to native vocal fold mucosa than were Teflon, cross-linked and uncross-linked collagen, and absorbable gelatin; this confirmed its candidacy as a biomechanically excellent vocal fold implant. Applying this knowledge to humans, Brandenburg and colleagues [57] demonstrated the usefulness of fat as an implant, and MRI studies have proven its durability, even years after injection. Concerns about the variability of resorption remain, and may be related, at least in part, to the ideal method of fat preparation, which has yet to be described [46].

Numerous ex vivo studies of candidate fillers have shown that HA possesses viscoelastic qualities closer to native vocal fold mucosa than do cross-linked collagen (Zyplast), micronized dermis (Cymetra), Teflon, gelfoam, and fat [58–60]. Chan and colleagues [61] also found that enzymatic degradation of HA significantly altered the viscoelastic properties of vocal fold mucosa, which suggests its importance in vocal fold cover mechanics.

In a prospective, randomized human trial of vocal fold fillers, Hertegard and colleagues [62] injected collagen or Hylan B gel (cross-linked HA) into one vocal fold in patients who had vocal fold atrophy or paresis. Forty-two patients were available for 2-year follow-up. Self-ratings and stroboscopic measures were improved in both groups. Less resorption was noted in the group that received Hylan B gel, which again suggests the usefulness of HA.

Characterization of scar

Fundamental understanding of the nature of vocal fold scar has been pursued in various animal models at different intervals after injury. Using a canine model, Rousseau and colleagues [63] performed histologic studies after cold instrument injury to the vocal folds, and found decreased elastin content with substantial disorganization of fibers. There was increased collagen deposition when compared with the noninjured side at 2 and 6 months after injury. Hirano and colleagues [64] also examined canine vocal folds at the same time interval after injury with cold instruments. Compared with the control vocal folds, fibronectin increased significantly in the SLP on the scarred vocal folds at 2 and 6 months; however, codeposition of collagen was observed only at 6 months. They concluded that fibronectin might be important in providing a scaffold for the deposition of other proteins, such as collagen.

In the rabbit model, Rousseau and colleagues [65] found results that were similar to earlier canine studies. Six months after stripping the vocal folds to the thyroarytenoid muscle, fragmented and disorganized elastin was noted along with increased collagen deposition, when compared with the noninjured side. Thibeault and colleagues [66] found a decrease in collagen and elastin deposition 60 days after similar injury in rabbits. As expected, however, there was more disorganization of collagen bundles and an increased stiffness of the injured side. In a study of rat vocal fold scarring at different time intervals, Tateya and colleagues [18] found less HA and more collagen types I and III than in the controls at all time points. Furthermore, they noted an active wound healing process in the first 2 months, which was followed by more modest remodeling. These studies help to solidify the notions that disorganized collagen deposition is a common event in early wound healing, that collagen deposition may be dependent on fibronectin, and that HA levels are reduced in injured animal vocal folds.

Molecular interventions

Given that the process of vocal fold wound healing is at the heart of scar modulation, the use of growth factors and stem cells has been investigated recently. In preliminary studies, Hirano and colleagues [67] found hepatocyte growth factor (HGF) and its receptor (c-met) on epithelial and gland cells of rat vocal folds. Their presence was most prominent during the re-epithelialization process 10 to 15 days after injury; HGF was localized to the fibroblasts of the lamina propria, which implicated those cells in the wound-healing process. To test the activity of these fibroblasts, canine lamina propria fibroblasts were cultured in vitro and subjected to HGF and transforming growth factor (TGF)-β1. Production of HA, collagen type I, and fibronectin were measured after treatment with the growth factors. TGF-β1 increased production of all molecules, whereas HGF increased only HA, did not change fibronectin levels, and reduced collagen type I. Thus, the profile of molecules that are favorable for reduction of scar is found with HGF stimulation of fibroblasts, and led to further investigations [68].

Again using cultured canine fibroblasts, Hirano and colleagues [69] found that the fibroblasts in Reinke's space were far more susceptible to influence by HGF than were the fibroblasts of the macula flava, which indicated locoregional control mechanisms. Although the same group found that multiple growth factors—HGF, TGF-β1, epidermal growth factor, and basic growth factor—increased the production of HA from cultured fibroblasts in vitro, the overall positive healing profile of HGF led to its use in interventional animal studies [70].

To evaluate the therapeutic effects of HGF, Hirano and colleagues [71] injured one vocal fold of 20 rabbits, and immediately injected them with HGF or saline. The group that was treated with HGF displayed less collagen deposition, less disorganized elastin, less tissue contraction, and less stiffness on rheologic and stroboscopic evaluation. Similarly in a canine model, HGF demonstrated improvement of aerodynamic and stroboscopic measures 6 months after injury when compared with vocal folds that were treated with saline or with simultaneous HGF and autologous vocal fold fibroblasts. Collagen deposition also was reduced, and tissue contraction was barely noticeable with HGF treatment [72].

Another promising development in the treatment of vocal fold scar has been the use of stem cells. Using a canine model, Chhetri and colleagues [73] made use of autologous cultured fibroblasts to test histologic and stroboscopic effects on injured vocal folds. Although histologic evaluation revealed an increased density of fibroblasts, collagen, and reticulin; a decreased density of elastin; and no change in HA, stroboscopic parameters mucosal waves became normal in four animals and near normal in the other four. Using cultured autologous mesenchymal stem cells in a canine model, Kanemaru and colleagues [42] also demonstrated that the injection of stem cells into injured vocal fold tissue helped to restore vocal fold morphology and histology. Mesenchymal stem cells were believed to persist in the tissues and to enhance nuclear staining of existing cell types, such as muscle.

Gene therapy also may be on the horizon for treatment of scar. Liu and colleagues [74] hypothesized that blocking the TGF-β receptor on fibroblasts using adenovirus transfection may alter would healing in rat dermis. They found a decrease in TGF-β production, a migration of fewer inflammatory cells to the wound, and a reduction of the size of the scar.

Summary

Treatment of sulcus vocalis and vocal fold scar are linked intimately to a stiffened and volumetrically deficient lamina propria. Open and endoscopic procedures with or without vocal fold fillers must be tailored to the needs of the individual patient. Often, combined and repeated treatments are necessary to enhance vocal outcomes. Extensive research has revealed the importance of restoration of HA and collagen in basic vocal fold architecture and function during phonation. As the homeostatic mechanisms of the lamina propria continue to be understood, new pathways, such as growth factors, stem cells, and gene therapy, may provide exciting avenues for this refractory problem.

Acknowledgments

I gratefully acknowledge the editing of Dr. Diane Bless and the administrative assistance of Delight Hensler.

References

[1] Ford CN, Inagi K, Khidr A, et al. Sulcus vocalis: a rational analytical approach to diagnosis and management. Ann Otol Rhinol Laryngol 1996;105(3):189–200.

[2] Itoh T, Kawasaki H, Morikawa I, et al. Vocal fold furrows. A 10-year review of 240 patients. Auris Nasus Larynx 1983;10(Suppl):S17–26.

[3] Sato K, Hirano M. Electron microscopic investigation of sulcus vocalis. Ann Otol Rhinol Laryngol 1998;107(1):56–60.

[4] Arnold GE. Dysplastic dysphonia: minor anomalies of the vocal cords causing persistent hoarseness. Laryngoscope 1958;68(2):142–58.

[5] Bouchayer M, Cornut G, Witzig E, et al. Epidermoid cysts, sulci, and mucosal bridges of the true vocal cord: a report of 157 cases. Laryngoscope 1985;95(9 Pt 1):1087–94.

[6] Van Caneghem D. L'etiologie de la corde vocale a sillon. Ann Mal Oreille Larynx Nez Pharynx 1928;47:121–30 [in French].

[7] Nakayama M, Ford CN, Brandenburg JH, et al. Sulcus vocalis in laryngeal cancer: a histopathologic study. Laryngoscope 1994;104(1 Pt 1):16–24.

[8] Hirano M, Yoshida T, Tanaka S, et al. Sulcus vocalis: functional aspects. Ann Otol Rhinol Laryngol 1990;99(9 Pt 1):679–83.

[9] Burns JA. Imaging the mucosa of the human vocal fold with optical coherence tomography. Ann Otol Rhinol Laryngol 2005;114(9):671–6.

[10] Mapping the visco-elastic properties of the vocal fold. Advances in quantitative laryngology, voice and speech research. Hamburg (Germany): 2003.

[11] Hertegard S. Viscoelasticity in scarred rabbit vocal folds after hyaluronan injection - short term results. Presented at the Annual Meeting of the American Academy of Otolaryngology-Head and Neck Surgery Foundation. New York, September 19–22, 2004.

[12] Klein A. In-vivo imaging of human vocal folds using optical coherence tomography. Boca Raton (FL): American Laryngological Association; May 13–16, 2005.

[13] Benninger MS, Alessi D, Archer S, et al. Vocal fold scarring: current concepts and management. Otolaryngol Head Neck Surg 1996;115(5):474–82.

[14] Ossoff RH, Werkhaven JA, Dere H. Soft-tissue complications of laser surgery for recurrent respiratory papillomatosis. Laryngoscope 1991;101(11):1162–6.

[15] Sataloff RT, Hawkshaw M, Hoover C, et al. Post-intubation vocal fold scar. Ear Nose Throat J 1997;76(3):128.

[16] Woo P, Casper J, Colton R, et al. Diagnosis and treatment of persistent dysphonia after laryngeal surgery: a retrospective analysis of 62 patients. Laryngoscope 1994;104(9):1084–91.

[17] Leonard RJ, Kiener D, Charpied G, et al. Effects of repeated stripping on vocal fold mucosa in cats. Ann Otol Rhinol Laryngol 1985;94(3):258–62.

[18] Tateya T, Tateya I, Sohn JH, et al. Histologic characterization of rat vocal fold scarring. Ann Otol Rhinol Laryngol 2005;114(3):183–91.

[19] Zeitels SM. Optimizing voice after endoscopic partial laryngectomy. Otolaryngol Clin North Am 2004;37(3):627–36.

[20] Steiner W. Results of curative laser microsurgery of laryngeal carcinomas. Am J Otolaryngol 1993;14(2):116–21.

[21] Lindestad PA, Hertegard S. Spindle-shaped glottal insufficiency with and without sulcus vocalis: a retrospective study. Ann Otol Rhinol Laryngol 1994;103(7):547–53.

[22] Poels PJ, de Jong FI, Schutte HK. Consistency of the preoperative and intraoperative diagnosis of benign vocal fold lesions. J Voice 2003;17(3):425–33.

[23] Dailey SH, Zeitels SM. The evaluation of benign glottic lesions: rigid telescopic stroboscopy vs. suspension microlaryngoscopy. J Voice (in press).

[24] Berry DA, Montequin DW, Tayama N. High-speed digital imaging of the medial surface of the vocal folds. J Acoust Soc Am 2001;110(5 Pt 1):2539–47.

[25] Rosen CA. Vocal fold scar: evaluation and treatment. Otolaryngol Clin North Am 2000;33(5):1081–6.

[26] Welham NV, Rousseau B, Ford CN, et al. Tracking outcomes after phonosurgery for sulcus vocalis: a case report. J Voice 2003;17(4):571–8.

[27] Pontes P, Behlau M. Treatment of sulcus vocalis: auditory perceptual and acoustical analysis of the slicing mucosa surgical technique. J Voice 1993;7(4):365–76.

[28] Netterville JL, Stone RE, Luken ES, et al. Silastic medialization and arytenoid adduction: the Vanderbilt experience. A review of 116 phonosurgical procedures. Ann Otol Rhinol Laryngol 1993;102(6):413–24.

[29] Postma GN, Blalock PD, Koufman JA. Bilateral medialization laryngoplasty. Laryngoscope 1998;108(10):1429–34.

[30] Koufman JA. Laryngoplasty for vocal cord medialization: an alternative to Teflon. Laryngoscope 1986;96(7):726–31.

[31] Cummings CW, Purcell LL, Flint PW. Hydroxylapatite laryngeal implants for medialization. Preliminary report. Ann Otol Rhinol Laryngol 1993;102(11):843–51.

[32] Zeitels SM, Mauri M, Dailey SH. Medialization laryngoplasty with Gore-Tex for voice restoration secondary to glottal incompetence: indications and observations. Ann Otol Rhinol Laryngol 2003;112(2):180–4.

[33] Koufman JA, Isaacson G. Laryngoplastic phonosurgery. Otolaryngol Clin North Am 1991; 24(5):1151–77.

[34] Su CY, Tsai SS, Chiu JF, et al. Medialization laryngoplasty with strap muscle transposition for vocal fold atrophy with or without sulcus vocalis. Laryngoscope 2004;114(6):1106–12.

[35] Ford CN, Bless DM, Campbell D. Studies of injectable soluble collagen for vocal fold augmentation. Rev Laryngol Otol Rhinol (Bord) 1987;108(1):33–6.

[36] Ford CN, Bless DM, Loftus JM. Role of injectable collagen in the treatment of glottic insufficiency: a study of 119 patients. Ann Otol Rhinol Laryngol 1992;101(3):237–47.

[37] Ford CN, Bless DM. Selected problems treated by vocal fold injection of collagen. Am J Otolaryngol 1993;14(4):257–61.

[38] Ford CN, Staskowski PA, Bless DM. Autologous collagen vocal fold injection: a preliminary clinical study. Laryngoscope 1995;105(9 Pt 1):944–8.

[39] Ford C, Bless DM. Collagen injection in the scarred vocal fold. J Voice 1987;1:116–8.

[40] Remacle M, Lawson G, Degols JC, et al. Microsurgery of sulcus vergeture with carbon dioxide laser and injectable collagen. Ann Otol Rhinol Laryngol 2000;109(2):141–8.

[41] Perceptual, instrumental and psychosocial outcomes after phonosurgery for sulcus vocalis. American Academy of Otolaryngology- Head and Neck Surgery; 2004; New York.

[42] Kanemaru S, Nakamura T, Omori K, et al. Regeneration of the vocal fold using autologous mesenchymal stem cells. Ann Otol Rhinol Laryngol 2003;112(11):915–20.

[43] Hsiung MW, Kang BH, Pai L, et al. Combination of fascia transplantation and fat injection into the vocal fold for sulcus vocalis: long-term results. Ann Otol Rhinol Laryngol 2004; 113(5):359–66.

[44] Hartl DM, Hans S, Vaissiere J, et al. Objective voice analysis after autologous fat injection for unilateral vocal fold paralysis. Ann Otol Rhinol Laryngol 2001;110(3):229–35.

[45] Hsiung MW, Lin YS, Su WF, et al. Autogenous fat injection for vocal fold atrophy. Eur Arch Otorhinolaryngol 2003;260(9):469–74.

[46] Mikus JL, Koufman JA, Kilpatrick SE. Fate of liposuctioned and purified autologous fat injections in the canine vocal fold. Laryngoscope 1995;105(1):17–22.

[47] Wexler DB, Jiang J, Gray SD, et al. Phonosurgical studies: fat-graft reconstruction of injured canine vocal cords. Ann Otol Rhinol Laryngol 1989;98(9):668–73.

[48] Dedo HH. A technique for vertical hemilaryngectomy to prevent stenosis and aspiration. Laryngoscope 1975;85(6):978–84.

[49] Brandenburg JH, Kirkham W, Koschkee D. Vocal cord augmentation with autogenous fat. Laryngoscope 1992;102(5):495–500.

[50] Sataloff RT, Spiegel JR, Hawkshaw MJ. Vocal fold scar. Ear Nose Throat J 1997;76(11):776.

[51] Neuenschwander MC, Sataloff RT, Abaza MM, et al. Management of vocal fold scar with autologous fat implantation: perceptual results. J Voice 2001;15(2):295–304.

[52] Tsunoda K, Baer T, Niimi S. Autologous transplantation of fascia into the vocal fold: long-term results of a new phonosurgical technique for glottal incompetence. Laryngoscope 2001; 111(3):453–7.

[53] Tsunoda K, Niimi S. Autologous transplantation of fascia into the vocal fold. Laryngoscope 2000;110(4):680–2.

[54] Tsunoda K, Takanosawa M, Niimi S. Autologous transplantation of fascia into the vocal fold: a new phonosurgical technique for glottal incompetence. Laryngoscope 1999;109(3): 504–8.

[55] Jiang JJ, Titze IR, Wexler DB, et al. Fundamental frequency and amplitude perturbation in reconstructed canine vocal folds. Ann Otol Rhinol Laryngol 1994;103(2):145–8.

[56] Chan RW, Titze IR. Viscosities of implantable biomaterials in vocal fold augmentation surgery. Laryngoscope 1998;108(5):725–31.

[57] Brandenburg JH, Unger JM, Koschkee D. Vocal cord injection with autogenous fat: a long-term magnetic resonance imaging evaluation. Laryngoscope 1996;106(2 Pt 1):174–80.

[58] Dahlqvist A, Garskog O, Laurent C, et al. Viscoelasticity of rabbit vocal folds after injection augmentation. Laryngoscope 2004;114(1):138–42.

[59] Klemuk SA, Titze IR. Viscoelastic properties of three vocal-fold injectable biomaterials at low audio frequencies. Laryngoscope 2004;114(9):1597–603.

[60] Chan RW, Titze IR. Hyaluronic acid (with fibronectin) as a bioimplant for the vocal fold mucosa. Laryngoscope 1999;109(7 Pt 1):1142–9.

[61] Chan RW, Gray SD, Titze IR. The importance of hyaluronic acid in vocal fold biomechanics. Otolaryngol Head Neck Surg 2001;124(6):607–14.

[62] Hertegard S, Hallen L, Laurent C, et al. Cross-linked hyaluronan versus collagen for injection treatment of glottal insufficiency: 2-year follow-up. Acta Otolaryngol 2004;124(10): 1208–14.

[63] Rousseau B, Hirano S, Scheidt TD, et al. Characterization of vocal fold scarring in a canine model. Laryngoscope 2003;113(4):620–7.

[64] Hirano S, Bless DM, Rousseau B, et al. Fibronectin and adhesion molecules on canine scarred vocal folds. Laryngoscope 2003;113(6):966–72.

[65] Rousseau B, Hirano S, Chan RW, et al. Characterization of chronic vocal fold scarring in a rabbit model. J Voice 2004;18(1):116–24.

[66] Thibeault SL, Gray SD, Bless DM, et al. Histologic and rheologic characterization of vocal fold scarring. J Voice 2002;16(1):96–104.

[67] Hirano S, Thibeault S, Bless DM, et al. Hepatocyte growth factor and its receptor c-met in rat and rabbit vocal folds. Ann Otol Rhinol Laryngol 2002;111(8):661–6.

[68] Hirano S, Bless D, Heisey D, et al. Roles of hepatocyte growth factor and transforming growth factor beta1 in production of extracellular matrix by canine vocal fold fibroblasts. Laryngoscope 2003;113(1):144–8.

[69] Hirano S, Bless DM, Massey RJ, et al. Morphological and functional changes of human vocal fold fibroblasts with hepatocyte growth factor. Ann Otol Rhinol Laryngol 2003;112(12): 1026–33.

[70] Hirano S, Bless DM, Heisey D, et al. Effect of growth factors on hyaluronan production by canine vocal fold fibroblasts. Ann Otol Rhinol Laryngol 2003;112(7):617–24.

[71] Hirano S, Bless DM, Rousseau B, et al. Prevention of vocal fold scarring by topical injection of hepatocyte growth factor in a rabbit model. Laryngoscope 2004;114(3):548–56.

[72] Hirano S, Bless DM, Nagai H, et al. Growth factor therapy for vocal fold scarring in a canine model. Ann Otol Rhinol Laryngol 2004;113(10):777–85.

[73] Chhetri DK, Head C, Revazova E, et al. Lamina propria replacement therapy with cultured autologous fibroblasts for vocal fold scars. Otolaryngol Head Neck Surg 2004;131(6): 864–70.

[74] Liu W, Chua C, Wu X, et al. Inhibiting scar formation in rat wounds by adenovirus-mediated overexpression of truncated TGF-beta receptor II. Plast Reconstr Surg 2005;115(3): 860–70.

ELSEVIER
SAUNDERS

Otolaryngol Clin N Am
39 (2006) 43–54

OTOLARYNGOLOGIC
CLINICS
OF NORTH AMERICA

Injection Laryngoplasty

Miriam A. O'Leary, MD,
Gregory A. Grillone, MD, FACS*

*Department of Otolaryngology–Head and Neck Surgery, Boston University Medical Center,
88 East Newton Street, D-608, Boston, MA 02118, USA*

History

Injection laryngoplasty is a continuously evolving procedure, and yet, it retains important principles that were established more than a century ago. Even the syringe that was designed by Bruening, the forefather of this technique, is still in use today. His experiments with injecting paraffin into the paraglottic space to medialize paralyzed vocal cords were published in 1911 [1,2]. The procedure was so riddled with complications, however, that it nearly died out in the early 1900s. Bruening's difficulties with inflammatory response to the injected substance, as well as migration and extrusion, remain challenges today. Forty years passed before another investigator effectively continued Bruening's work. Arnold experimented with injection into the thyroarytenoid muscle using cartilage particles and bovine bone dust, and used the theory that biologic materials would induce less tissue reaction and would be tolerated better than synthetic ones [1]. Arnold was correct, but he encountered the other chief problem that continues to trouble researchers today: resorption of injected material with loss of the desired effect on the vocal cords.

The next milestone in the history of injection laryngoplasty was the use of polytetrafluoroethylene (Teflon), which was introduced in the 1960s. This remains a tool in the laryngologist's armamentarium, although its pitfalls and complications are well documented in the literature. These are discussed later in more detail. The double-edged sword of Teflon is its permanence in tissue once it is injected. The subsequent developments in vocal cord injection allowed otolaryngologists to envision this procedure not only as a permanent alteration, but also as a temporizing measure. Gelatin (Gelfoam), introduced in the 1970s, was the diametric opposite of Teflon, and lasted

---

* Corresponding author.
E-mail address: gregory.grillone@bmc.org (G.A. Grillone).

0030-6665/06/$ - see front matter © 2005 Elsevier Inc. All rights reserved.
doi:10.1016/j.otc.2005.10.008   *oto.theclinics.com*

for only 4 to 6 weeks in the thyroarytenoid muscle [1]. It is still a useful tool clinically, but is not discussed here.

It is interesting that many of the materials that have been studied in the past several decades are borrowed from the field of facial plastics. Bovine collagen was introduced in the 1980s after many years of use by aesthetic surgeons [3,4]. This was the first substance that was proposed to have mechanical and physiologic effects on the tissues of the vocal fold [5]. In addition, laryngologists used the characteristics of this biologic graft to address the question of how to improve the mobile, but atrophied, vocal fold. This has blossomed into a huge interest within injection laryngoplasty, and has been the source of several exciting discoveries.

The main pitfall of bovine collagen, hypersensitivity, led to experimentation with autologous collagen. As expected, this often is prohibitively expensive and time consuming, so attention turned to banked cadaveric tissues. These include acellular dermis (Alloderm, LifeCell Corp., Branchburg, NJ) and a micronized formulation (Cymetra, LifeCell Corp. Branchburg, NJ) that still enjoy popularity among researchers and clinicians. Easily obtainable autologous tissues (ie, fascia and fat) began to appear in studies during the 1990s. Their physiologic properties are even more compatible with native vocal fold than are those of bovine collagen, and led to more experiments with mobile, but scarred or atrophied, vocal cords. The ideal injectable substance remains elusive.

The two most recent developments in injectable materials emphasize the increasingly divergent applications of injection laryngoplasty (ie, medializing a paralyzed or paretic cord versus restoring a vibratory membrane in a scarred or atrophied cord). Hydroxylapatite (HA) and hyaluronan attempt to address these two applications, respectively. Long-term results will not be available soon, but the early outcomes are promising, and ensure that injection laryngoplasty will maintain its place in phonosurgery for the foreseeable future.

Materials

Many of the advances in injection laryngoplasty have arisen from novel materials rather than new techniques. Comparison of these substances (Table 1) elucidates many of the issues that are considered by the laryngologist as he or she evaluates a patient for injection laryngoplasty. Teflon still has its place in the field of injection laryngoplasty, namely for the permanent medialization of a paralyzed vocal cord. Livesey and Carding [6], among other investigators, demonstrated its effectiveness in restoring effective glottic closure for unilateral cord paralysis. Teflon's permanence in tissue has been verified by multiple investigators. Problems arise from the technical challenge of injecting this nonviscous substance, which requires a large gauge needle, and therefore is difficult to place precisely in the millimeters-thick layers of the vocal fold. In Chang and Chang's [7] series, poor voice

Table 1
Comparison of materials for injection laryngoplasty

Material	Location of injection	Amount injected	Duration	Viscosity	Needle gauge	FDA Approval
Teflon	Lateral to vocal ligament	Exact amount	Permanent	Low	18	Yes
Bovine collagen	Lateral to vocal ligament or in vibratory membrane	Overinject	6 months	High	27	No
Human collagen	Lateral to vocal ligament or in vibratory membrane	Overinject	6 months	High	27–30	No
Cymetra	Lateral to vocal ligament	Overinject	6–9 months	Low	22	Yes
Fascia	Lateral to vocal ligament or in vibratory membrane	Overinject	3 months	High	18–22	NA
Fat	Lateral to vocal ligament or in vibratory membrane	Overinject	3 months	High	18–22	NA
Hydroxylapatite	Lateral to vocal ligament	Slightly overinject	2 years	Low	26	Yes
Hyaluronic acid	In vibratory membrane	Slightly overinject	2 years	High	26	No

Abbreviations: FDA, U.S. Food and Drug administration; NA, not applicable.

outcome occurred only when Teflon was injected in the wrong amount (overfilling, impairing effective closure) or location (superficial injection stiffening the vibratory membrane). Their patients had no Teflon granulomas; however, this is a known phenomenon, even with flawless technique [8]. Voice often remains poor despite removal of these granulomas [2]. There also are reports of Teflon particles migrating within the tissues [1]. Clearly, Teflon should not be used for patients who have atrophied cords or mobile vocal cords that are scarred.

Silicone, as an injectable substance, has been studied much less frequently than have many of the other substances described here. Therefore, long-term results are unavailable. In theory, as a stable nonviscous material, it will medialize a paralyzed vocal cord permanently. One of the formulations that is used consists of silicone microspheres suspended in a water-soluble "carrier gel," namely polymethylsiloxane elastomer (Bioplastique, Uroplasty BV, Geleen, The Netherlands) [9]. The gel is excreted by the body, whereas the microspheres remain in place. This injectable substance is unique in that its texture is similar to cartilage. It is purported to be nonporous and to induce minimal tissue inflammation [10]. Hirano and colleagues [11] demonstrated significant improvement in voice quality and objective measurements of phonation after injection of paralyzed cords with silicone. Alves and colleagues [12] obtained similar results, and were able to demonstrate sustained effect over 6 months.

Bovine collagen has been well studied for more than 2 decades. Unlike most of the other materials that are discussed here, it has been applied successfully to scarred/atrophied cords and immobile cords. This was demonstrated elegantly by Courey [13]. Ford and colleagues [3,4,14–16] published several studies on scarred, atrophied, or otherwise damaged vibratory membranes that they treated with bovine collagen. Their results demonstrated subjective and objective improvements in phonation that were sustained over several months. Notably, patients who had one, rather than two, damaged vocal folds experienced superior outcomes. They postulated that this xenograft promotes native production of collagen; at the same time, it stimulates native collagenase activity, which leads to tissue remodeling, and ultimately, "softening" of scar. This remains to be proven definitively. Hertegard and colleagues [17] showed that bovine collagen has viscoelastic properties that are similar to the rabbit vocal fold, which again supports its use to restore the vibratory membrane. It can be injected through a 27-gauge needle, which allows the precision that is needed to inject the superficial lamina propria.

Experiments with bovine collagen in paralyzed vocal cords also showed efficacy. Investigators achieved good outcomes with transcutaneous [18] and transoral [19] techniques. Some studies showed more subjective, than objective, improvement (ie, patient surveys indicated better outcomes than have measurements of maximum phonatory time, fundamental frequency, jitter, and shimmer) [5,14]. Hoffman and colleagues [20] found bovine collagen injection to be a useful adjunct to medialization laryngoplasty when further improvements in voice were desired. The material lasts approximately 6 months in the plane of the thyroarytenoid muscle [10,13]. This is beneficial to the patient whose vocal cord function may recover over time; however, a more long-term solution is necessary for most patients. Another major problem that is associated with the use of bovine collagen is the risk of hypersensitivity. Patients must undergo skin testing before injection; furthermore, patients may experience an adverse reaction despite a normal skin test [1,10,21]. Cross-linked preparations of this substance are associated with a lower risk of hypersensitivity [4]. Finally, it is necessary to overinject by approximately 20% to 30% because some resorption will occur soon after injection [22].

Autologous collagen was developed to avoid the possibility of hypersensitivity. This material is obtained by harvesting skin from the patient, and processing it to obtain collagen from the dermal elements. Approximately 5 cm^2 of skin yields 1 mL of injectable collagen [10]. The injection is tolerated well and provides results that are comparable to bovine collagen, in terms of voice outcome, duration of effect, and degree of resorption [1,10,15,23]; however, preparation of the final product can take several weeks and is extremely expensive. This essentially negates the advantage of better biocompatibility, and autologous collagen has not been used widely in injection laryngoplasty.

Acellular dermis (Alloderm) and its micronized form (Cymetra) are also borrowed from our plastic surgery colleagues. The removal of all cells from cadaveric dermis results in a graft with low immunogenicity [9,10,24]. At the same time, the matrix of dermal components facilitates fibrous ingrowth and angiogenesis after injection [13]. This advantageous combination of properties presumably creates a stable, long-lasting implant. Lundy and colleagues [25] attained results with Cymetra that were comparable to type I thyroplasty, as measured by multiple perceptual, stroboscopic, acoustic, and aerodynamic parameters; however, validation of their results is lacking in the literature. Karpenko and colleagues [26] found that voice improvements were not maintained over a 3-month period for unilateral vocal cord paralysis. The authors have found that Cymetra gives favorable voice results. Although the effect can be short-lived, this can be overcome by adding "booster" injections as necessary. Also, as the authors have gained more experience with using this substance, they have found that overinjection and overcorrection results in longer lasting effects.

Over the past 5 years, several investigators have published their experience with injecting fascia into scarred and paralyzed vocal cords [27–32]. Overall, subjective and objective measures of voice show improvement that is maintained over approximately 1 year. The degree and speed of resorption vary among these reports. In addition, fascia has not been compared with other injectable materials in the literature, so it is difficult to assess its place within the field. In an animal study, Duke and colleagues [30] showed similar graft yield and duration between fascia and fat injection.

Fat is a much more popular autologous graft. Numerous studies have demonstrated its usefulness in immobile and atrophied/scarred cords [32–43]. Advantages of this technique include abundant availability of material, uncomplicated harvest, and minimal graft preparation. Like fascia, fat has excellent biocompatibility as a graft, and causes minimal inflammatory reaction. A histologic analysis by Sasai and colleagues [33] demonstrated viable, normal-appearing adipocytes and minimal surrounding inflammatory response 1 and 3 years after injection. The clinical effects of fat injection are not as long-lived.

The viscoelastic properties of fat are similar to those of the vocal cord lamina propria. A publication by Chen and colleagues [34] showed that patients who had atrophy or sulcus vocalis had improved vocal fold edge linearity, vibration amplitude, and mucosal wave excursion after fat injection into the lamina propria. Hsiung and colleagues [43] showed similar effect on acoustic and stroboscopic characteristics for paralyzed and atrophied cords that were treated with fat injection. The two drawbacks to the use of fat are the need to overcorrect to account for resorption, and the short and unpredictable duration of effect. For the patient who may recover mobility of a paretic cord, fat injection is an excellent choice to restore voice and glottic competence early in their course.

HA, which is the mineral component of bone, actually assumes a texture that is similar to soft tissue in its injectable form [10]. There are high hopes that HA will match the durability of Teflon, without the tendency to foreign body reactions, migration, and extrusion. Much work remains to be done to demonstrate this; however, studies show stability over 2 years and an overall mild inflammatory response (although foreign body giant cell reactions occasionally have been reported) [1,10,44]. HA has provided good vocal fold closure in paralyzed cords without altering their normal mucosal wave. It also has been applied in presbylaryngis, Parkinson's disease, and abductor spasmodic dysphonia with good subjective results. The carrier gel for the HA microspherules is water-based and resorbs quickly after injection, so a small degree of over overcorrection is necessary [45].

Hyaluronic acid is the subject of several recent publications. This organic molecule, which is common to all species, offers excellent biocompatibility; histologic studies show recruitment of fibroblasts and ingrowth of new connective tissue with no inflammatory reaction [46,47]. In addition, hyaluronic acid has the closest match to native vocal cord viscoelasticity of any substance that has been evaluated to date [17,48]. In a compelling study by Tateya and colleagues [49], vocal cord scar was induced in rats; subsequent histologic examination of these cords, compared with normal ones, revealed a decrease in hyaluronic acid and an increase in fibronectin and collagen types I and III. Tateya and colleagues' work lends credence to the further evaluation of hyaluronic acid injections for scarred or traumatized vocal cords. Another favorable property of hyaluronic acid is that it binds water, and thus, loses less volume over time [10], although some resorption has been noted [50]. A large study by Hertegard and colleagues [50,51] demonstrated efficacy for immobile and atrophied cords that was maintained over 2 years. Additionally, they showed that hyaluronic acid was superior to bovine collagen in preserving vibration amplitude and glottal area variations at the vocal fold edge.

Finally, one of the most recent and interesting developments in injection laryngoplasty has been the use of fibroblast growth factor (FGF). Hirano and colleagues [52] have injected FGF into animal models of atrophied cords. They based this study on their previous in vitro work, in which FGF induced hyaluronic acid production and decreased collagen synthesis (ie, FGF reversed processes that contribute to atrophy). The in vivo study shows a promising increase in hyaluronic acid content of the lamina propria, but no effect on collagen. Undoubtedly, this work will be continued based on these enticing results. If FGF proves to be successful, it will further the current trend of addressing the root causes of vocal cord dysfunction.

Technique

In one sense, injection laryngoplasty is the "minimally invasive" form of medialization laryngoplasty. Typically, no external incisions are made, and injections can be performed in a variety of settings, depending on several factors, including the goal of the procedure, the need to overinject versus fill the defect precisely, patient comfort and anatomy, and physician skill. Laryngologists have the luxury of multiple options when planning an injection laryngoplasty.

The classic approach is suspension microlaryngoscopy (SML). This is the least technically difficult method because the patient is positioned optimally, and the view of the glottis is magnified. Options for anesthesia include a small endotracheal tube or jet ventilation. The key disadvantage of this technique is that the patient is unable to phonate during the procedure and provide immediate feedback as to the vocal quality after injection. This is more of an issue for materials that do not resorb, because they must be injected in the precise amount. These are described in Table 1, and include Teflon and HA. It is easier to judge the degree of correction if the patient can phonate during the procedure. For grafts that must be overinjected to account for subsequent resorption (including collagen, fascia, and fat, and in the authors' experience, Cymetra), SML is a good technique because injection is judged by careful visualization more than by the sound of the voice. Some patients, such as those who have an anteriorly placed larynx or poor head extension, may be difficult to expose using this technique. In those cases, alternative techniques must be used. Furthermore, some laryngologists, including Ford and colleagues [53], argued that even if exposure is not a problem, proper positioning for SML distorts laryngeal anatomy "so that it can be difficult to precisely gauge the anatomic effect of injected materials."

Transoral techniques in the sitting, awake patient are common. Initially, they were performed with indirect laryngoscopy, but flexible fiberoptic videolaryngoscopy typically is used now for visualization. If indirect laryngoscopy is used, an assistant or the patient must pull the tongue forward to improve the view of the glottis; this may add to patient discomfort. The ability of the patient to phonate during the procedure has many benefits. Ford and colleagues [53] argued that more precise placement is possible, and thus, smaller doses of graft are used. In addition, the technology of videolaryngostroboscopy has raised the standards tremendously for fine-tuning laryngoplasty, which is possible with an awake patient [54]. The obvious disadvantages to this procedure are the technical challenge and the inability of some patients to tolerate it. Typically, an anesthetic, such as benzocaine spray, is applied to the hypopharynx before the procedure. Then under direct vision, a curved applicator is used to apply topical 4% lidocaine to the epiglottis, false vocal folds, and glottis. Anesthesia must be sufficient to allow the end of the injection apparatus to retract the epiglottis anteriorly [20];

however, there is a fine balance to be achieved with topical anesthesia. Over-zealous application causes significant pooling of secretions in the hypophar-ynx and glottis, which hinders one's view, causes frequent swallowing and coughing during the procedure, and risks aspiration.

Transcutaneous techniques that use indirect mirror laryngoscopy or flex-ible videolaryngoscopy for visual guidance are popular among many laryng-ologists. These can be performed in the awake patient in the sitting position as an office procedure, or in the supine position under general anesthesia. The outpatient approaches are particularly beneficial for patients who are poor surgical candidates or who may not tolerate awake transoral injections because of a brisk gag reflex. Typically, the transcutaneous technique is painless. Disadvantages include more limited access to the vocal cords. Berke and colleagues [55] described two approaches from the anterior neck. The halfway point between the superior notch and inferior border of the thyroid cartilage correlates to the superior surface of the true vocal folds; thus, the transcartilaginous injection is placed inferior to this halfway point. In some patients, calcification of the thyroid cartilage precludes the use of this approach. In these instances, placement of the needle through the cricothyroid membrane is an alternative, although this requires signifi-cant angling of the needle superiorly to reach the true cords. Again, Ford and Bless [4] emphasized that the use of videolaryngostroboscopy in trans-cutaneous (and transoral) techniques "affords the best assessment of glottic function and correlates well with vocal quality." They and many other lar-yngologists cite maximum phonation time and transglottic airflow as the most precise measures of glottic efficiency. In the authors' hands, the trans-cutaneous approach is accomplished best in the operating room under seda-tion or general anesthesia using a laryngeal mask airway (LMA). General anesthesia with the LMA is useful in patients who do not tolerate sedation, and can be used routinely if the material being injected requires overcorrec-tion. A fiberoptic laryngoscope, coupled to a three-chip camera and video monitor, is passed through the LMA to provide an excellent view of the vo-cal cords during injection. A small skin incision is made over the thyroid cartilage, and a small hole is drilled in the cartilage, similar to the technique that was described by Gray and colleagues [56]. This provides better control of the needle and the ability to angle the needle slightly as necessary, which allows more precise deposition of the material.

Regardless of the approach to the vocal cords, certain principles of injec-tion hold true. To medialize an immobile cord, the injection must be placed in the paraglottic space or the medial or lateral aspect of the thyroarytenoid muscle, depending on the material used. The paraglottic space is bound me-dially by the conus elasticus and vocal ligament, and laterally by the inner perichondrium of the thyroid and cricoid cartilages; it accommodates an in-jected volume of approximately 0.76 mL [13]. Courey [1] suggested "stair stepping" the path of this type of injection so that the entry site into the mu-cosa does not align with the entry site through the vocal ligament; this minimizes extrusion of the material through the injection site. Injecting lateral to the tip of the vocal process allows the vocal process to rotate medially. The remainder of the vocal cord can be aligned by injecting lateral to the middle portion of the thyroarytenoid muscle.

For bowing or atrophy of a mobile cord, injection into the body of the thyroarytenoid muscle (just under the vocal ligament) corrects the patient's troublesome glottic insufficiency; this region has a capacity of approximately 0.21 mL. To treat a damaged vibratory membrane, injection must be placed in the uniquely architectured, trilayered lamina propria. Because this structure is only 1 to 1.5 mm thick, the material must be injected with a small needle. This affects the choice of material (see Table 1), and makes general anesthesia, with an optimally positioned patient and a magnified view, essential. Typically, the first injection is just anterior to the vocal process and deep to the vocal ligament; this minimizes the amount of material that is needed to accomplish the task. The second injection is placed in the anterior third of the vibratory membrane to complete alignment of the cord, but it is critical to avoid overcorrection or an anterior "bulge." For mobile cords, injection laterally in the thyroarytenoid muscle or paraglottic space can stiffen the cord and impair native movement, and thus, is contraindicated.

Indications

Bruening designed injection laryngoplasty for the patient who had a paralyzed vocal cord [57]. Advances in laryngology have made it possible to diagnose other, more subtle, causes of dysphonia. These conditions fall under two categories: cords that cannot adequately adduct but have normal vibratory membranes, and cords that have damaged vibratory membranes but can adduct fully. The list of conditions lengthens regularly, but the most common entities include vocal cord atrophy; bowing; abductor spasmodic dysphonia; neurologic disorders, like Parkinson's; vibratory membrane scarring; phonotrauma; or effects of reflux and radiation. It is generally agreed that a course of speech therapy is indicated before performing injection for any of these conditions.

The immobile cord can cause troublesome symptoms, including ineffective cough, aspiration, breathy hoarseness, vocal fatigue, poor oxygenation, and dyspnea on exertion [1]. The damaged vibratory membrane leads primarily to vocal complaints, whereas swallowing, cough, and valsalva usually are unaffected. These patients may complain of dyspnea because of excessive air loss during phonation. Courey [1] stated that laryngologists are becoming more successful in addressing the primary etiology of a patient's vocal cord dysfunction—rather than using a generic approach to all glottic insufficiency; this will lead to more predictable, and less variable, results. The usefulness of injection laryngoplasty will continue to improve as we improve our understanding of, and ability to manipulate, vocal cord pathology.

Summary

A century after its inception, injection laryngoplasty remains an area of continual study and exciting advancements. It is challenging to evaluate the literature on this topic for several reasons. In 2004, Behrman [58] wrote a comprehensive analysis of outcomes and efficacy data that were related to paralytic dysphonia. Many of her observations hold true for the body of literature regarding injection laryngoplasty. The subjective and objective measurements of voice outcome vary significantly among reports. Perhaps more importantly, few studies have compared materials or techniques directly with each other. Finally, patients who have scarred cords often are included in the same study group as patients who have paralyzed cords. The two problems have markedly different etiologies, and require diagnostic and therapeutic approaches that are directed at those etiologies. Clearly, much work remains to be done before we provide our patients with more evidence-based recommendations. The yield of recent investigations and the new questions that were raised by them guarantee that injection laryngoplasty will have a role in operative laryngology for years to come.

References

[1] Courey MS. Injection laryngoplasty. Otolaryngol Clin N Am 2004;37:121–38.
[2] Fewins J, Simpson B, Miller FR. Complications of thyroid and parathyroid surgery. Otolaryngol Clin North Am 2003;36:189–206.
[3] Ford CN, Bless DM. A preliminary study of injectable collagen in human vocal fold augmentation. Otolaryngol Head Neck Surg 1986;94(1):104–12.
[4] Ford CN, Bless DM. Clinical experience with injectable collagen for vocal fold augmentation. Laryngoscope 1986;96(8):863–9.
[5] Bjorck G, D'Agata L, Hertegard S. Vibratory capacity and voice outcome in patients with scarred vocal folds treated with collagen injections—case studies. Logoped Phoniatr Vocol 2002;27(1):4–11.
[6] Livesey JR, Carding PN. An analysis of vocal cord paralysis before and after Teflon injection using combined glottography. Clin Otolaryngol Allied Sci 1995;20(5):423–7.
[7] Chang HP, Chang SY. Morphology and vibration pattern of the vocal cord after intracordal Teflon injection: long-term results. Zhonghua Yi Xue Za Zhi (Taipei) 1997;60(1):6–12.
[8] Nakayama M, Ford CN, Bless DM. Teflon vocal fold augmentation: failures and management in 28 cases. Otolaryngol Head Neck Surg 1993;109(3):493–8.
[9] Injectable fillers for soft tissue augmentation. Facial Plastic Surgery Network. Available at: http://www.facialplasticsurgery.net/injectable_fillers.htm. Accessed June 8, 2005.
[10] Owens JM. Soft tissue implants and fillers. Otolaryngol Clin North Am 2005;38:361–9.
[11] Hirano M, Tori K, Tanaka S, et al. Vocal function in patient with unilateral vocal cord paralysis before and after silicone injection. Acta Otolaryngol 1995;115(4):553–9.
[12] Alves CB, Loughran S, MacGregor FB, et al. Bioplastique medialization therapy improves the quality of life in terminally ill patients with vocal cord palsy. Clin Otolaryngol Allied Sci 2002;27(5):387–91.
[13] Courey MS. Homologous collagen substances for vocal fold augmentation. Laryngoscope 2001;111(5):747–58.

[14] Ford CN, Bless DM. Selected problems treated by vocal fold injection of collagen. Am J Otolaryngol 1993;14(4):257–61.

[15] Ford CN, Staskowski PA, Bless DM. Autologous collagen vocal fold injection: a preliminary clinical study. Laryngoscope 1995;105(9):944–8.

[16] Ford CN, Bless DM, Loftus JM. Role of injectable collagen in the treatment of glottic insufficiency: a study of 119 patients. Ann Otol Rhinol Laryngol 1992;101(3):237–47.

[17] Hertegard S, Dahlqvist A, Laurent C, et al. Viscoelastic properties of rabbit vocal folds after augmentation. Otolaryngol Head Neck Surg 2003;128(3):401–6.

[18] Sagawa M, Sato M, Fujimura S, et al. Vocal fold injection of collagen for unilateral vocal fold paralysis caused by chest diseases. J Cardiovasc Surg (Torino) 1999;40(4):603–5.

[19] Montgomery P, Sharma A, Qayyum A, et al. Direct phonoplasty under local anesthetic. J Laryngol Otol 2005;119(2):134–7.

[20] Hoffman H, McCabe D, McCullough T, et al. Laryngeal collagen injection as an adjunct to medialization laryngoplasty. Laryngoscope 2002;112(8):1407–13.

[21] Anderson TD, Sataloff RT. Complications of collagen injection of the vocal fold: report of several unusual cases and review of the literature. J Voice 2004;18(3):392–7.

[22] Remacle M, Dujardin JM, Lawson G. Treatment of vocal fold immobility by glutaraldehyde-cross-linked collagen injection: long-term results. Ann Otol Rhinol Laryngol 1995;104(6):437–41.

[23] Remacle M, Lawson G, Delos M, et al. Correcting vocal fold immobility by autologous collagen injection for voice rehabilitation. A short-term study. Ann Otol Rhinol Laryngol 1999; 108(8):788–93.

[24] Sengor A, Aydin O, Mola F, et al. Evaluation of alloderm and autologous skin in quadriceps muscles of rats for injection laryngoplasty. Eur Arch Otorhinolaryngol 2005;262(2):107–12.

[25] Lundy DS, Casiano RR, McClinton ME, et al. Early results of transcutaneous injection laryngoplasty with micronized acellular dermis versus type-I thyroplasty for glottic incompetence dysphonia due to unilateral vocal fold paralysis. J Voice 2003;17(4):589–95.

[26] Karpenko AN, Dworkin JP, Meleca RJ, et al. Cymetra injection for unilateral vocal cord paralysis. Ann Otol Rhinol Laryngol 2003;112(11):927–34.

[27] Rihkanen H, Lehikoinen-Soderlund S, Reijonen P. Voice acoustics after autologous fascia injection for vocal fold paralysis. Laryngoscope 1999;109(11):1854–8.

[28] Rihkanen H. Vocal fold augmentation by injection of autologous fascia. Laryngoscope 1998;108(1):51–4.

[29] Tsunoda K, Baer T, Niimi S. Autologous transplantation of fascia into the vocal fold: long-term results of a new phonosurgical technique for glottal incompetence. Laryngoscope 2001; 111(3):453–7.

[30] Duke SG, Salmon J, Blalock PD, et al. Fascia augmentation of the vocal fold: graft yield in the canine and preliminary clinical experience. Laryngoscope 2001;111(5):759–64.

[31] Hsiung MW, Kang BH, Pai L, et al. Combination of fascia transplantation and fat injection into the vocal fold for sulcus vocalis: long-term results. Ann Otol Rhinol Laryngol 2004; 113(5):359–66.

[32] Rihkanen H, Reijonen P, Lehikoinen-Soderlund S, et al. Videostroboscopic assessment of unilateral vocal fold paralysis after augmentation with autologous fascia. Eur Arch Otorhinolaryngol 2004;261(4):177–83.

[33] Sasai H, Watanabe Y, Muta H, et al. Long-term histological outcomes of injected autologous fat into human vocal folds after secondary laryngectomy. Otolaryngol Head Neck Surg 2005;132(5):685–8.

[34] Chen YY, Pai L, Lin YS, et al. Fat augmentation for nonparalytic glottic insufficiency. ORL J Otorhinolaryngol Relat Spec 2003;65(3):176–83.

[35] Shindo ML, Zaretsky LS, Rice DH. Autologous fat injection for unilateral vocal fold paralysis. Ann Otol Rhinol Laryngol 1996;105(8):602–6.

[36] Chang HP, Chang SY. Autogenous fat intracordal injection as treatment for unilateral vocal palsy. Zhonghua Yi Xue Za Zhi (Taipei) 1996;58(2):114–20.

[37] Cantarella G, Mazzola RF, Domenichini E, et al. Vocal fold augmentation by autologous fat injection with lipostructure procedure. Otolaryngol Head Neck Surg 2005; 132(2):239–43.
[38] Umeno H, Shirouzu H, Chitose S, et al. Analysis of voice function following autologous fat injection for vocal fold paralysis. Otolaryngol Head Neck Surg 2005;132(1):103–7.
[39] Sato K, Umeno H, Nakashima T. Autologous fat injection laryngohypopharyngoplasty for aspiration after vocal fold paralysis. Ann Otol Rhinol Laryngol 2004;113(2):87–92.
[40] Hsiung MW, Lin YS, Su WF, et al. Autogenous fat injection for vocal fold atrophy. Eur Arch Otorhinolaryngol 2003;260(9):469–74.
[41] McCullough TM, Andrews BT, Hoffman HT, et al. Long-term follow-up of fat injection laryngoplasty for unilateral vocal cord paralysis. Laryngoscope 2002;112(7):1235–8.
[42] Brandenburg JH, Kirkham W, Koschkee D. Vocal cord augmentation with autogenous fat. Laryngoscope 1992;102(5):495–500.
[43] Hsiung MW, Woo P, Minasian A, et al. Fat augmentation for glottic insufficiency. Laryngoscope 2000;110(6):1026–33.
[44] Chhetri DK, Jahan-Parwar B, Hart SED, et al. Injection laryngoplasty with calcium hydroxlapatite gel in an in vivo canine model. Ann Otol Rhinol Laryngol 2004;113(4): 259–64.
[45] Belafsky PC, Postma GN. Vocal fold augmentation with calcium hydroxylapatite. Otolaryngol Head Neck Surg 2004;131(4):351–4.
[46] Borzacchiello A, Mayol L, Garskog O, et al. Evaluation of injection augmentation treatment of hyaluronic acid based materials on rabbit vocal folds viscoelasticity. J Mater Sci Mater Med 2005;16(6):553–7.
[47] Hallen L, Johansson C, Laurent C. Cross-linked hyaluronan (Hyalan B gel): a new injectable remedy for treatment of vocal fold insufficiency – an animal study. Acta Otolaryngol 1999; 119(1):107–11.
[48] Piacquadio D, Jarcho M, Goltz R. Evaluation of hyalan b gel as a soft-tissue augmentation implant material. J Am Acad Dermatol 1997;36(4):544–9.
[49] Tateya T, Tateya I, Sohn JH, et al. Histologic characterization of rat vocal fold scarring. Ann Otol Rhinol Laryngol 2005;114(3):183–91.
[50] Hertegard S, Hallen L, Laurent C, et al. Cross-linked hyaluronan versus collagen for injection treatment of glottal insufficiency: 2-year follow-up. Acta Otolaryngol 2004;124(10): 1208–14.
[51] Hertegard S, Hallen L, Laurent C, et al. Cross-linked hyaluronan used as augmentation substance for treatment of glottal insufficiency: safety aspects and vocal fold function. Laryngoscope 2002;112(12):2211–9.
[52] Hirano S, Nagai H, Tateya I, et al. Regeneration of aged vocal folds with basic fibroblast growth factor in a rat model: a preliminary report. Ann Otol Rhinol Laryngol 2005; 114(4):304–8.
[53] Ford CN, Roy N, Sandage M, et al. Rigid endoscopy for monitoring indirect vocal fold injection. Laryngoscope 1998;108:1584–6.
[54] Arad-Cohen, et al. Office-based direct fiberoptic laryngoscopic surgery. Operative Techniques in Otolaryngology Head and Neck Surgery 1998;9:238–42.
[55] Berke GS, Gerratt B, Kreiman J, et al. Treatment of Parkinson hypophonia with percutaneous collagen augmentation. Laryngoscope 1999;109(8):1295–9.
[56] Gray SD, Bielamowicz SA, Titze IR, et al. Experimental approaches to vocal fold alteration: introduction to the minithyrotomy. Ann Otol Rhinol Laryngol 1999;108(1):1–9.
[57] Rosen CA. Phonosurgical vocal fold injection—indications and technique. Operative Techniques in Otolaryngology Head and Neck Surgery 1998;9:203–9.
[58] Behrman A. Evidence-based treatment of paralytic dysphonia: making sense of outcomes and efficacy data. Otolaryngol Clin North Am 2004;37:75–104.

ELSEVIER
SAUNDERS

Otolaryngol Clin N Am
39 (2006) 55–75

OTOLARYNGOLOGIC
CLINICS
OF NORTH AMERICA

Practical Applications of Laryngeal Framework Surgery

Hans F. Mahieu, MD, PhD

*Department of Otolaryngology/Head and Neck Surgery, Vrije Universiteit Medisch Centrum,
De Boelelaan 1117, Amsterdam 1081 HV, The Netherlands*

Phonosurgery is defined by the International Association of Phonosurgery as any type of surgery that is performed with the aim of improving or changing voice or speech. This definition implies that the goal of phonosurgery is to restore function rather than normal anatomy. The subgroup of phonosurgical techniques that demonstrate this concept most clearly is laryngeal framework surgery (LFS), which is based on concepts of the physiology of phonation and laryngeal biomechanics and is by definition a functional type of surgery.

One of the important aspects of LFS is that these procedures are performed under local anesthesia to enable intraoperative voice monitoring, which allows the surgeon to fine-tune the voice and thus obtain the best functional result. Another important aspect of LFS is that surgical damage to the vocal folds is avoided by directing the intervention to the cartilaginous structures attached to the vocal folds rather than the vocal folds themselves. By changing the shape or position of some of the laryngeal cartilages and thus providing biomechanical compensation for the phonatory dysfunction, many types of dysphonia can be corrected without jeopardizing the delicate structure of the vocal folds and without inadvertently changing the mass, volume, or stiffness of the vocal folds.

Some types of laryngeal framework surgery have already been suggested decades ago. For example, in 1915, Payr [1] described an anteriorly pedicled transverse, U-shaped cartilage flap in the thyroid ala, which was depressed inwardly to medialize the vocal fold. The effect, however, was limited, probably because the anterior pedicle restricted adequate medialization and because fixing the cartilage flap in the desired position proved difficult and uncertain [2]. Despite several other efforts, the concept of LFS remained fragmentary until Isshiki and colleagues [3] presented their innovative ideas

E-mail addresses: hf.mahieu@vumc.nl; h.mahieu@meandermc.nl

for correcting several types of dysphonia in 1974. The authors describe several different types of LFS, which were termed "thyroplasties." Over the years Isshiki and coworkers [4–8] molded these thyroplasties into a versatile set of phonosurgical techniques that are performed widely today and that have enabled surgeons to achieve such good results in the treatment of many different types of dysphonia.

The nomenclature of LFS procedures has been the subject of many heated discussions among phonosurgeons. Isshiki and colleagues have described four types of thyroplasties, but except for thyroplasty type 1 (the medialization thyroplasty), the descriptions of the other types have often led to confusion and are frequently not followed according to the original definition. A practical suggestion toward the standardization of LFS has been presented by the European Laryngological Society, in collaboration with others [9].

The Society has defined LFS as a group of surgical procedures performed on the laryngeal skeleton or inserting muscles for the correction of vocal-fold position or tension. Laryngoplasty is a term that is often used more or less synonymously with laryngeal framework surgery but refers, in fact, to the surgical procedure per se. Thyroplasty is defined as a subgroup of LFS and refers exclusively to procedures performed on the thyroid cartilage.

Four function-oriented types of LFS can be distinguished according to the intended purpose of the surgery and to the underlying pathogenesis of the dysphonia:

- Approximation LFS are procedures designed to correct incomplete glottal closure by medialization of the vocal folds. These procedures include medialization thyroplasty, arytenoid adduction, and arytenopexy [10].
- Expansion LFS are procedures designed to correct overly tight glottal closure by lateralization of the vocal folds. These procedures include lateralization thyroplasty and other procedures aimed at vocal-fold abduction. Procedures to widen the glottis to improve the airway are not considered phonosurgical procedures and are beyond the scope of this article.
- Tensioning LFS are procedures designed to correct the tension of overly flaccid vocal folds or to correct an excessively low-pitched voice by increasing the tension of the vocal folds. These procedures include cricothyroid approximation, cricothyroid subluxation [10], and elongation thyroplasty.
- Relaxation LFS are procedures designed to correct overly tensed or stiff vocal folds or to correct an excessively high-pitched voice by reducing the tension of the vocal folds. These procedures include shortening thyroplasties.

Because approximation LFS procedures form the mainstay of LFS (comprising approximately 70% of the author's series of more than 400 LFS interventions), these procedures are discussed more extensively in this report than the other LFS procedures. Some information concerning surgical technique is presented here but for more detailed instructions the reader is referred to textbooks concerning these issues [7,11].

Approximation laryngeal framework surgery

The most common indication for LFS is the correction of incomplete glottal closure resulting from vocal-fold paralysis, presbyphonia, vocal-fold atrophy, previous glottic tumor resection, abductor spasmodic dysphonia, or other causes.

Medialization thyroplasty (Fig. 1) involves medializing a "window" cut into the thyroid cartilage at the level of the vocal fold. It is a very effective and easy surgical procedure used to correct incomplete closure in the anterior or mid portion of the glottis. This procedure can be performed bilaterally if necessary, without compromising the airway. Furthermore this procedure will not interfere with the recovery of vocal-fold mobility.

Arytenoid adduction (Fig. 2) involves medializing the vocal process and, consequently, the posterior part of the vocal fold by sutures tied around the muscular process that pull in the direction of traction that is naturally exerted on the arytenoids by the lateral cricoarytenoid muscle. It is an effective but technically more difficult surgical procedure used to correct incomplete closure in the more posterior part of the glottis. This procedure can only be performed unilaterally because a bilateral procedure will severely compromise the airway. Although the recovery of vocal-fold mobility has been reported after arytenoid adduction (Maragos, personal communication, 2003), interference with full recovery is to be expected. Arytenoid adduction

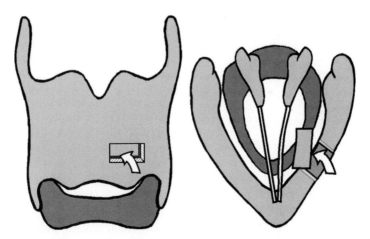

Fig. 1. Medialization thyroplasty. The impression of a cartilage window (*arrows*) results in medialization of vocal fold. (left) view from front. (right) view from above.

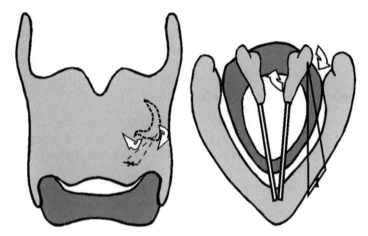

Fig. 2. Arytenoid adduction. Sutures tied around the muscular process of the arytenoids (*arrows*) are pulled in an anterior direction, consequently adducting the vocal process and the vocal fold attached to it. (left) view from front. (right) view from above.

is usually not performed as an isolated procedure but is typically combined with a medialization thyroplasty to correct glottal gaps that involve the anterior and middle as well as the posterior glottis.

The combination of arytenoid adduction and medialization thyroplasty is much more challenging but is also much more effective in correcting large glottal gaps than medialization thyroplasty alone. In the present author's series, approximately 30% of the approximation LFS procedures involved arytenoid adduction. The voice result obtained with arytenoid adduction combined with medialization thyroplasty is significantly better than with medialization thyroplasty alone, in terms of maximum phonation time (MPT) (MPT gain 8.2 seconds versus 2.6 seconds) and dynamic range (dynamic range gain 8.6 dB versus 5.9 dB). Because the patient group that underwent medialization thyroplasty alone had less severe dysphonia to start with, the end result of both groups was the same (MPT 14.2 seconds and dynamic range 22.8 dB). Both procedures have proven to result in stable long-term voice outcomes.

Medialization thyroplasty

Medialization thyroplasty is based on the concept that medial displacement of a cartilage window cut into the thyroid ala at the level of the vocal fold will medialize that vocal fold (Fig. 3). The surgical landmarks for the thyroplasty type 1 procedure are the thyroid notch (Fig. 3A), the midline point (Fig. 3B) of the lower margin of the thyroid ala, the midway point (Fig. 3C) between the two former landmarks (determined with a caliper), which coincides with the position of the anterior commisure (the so called "vocal-fold line") (Fig. 3E) drawn from the point marking the anterior

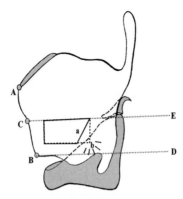

Fig. 3. Design of the cartilage window. The surgical landmarks for the thyroplasty type 1 procedure are the thyroid notch (*A*), the midline point (*B*) of the lower margin of the thyroid ala, the midway point (*C*) between the two former landmarks (determined with a caliper), which coincides with the position of the anterior commisure, the so called "vocal-fold line" (*E*) drawn from the point marking the anterior commisure in the posterior direction. This line marks the level of the vocal fold and runs parallel to an imaginary straight line (*D*) along the lower margin of the thyroid ala, from the anterior point (*B*) to the lower thyroid ala margin just in front of the inferior horn. Dashed box, a, oblique posterior margin of cartilage window; b, posteroinferior corner of rectangular window, which cannot be medialized because of the underlying cricoid. (lateral view)

commisure in the posterior direction. This line marks the level of the vocal fold and runs parallel to an imaginary straight line (Fig. 3D) along the lower margin of the thyroid ala, from the anterior point (Fig. 3B) to the lower thyroid ala margin, just in front of the inferior horn.

A cartilage window is designed on the thyroid ala, starting 4 to 5 mm from the midline. The upper margin of the cartilage window coincides with the vocal-fold line, adjusted to the individual's dimensions (approximately 4–5 × 8–10 mm in females and 5–6 × 10–12 mm in males). A patent lower rim of thyroid cartilage must be maintained just below the window. The posterior margin of the cartilage window is designed slightly oblique (Fig. 3a) because the cricoid cartilage is located medial to the posteroinferior part of the thyroid ala and can prevent medialization if the cartilage window extends too far posteriorly (Fig. 3b).

The perichondrium overlying the cartilage window is incised, elevated, and removed. The cartilage window is then cut with either a number 15 or 11 knife blade in young or female patients. In cases in which the cartilage is calcified, a drill with fine cutting burr is used. In highly calcified larynges, it can be helpful to first drill multiple small holes along the margins of the window and later connect these holes to complete the cartilage cuts.

The last attachments are freed with a small Rosen dissector or freer. The inner perichondrium is elevated widely and carefully from the inner cartilage surface around the cartilage window, especially posteriorly, to enable adequate medialization of the cartilage window.

The cartilage window is depressed inwardly to various depths while the patient phonates to determine the optimal degree of vocal-fold medialization under fiber-optic and voice monitoring. Often, more medialization is required posteriorly and inferiorly than superiorly and anteriorly. Special care should be taken not to overcorrect anteriorly. Before testing the voice, the surgeon must assure that the patient's head and neck are in a neutral position. It is advisable to have the patient phonate at different intensities and frequencies and to include a short phrase of connected speech to accurately assess voice quality. The present author prefers either a silastic wedge (Fig. 4), a plug (Fig. 5), or occasionally only sutures (Fig. 6) for fixation of the cartilage window in the optimal position. The material chosen depends on the required degree of medialization. The wedge or plug can be carved according to the requirements from a block of medical-grade silastic. A snug-fitting wedge that requires no further fixation is preferred. The silastic block may come in several degrees of stiffness, depending on the manufacturer. The silastic with the highest degree of stiffness is preferred for adequate medialization and fixation.

Contrary to the often recommended practice of removing the cartilage window [12,13], this author prefers to preserve the cartilage window as a buttress against endolaryngeal extrusion of the silastic implant. Furthermore, in the present author's experience, in the exceptional cases that require revision surgery, repositioning of the vocal fold is much more difficult if the cartilage has been removed during the initial surgery because of more extensive fibrosis.

At the completion of the approximation LFS procedure, the cricoid and thyroid cartilages are approximated manually to determine whether applying vocal-fold tension by means of cricothyroid approximation will further improve the voice. If this is indeed the case, an additional cricothyroid approximation can be performed.

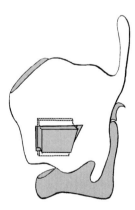

Fig. 4. Cartilage window medialized by silastic wedge, carved to fit, with inferior and superior flanges on the inside of the thyroid cartilage for retention. (lateral view)

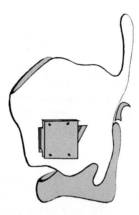

Fig. 5. Cartilage window medialized by silastic plug, carved to fit, with inferior and superior flanges sutured to the outside of the thyroid cartilage for fixation. (lateral view)

Special considerations and pitfalls in medialization thyroplasty

Local anesthesia versus general anesthesia

Considering the major impact that even minor changes in the position and medialization of the cartilage window can have on the voice, voice monitoring during the surgical procedure is considered a "conditio sine qua non." General anesthesia is therefore not recommended, and premedication should be minimized to avoid oversedation and to allow adequate phonation on request. This author's preference for premedication is morphine, 10 mg, and atropine, 0.5 mg, administered intramuscularly 30 minutes before surgery. Some surgeons prefer not to administer atropine because the resulting dryness of the mucosa may interfere with voice production. The reduction of saliva secretion and consequently reduction of swallowing movements during surgery, however, in this author's opinion, justify its use. The

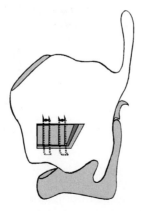

Fig. 6. Cartilage window medialized by sutures, keeping the window slightly impressed. (lateral view)

considerations mentioned above hold true for all types of laryngeal framework surgery.

Design of the cartilage window

The two errors made most frequently in designing the cartilage window consist of placing or extending the cartilage window too high and too posteriorly, especially in the posterior lower corner of the window.

The window should be placed parallel to an imaginary line along the lower border of thyroid ala. Because the thyroid ala is highly variable in shape and inferior extension, it is not always easy to project an imaginary line along the lower border of the thyroid ala. Adequate exposure of the lower thyroid ala border and the identification of the inferior thyroid horn can prevent this error. If the cartilage window is created too high, medialization will occur at the level of the ventricular fold instead of at the glottic level. This is recognized by insufficient voice improvement and is confirmed on fiber-optic laryngeal examination.

Because of the position of the cricoid cartilage medial to this area, the medialization of the cartilage window will be impeded posteriorly, resulting in insufficient voice improvement. Resecting the lower posterior corner of the cartilage window will correct this condition.

Fixation of the cartilage window in the optimal position

Usually the carved silastic implant enables excellent control over the degree and area of medialization of the vocal fold and guarantees sufficient fixation of the cartilage window in the optimal medialized position. Occasionally, an additional fixation of the cartilage window and the silastic wedge is required, which can be achieved with nylon 4-0 or Gore-Tex 5 sutures.

Many prefabricated implants have been developed, some with a posterior extension to correct a posterior gap. This author prefers to perform an arytenoid adduction rather than trying to insert an implant with a very large posterior extension. Most prefabricated implants, with the exception of Friedrich's titanium implant (Heinx Kurz GmbH Medizintechnik, Dusslingen, Germany) [14], have the disadvantages of not being able to be tailored to the situation and the patient's needs. The different sizes available for most prefabricated implants, in this author's opinion, do not cover the entire range of what is required for an optimal voice result in every patient. Also, the presently advocated use of a Gore-Tex sheet [10], in the present author's hands, enables less direct control over the degree and area of medialization than an individually carved silastic wedge or plug.

Edema

Occasionally, endolaryngeal edema can occur during the procedure, which can interfere with voice monitoring. In such cases, a slight overcorrection is required. It is therefore important to distinguish between the voice associated with edema and the voice associated with overcorrection. Edema will result in a rough and unstable voice, whereas overcorrection results in a "pressed" voice quality. Severe edema that interferes with the airway has not been observed in the present author's experience. Mild postoperative vocal-fold edema is a normal finding and usually requires no treatment.

Undercorrection and overcorrection

Voice monitoring during laryngeal framework surgery should be performed with the patient's head and neck lying in a comfortable and neutral position to prevent under- or overcorrection. Overcorrection at the subglottis, glottis, or supraglottis level is recognized by a pressed, hyperkinetic, and rough voice quality; sometimes a protruding ventricular fold can be seen at laryngoscopy as a sign of medialization at the supraglottis rather than the glottis level. If the surgeon is in doubt as to whether the optimal degree of medialization has been achieved, the silastic wedge should be removed and remodeled. If the result is not satisfying, arytenoid adduction should be considered. Voice tasks during monitoring should include spoken text as well as sustained vowels at several pitch levels in order detect under- or overcorrection.

Implant extrusion

Endolaryngeal extrusion of the silastic implant has never been observed in thyroplasty techniques that preserve the cartilage window. Cases of endolaryngeal extrusions have been reported after techniques in which the cartilage window is removed have been used [15–19].

Arytenoid adduction

Arytenoid adduction is based on the concept that the vocal fold can be medialized by placing sutures through the muscular process of the arytenoid and pulling these sutures in the same direction as the lateral cricoarytenoid muscle would exert traction.

The surgical landmarks for the arytenoid adduction (Fig. 7) are the vocal-fold line (Fig. 7E) (also see landmarks for medialization thyroplasty), the posterior margin of the thyroid ala, the upper horn of the thyroid ala, the lower horn of the thyroid ala, the cricothyroid joint, the posterolateral surface of the cricoid cartilage, the cricoarytenoid joint, the muscular process of the arytenoid cartilage, a vertical line (Fig. 7F) at the junction of the anterior and middle third of the thyroid ala, a vertical line (Fig. 7G) at the junction of the anterior and the posterior half of the thyroid ala, and points of exit (Fig. 7H and I) for the sutures along the two vertical lines, located below the line marking the level of the vocal fold.

After exposing the thyroid ala cartilage, the posterior margin is exposed over its entire length, elevating and sectioning the thyropharyngeal musculature. Elevation of the perichondrium is continued around the posterior margin to the inner surface of the thyroid cartilage. Adequate exposure of

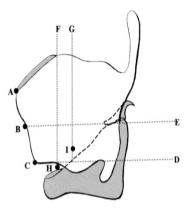

Fig. 7. The surgical landmarks are the thyroid notch (*A*), the midline point (*C*) of the lower margin of the thyroid ala, the midway point (*B*) between the two former landmarks (determined with a caliper), which coincides with the position of the anterior commisure, the so called "vocal-fold line" (*E*) running parallel to an imaginary straight line (*D*) along the lower margin of the thyroid ala. Estimation of the points of exit of the arytenoid adduction suture at point (*I*), well below the vocal-fold line (*E*), usually in the posterior part of the cartilage window if the procedure is performed in combination with medialization thyroplasty, and (*H*), just below the lower border of the thyroid, at the junction (*F*) of the anterior third and posterior two thirds of the thyroid ala. (lateral view)

the arytenoid region requires that the cricothyroid joint be dislocated. The superior horn of the thyroid cartilage is also cut.

While dislocating the cricothyroid joint and later, while locating and approaching the muscular process of the arytenoid, efforts should be made to preserve the recurrent laryngeal nerve, which runs just posteriorly to the cricothyroid joint and enters the larynx between the cricothyroid joint and the cricoarytenoid joint. Although in most cases in which arytenoid adduction is indicated, the underlying cause of the dysphonia will be a recurrent nerve palsy, very often a subclinical reinnervation has taken place, which is insufficient to restore laryngeal mobility but which may provide the musculature with sufficient tonicity to positively influence voice quality.

After dislocating the cricothyroid joint and resecting the upper thyroid horn, the posterior thyroid margin can be rotated anteromedially, thus exposing the arytenoid region (occasionally, partial resection of the posterior part of the thyroid ala is required in males for a better exposure). The arytenoid cartilage can then be palpated through the surrounding musculature. The line on the thyroid ala representing the level of the vocal fold will point in the direction of the muscular process of the arytenoid, which is approximately on the same level as the vocal fold. The cricoarytenoid joint is approached by following the posterolateral surface of the cricoid cartilage upward from the dislocated cricothyroid joint. The articular facet of the cricoarytenoid joint is located on the superior lateral ridge of the cricoid plate, approximately 1 cm (females) to 1.5 cm (males) cranially from the cricothyroid joint. During this part of the procedure, it is essential to stay on the solid cricoid cartilage surface to prevent entering the piriform sinus, which overlies the muscular process. The cricoarytenoid joint is opened slightly for a sure identification and to exclude cricoarytenoid joint fixation. Observance of the white, glistening articular facet confirms identification of the joint. Care should be taken not to open the joint too widely to avoid later dislocation.

Usually two sutures are passed through the muscular process from above, exiting through the cricoarytenoid joint. A Gore-Tex 5 or nylon 4-0 suture is used for this purpose. Which one of the sutures has the best grip on the arytenoid can be tested under fiber-optic control. This suture is tied loosely around the muscular process in such a way that both ends stay long enough to be pulled anteriorly in the general direction of the lateral cricoarytenoid muscles. This will result in the rotation of the vocal process medially, thus medializing the vocal fold. With a straight needle, these sutures are passed forward along the inside of the thyroid ala, taking precaution not to breach the inner perichondrium of the thyroid ala until the point of exit has been reached. One point of exit will be in the posterior part of the medialization cartilage window, at approximately the level of vertical line (Fig. 7G); the other point of exit is in the cricothyroid space just below the rim of the cartilage window at the level of vertical line (Fig. 7F).

The suture is tied on the outer surface of the thyroid ala, again under phonatory control to decide the optimal degree of traction. Usually, only mild and subtle traction is required. Care should be taken not to pull too hard. Usually, only one suture is required to achieve a good result. The other suture is not passed anteriorly and only plays a role in case of over-correction or arytenoid dislocation, when it can be used to pull the arytenoid slightly back toward its original position or to slightly tilt the muscular process downward and consequently the vocal process slightly upward. Over-correction is recognized by the pressed, hyperkinetic, and sometimes breathy voice quality and the endoscopic laryngeal image.

At the end of the procedure, the lower thyroid horn is again sutured to the cricoid. Usually, the thyroid horn is attached to the cricoid ventral to its previous articulation, much like the cricothyroid subluxation procedure described by Zeitels [10], thus also correcting for the loss of tension that often accompanies severe glottal insufficiency.

Special considerations and pitfalls in arytenoid adduction

Exposure of the cricoarytenoid area and approach to the muscular process

In the present author's hands, the procedure described above, as described originally by Isshiki [4], still represents the safest and most reliable method to approach the muscular process. However, the obvious consequence is disruption of the cricothyroid joint. This disruption can be justified because cricothyroid function is usually already hampered in cases for which arytenoid adduction is indicated. Furthermore, tension on the affected vocal fold is restored by the modification of suturing the inferior horn of the thyroid to the cricoid. Maragos [20] has described an elegant approach to the cricoarytenoid area by resecting a semicircular window in the posterior part of the thyroid ala. This eliminates the need to dislocate the cricothyroid joint and sever the superior thyroid horn. However, the identification of the cricoarytenoid joint can prove difficult without the landmark of the opened cricothyroid joint. Furthermore, if the posterior semicircular window is not designed perfectly, there is an increased risk of fracturing the thyroid ala, especially if the medialization thyroplasty window is created first, as is the present author's practice.

Identification of the cricoarytenoid joint

Identifying the cricoarytenoid joint can be difficult. When dissecting (for the most part bluntly) from the cricothyroid joint in a craniomedial direction, the cricoarytenoid will be found approximately 1.5 cm from the cricoarytenoid joint. Usually the muscular process of the arytenoid can be palpated at this stage as well.

The cricoarytenoid joint is opened slightly for positive identification, to exclude fixation and, if necessary, to cut adhesions . Opening this joint too widely will result in posterior instability of the arytenoid. If this occurs, the additionally placed suture can be fixed to the lower part of the posterior thyroid ala border. This will stabilize the arytenoid joint posteriorly preventing dislocation anteriorly.

Recurrent laryngeal nerve

The recurrent laryngeal nerve is at risk during the approach to the cricoarytenoid joint. Damage to the nerve may increase the dysphonia during the surgery, probably as a result of the loss of tonicity that was generated by subclinical or inappropriate innervation (or in cases of joint fixation even normal innervation!). Therefore, the recurrent laryngeal nerve, passing just posteriorly to the cricothyroid joint, should be preserved whenever possible.

Edema

Significant edema of the arytenoid region can be observed during and after arytenoid adduction, especially in the case with ankylosis of the cricoarytenoid joint, where special effort is required to mobilize the arytenoid. Usually, this will not compromise the airway, but occasionally steroid medication must be administered. Arytenoid adduction performed as an outpatient procedure is not advisable in any case. Emergency tracheotomies have been reported after arytenoid adduction. Edema usually does not develop immediately and therefore typically does not interfere with voice monitoring.

Future intubation

In the present author's experience, the most frequent settings in which revision surgery is indicated after approximation LFS (medialization thyroplasty as well as arytenoids adduction) occurs in patients who have undergone endotracheal intubation, even many years after successfully undergoing approximation LFS. Patients should be informed that after approximation LFS, endotracheal intubation may cause voice deterioration. They are advised to inform the anesthetist that intubation is best performed with a small diameter tube or a laryngeal mask airway.

Timing of approximation laryngeal framework surgery

The cause of dysphonia is a very important factor in timing, especially if the dysphonia is the result of a recurrent laryngeal or vagus nerve paralysis. In the case of mobile vocal folds, as for instance in severe presbyphonia, there is no reason for delaying the surgery because there is no chance of spontaneous recovery or compensation. Laryngeal framework surgery can therefore be planned immediately in all cases of glottic insufficiency with bilateral vocal-fold mobility, when voice therapy remains unsuccessful or is not indicated. In the case of unilateral immobility, the strategy will depend on the cause of the vocal-fold immobility.

If, in the case of paralysis, there is continuity of the nerve (eg, idiopathic paralysis) or it is believed to be intact, spontaneous recovery of function may be expected up to 1 year after the onset of the paralysis. Therefore it is advisable to plan a surgical treatment no sooner than 1 year after onset, unless other factors prevail.

If the paralysis is a result of a severed nerve without reconstruction (eg, resection of vagus nerve tumor, resection of the recurrent nerve because of thyroid malignancy, and other causes), no spontaneous recovery of function can be expected. In these circumstances, laryngeal framework surgery can be taken into consideration sooner. If, in such cases, the glottic insufficiency is relatively small, it is worthwhile to wait for compensation of the unaffected vocal fold to occur. Voice therapy can be advised during this period, but in the present author's opinion, therapy will not stimulate compensation. If compensation has not been achieved sufficiently within 6 months, surgical treatment can be planned.

If the dysphonia is a result of trauma, it is advisable to wait at least 6 months before framework surgery is contemplated. By that time, scar tissue will have matured. If the glottic insufficiency is a result of a fixed cricoarytenoid joint, there is no reason to postpone surgical treatment. Laryngeal electromyography is very helpful in differentiating between laryngeal paralysis and fixation of the cricoarytenoid joint.

In patients who have recurrent laryngeal nerve paralysis as a result of an intrathoracic malignancy, laryngeal framework surgery is usually performed as soon as is convenient for the patient because of the short life expectancy of these patients. In this category of patients, especially if they are in a poor general condition, vocal-fold augmentation by means of intracordal injection can be considered a reasonable alternative.

The degree of dysphonia can influence the timing of laryngeal framework surgery as well. If the degree of dysphonia is very significant, this author tends to operate sooner than 1 year after the onset; however, the patient must then realize that the performance of an arytenoid adduction is likely to interfere with the chance of spontaneous recovery.

Sometimes patients have other complaints related to laryngeal dysfunction, such as aspiration from vagal nerve palsy or hyperventilation as a result of the large airflow during phonation. These factors also can influence the surgeon to perform surgery sooner than 1 year after the onset of the palsy. In cases of severe aspiration, arytenoid adduction is effective in helping to prevent aspiration. In selected cases, professional and social factors may influence the surgeon to intervene sooner as well.

Approximation laryngeal framework surgery versus injection augmentation for paralytic dysphonia

Until several years ago, the method most frequently applied to correct paralytic dysphonia was endolaryngeal injection of soluble substances, such as Teflon, silicone, or collagen [21–25]. More recently, autologous fat, calcium hydroxyl-appetite, autologous fascia, and hyaluronic acid derivatives have been used to augment the paralytic vocal fold [26–28]. Treatments with injectable substances are quick and apparently simple procedures, but they are associated with some disadvantages compared with approximation LFS procedures, such as: (1) the mass, volume, and stiffness of the injected vocal fold is influenced by the injected substances. Such changes in vocal-fold mass, volume, and stiffness negatively influence the vibratory properties of the vocal fold, which can result in a poor voice, despite a better glottal closure; (2) the distribution of the injected substance is difficult to control. The substance will spread according to the path of least resistance, rather than to the area requiring augmentation; (3) the treatment is irreversible. Overinjection is difficult to correct and generally requires partial resection of the vocal fold resulting in severe dysphonia; (4) if the procedure is performed under general anesthesia, as many endolaryngeal injection procedures are, voice monitoring during the procedure is not possible. Consequently, it is difficult to estimate the proper amount of substance to be injected, and the voice outcome can be no more than a calculated guess; (5) some materials (eg, collagen and fat) are subject to partial absorption so that initial overcorrection is required, and repeated injections may be necessary. Other materials (eg, silicone and Teflon) are known to migrate; (6) often, vocal-fold palsy is associated with a difference in the height of the two vocal folds (vertical shift), which may be difficult to detect (special attention to the position of both vocal processes is required to diagnose this asymmetry in the videolaryngostroboscopic image). Such a difference in height usually cannot be corrected by vocal-fold injection; and (7) a considerable number of complications [29–31] and local tissue reactions attributable to the injected substances have been described, especially with Teflon, rendering this material obsolete for endolaryngeal injection. The injection of autologous fat seems to present fewer complications. On the other hand, the technique of injection augmentation also has some appealing qualities, including relative technical ease, low cost, and wide availability in many clinical settings.

In this author's opinion, these injection augmentation techniques should be considered as part of a complimentary armamentarium with LFS. The dysphonic patient requires an individualized approach tailored to his or her type of dysphonia and vocal demands. The modern phonosurgeon should therefore be versatile and skilled in the use of different, often complimentary, phonosurgical techniques.

Expansion laryngeal framework surgery

The most important indication for expansion LFS is adductor spasmodic dysphonia (ADSD) [8,32]. Although botulinum toxin is still considered the gold standard for the treatment of ADSD [33]; however, some patients, particularly young individuals, are appalled by the prospect of life-long, repeated botulinum injections, some patients demonstrate a decreased response to the injections, and some find it difficult to accept the periodic voice changes that accompany the initial paresis and the inevitable recurrence of spasmodic symptoms after several months.

Expansion LFS or lateralization thyroplasty (Fig. 8), consists of a lateralization of both thyroid ala after a vertical midline cartilage incision and

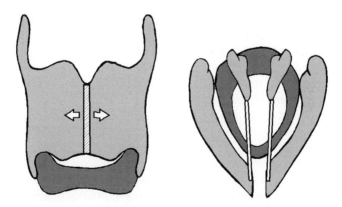

Fig. 8. Lateralization thyroplasty. Anterior separation of both thyroid ala results in anterior lateralization of both vocal folds and consequently in an anterior incomplete glottis closure (*arrows*). (left) view from front. (right) view from above.

consequently an anterior lateralization of both vocal folds. This procedure prevents the occurrence of spasmodic pressed phonation. The aim of this procedure is to enable phonation with less effort. The resulting voice will have a certain degree of breathiness as a result of the intentionally created anterior gap. The voice will never be as good as during the optimal period in the botulinum toxin cycle, but the result will be permanent, and speaking will require less effort.

Worldwide experience with expansion LFS is rapidly increasing. In the present author's personal series of 12 cases with a maximum follow-up of more than 5 years, the results are very promising. Careful patient selection and counseling are essential because of the inevitable breathy voice quality. Patients who are not familiar with botulinum toxin injections and request expansion LFS are advised to undergo botulinum toxin injections at least once before deciding on the surgical option. In this author's practice, most ADSD patients are still being treated with botulinum toxin injections, and expansion LFS is reserved for extraordinary cases of botulinum toxin failure.

Tensioning laryngeal framework surgery

Excessively lax vocal folds (eg, resulting from a superior laryngeal nerve palsy) may result in a weak, hoarse, and usually low-pitched voice. Diminished and asymmetrical vocal-fold tension, as may accompany vocal-fold palsy, may contribute to the breathy voice quality and can result in diplophonia. Furthermore, androphonia resulting from hormonal medication and gender dysphonia in male-to-female transsexual patients are characterized by low-pitched voice. Voice therapy is the mainstay of treatment for gender dysphonia, but additional tensioning LFS can be helpful in raising the habitual vocal pitch.

Normally, the tension of the vocal folds and consequently the vocal pitch are determined largely by the action of the cricothyroid and vocalis muscles, which act more or less as antagonists. Contraction of the cricothyroid muscles results in (1) anterior approximation of the cricoid and thyroid (pars recta of the cricothyroid muscles [Fig. 9 left]) cartilages and (2) anterior displacement of the thyroid cartilage in relation to the cricoid cartilage (pars oblique fibers of the cricothyroid muscles [Fig. 9 right]). As a consequence, the anterior commisure is displaced anteriorly and caudally, which results in displacing the vocal folds in the position for falsetto phonation: stretched, thinned, and stiffened, resulting in a high vocal pitch.

The simplest and most frequently applied tensioning LFS procedure is cricothyroid approximation (Fig. 10), which mimics the configuration of the vocal folds during falsetto phonation [6,34]. During this procedure, cricoid and thyroid cartilages are approximated anteriorly by strong sutures, two on each side. The most lateral sutures are placed near the midline on the cricoid and laterally on the thyroid, running in the direction of the

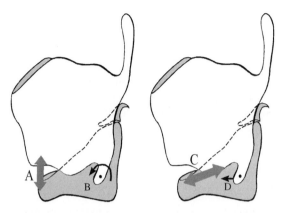

Fig. 9. (*left*) Contraction of the pars recta of the cricothyroid muscles (*A*) results in a downward rotation (*B*) of the thyroid, closing the cricothyroid visor anteriorly. (*right*) Contraction of the pars obliqua of the cricothyroid muscles (*C*) results in anterior displacement of the thyroid (*D*). (lateral view)

oblique fibers of the cricothyroid muscle to obtain cricothyroid approximation as well as anterior thyroid displacement. Because of the strong tension on the sutures, especially in gender dysphonia cases, the sutures are tied over a Gore-Tex bolster (cut from a 2-mm thick Gore-Tex patch) to avoid the sutures from pulling through.

In the present author's series of male-to-female transsexual patients, forming the largest patient group to undergo tensioning LFS, the preoperative habitual speaking pitch was 128 Hz, which is well within the normal range of the male habitual pitch (98–131 Hz). The mean postoperative habitual pitch was 191 Hz, which is well within the normal range of the female habitual pitch (174–262 Hz).

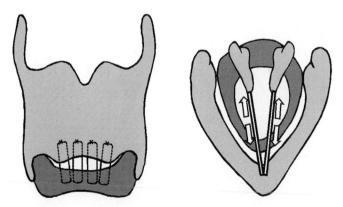

Fig. 10. Cricothyroid approximation. Sutures approximating cricoid and thyroid anteriorly results in increased tension (arrows) and consequently in a raise in pitch. (left) view from front. (right) view from above.

Cricothyroid subluxation as described by Zeitels [10] essentially mimics the anterior displacement of the thyroid, also with the aim of increasing the tension of the vocal folds. The timing of laryngeal framework surgery for vocal-fold tension is less strict than it is for approximation LFS and depends much more on the progress obtained with voice therapy. In the case of transsexual gender dysphonia, pitch-raising surgery is often postponed until all gender reassignment surgery has been performed, to reduce the risk of voice deterioration after intubation.

Relaxation laryngeal framework surgery

The indications for relaxation LFS are few [11]. Mutational dysphonias unresponsive to voice therapy and female-to-male transsexuals with a persistent high-pitched voice despite adequate hormonal substitution are two indications for this pitch-lowering procedure [7]. Also, some patients with congenital voice disorders, vocal-fold atrophy, or scarred and stiff vocal folds may benefit from relaxation LFS combined with medialization thyroplasty. Relaxation LFS can be performed unilaterally or bilaterally and consists of the excision of a vertical strip of cartilage at the junction of the anterior and middle third of the thyroid ala (Fig. 11). The anterior and posterior parts of the thyroid ala are sutured together again. Consequently, the vocal fold will become shorter and more lax, thereby reducing the vocal pitch. It is important to align the anterior and posterior parts of the thyroid ala in such a way that the vocal-fold line remains straight, to avoid level differences of the vocal folds. Good and long-lasting results can be obtained for patients requiring a lowering of the vocal pitch. Dysphonia because of atrophic or scarred vocal folds usually improves with regard to the effort required to speak but less with regard to overall voice quality.

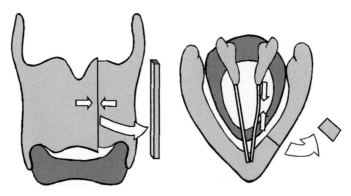

Fig. 11. Relaxation thyroplasty. Excision of a vertical strip of cartilage (*large arrows*) results shortening of the vocal fold (*small arrows*) and consequently in reduction of vocal-fold tension. (left) view from front. (right) view from above.

Perioperative care for laryngeal framework surgery

Thirty minutes before surgery, an intramuscular premedication of atropine sulfate (0.5 mg) and morphine (10 mg) is administrated. In the operating theater, the patient is placed in the supine position with the head extended but in a comfortable position that can be maintained for 1 to 2 hours. Rolled sheets can be placed beneath the shoulders to support the extended neck position. An intravenous drip with saline 0.9% is maintained throughout the procedure to enable the administration of medication intravenously if so required. Vital signs are monitored throughout the procedure by means of pulse-oximetry and heart rate monitoring apparatus. Drapes are positioned over a bar placed 10 cm above the patient's chin, leaving the nose and mouth free for access to the fiber-optic endoscope, which is used during several stages of the procedure to monitor the vocal folds. The surgeon may view the larynx on the video monitor during the procedure. The changes in quality of the voice, however, are the most important parameters to assess during the surgery.

Local anesthesia is given using 1% lidocaine hydrochloride with 0.001% epinephrine, 10 to 20 mL. Prophylactic antibiotic treatment given at the start of the surgery and is continued for 5 days. Wound drainage to reduce the risk of airway obstruction from hematoma is mandatory for all LFS procedures, with the exception of isolated cases of cricothyroid approximation or cricothyroid subluxation.

In the present author's opinion, LFS should not be performed as a day surgery because of the potential risk for airway compromise. Again, an exception can be made for isolated cricothyroid approximation or cricothyroid subluxation cases because these procedures do not involve cutting or otherwise manipulating the laryngeal framework apart from the external sutures, and thus the risk of endolaryngeal hematoma is negligible.

Postoperatively, the period in which to rest the voice ranges from 2 to 4 days, depending on the laryngoscopic findings. Rarely, steroid administration is required for postoperative endolaryngeal swelling. Codeine may be administered postoperatively in case of excessive coughing or throat clearing.

In this author's opinion, postoperative voice therapy, if indicated, should start no sooner than 2 months after surgery. The instability of the voice associated with reactive postoperative swelling and readjustment of the neuromuscular system to the new laryngeal situation should not be burdened too soon with intensive voice therapeutic training.

Summary

LFS procedures enable functionally monitored correction of vocal-fold position as well as vocal-fold tension, without jeopardizing the delicate structure of the vocal folds, producing good results with few and usually minor complications. Modern phonosurgery requires versatile surgeons to adequately comply with the demands of dysphonic patients. The different types of LFS are rewarding but occasionally demanding procedures, which should be part of the armamentarium of the phonosurgeon.

References

[1] Payr E. Plastik am Schildknorpel zur Behebung der Folgen einseitiger Stimmbandlähmung. Dtsch Med Wochenschr 1915;41:1264–70.
[2] Seiffert A. Operative Wiederherstellung des Glottisschlusses bei einseitiger Recurrenslahmung und Stimmbanddefekten. Archiv Ohren-Nasen-Kehlkopfheilkunde 1942;152:366–8.
[3] Isshiki N, Morita H, Okamura H, et al. Thyroplasty as a new phonosurgical technique. Acta Otolaryngol 1974;78:451–7.
[4] Isshiki N, Tanabe M, Sawada M. Arytenoid adduction for unilateral vocal cord paralysis. Arch Otolaryngol 1978;140:555–8.
[5] Isshiki N. Recent advances in phonosurgery. Folia Phoniatr Logop 1980;32:119–54.
[6] Isshiki N, Taira T, Tanabe M. Surgical alteration of the vocal pitch. J Otolaryngol 1983;12: 335–40.
[7] Isshiki N. Phonosurgery, theory and practice. Tokyo: Springer Verlag; 1989.
[8] Isshiki N, Haji T, Yamamoto Y, et al. Thyroplasty for adductor spasmodic dysphonia: further experiences. Laryngoscope 2001;111:615–21.
[9] Friedrich G, de Jong FI, Mahieu HF, et al. Laryngeal framework surgery: a proposal for classification and nomenclature by the Phonosurgery Committee of the European Laryngological Society. Eur Arch Otorhinolaryngol 2001;258:389–96.
[10] Zeitels SM. New procedures for paralytic dysphonia: adduction arytenopexy, Goretex medialization laryngoplasty, and cricothyroid subluxation. Otolaryngol Clin North Am 2000;33:841–54.
[11] Mahieu HF. Laryngeal framework surgery. In: Ferlito A, editor. Diseases of the larynx. London: Arnold; 2000. p. 437–73.
[12] Montgomery WW, Montgomery SK. Montgomery thyroplasty implant system. Ann Otol Rhinol Laryngol 1997;170(Supp l):S1–16.
[13] Flint PW, Cummings CW. Phonosurgical procedures. In: Cummings CW, Frederickson JM, Harker LA, et al, editors. Otolaryngology head and neck surgery. 3rd edition. St Louis (MO): Mosby; 1998. p. 2078–9.
[14] Friedrich G. Titanium vocal fold medializing implant: introducing a novel implant system for external vocal fold medialization. Ann Otol Rhinol Laryngol 1999;108:79–86.
[15] Tucker HM. Complications of laryngeal framework surgery for phonation disorders. Operative Techniques in Otolaryngology-Head and Neck Surgery. 1993;4:232–5.
[16] Netterville JL, Stone RE, Luken ES, et al. Silastic medialization and arytenoid adduction: the Vanderbilt experience: a review of 116 phonosurgical procedures. Ann Otol Rhinol Laryngol 1993;102:413–24.
[17] Cotter CS, Avidano MA, Crary MA, et al. Laryngeal complications after type 1 thyroplasty. Otolaryngol Head Neck Surg 1995;113:671–3.
[18] Halum SL, Postma GN, Koufman JA. Endoscopic management of extruding medialization laryngoplasty implants. Laryngoscope 2005;115:1051–4.
[19] Woo P, Pearl AW, Hsiung MW, et al. Failed medialization laryngoplasty: management by revision surgery. Otolaryngol Head Neck Surg 2001;124:615–21.
[20] Maragos NE. The posterior thyroplasty window: anatomical considerations. Laryngoscope 1999;109:1228–31.
[21] Harries ML. Unilateral vocal fold paralysis: a review of the current methods of surgical rehabilitation. J Laryngol Otol 1996;110:111–6.
[22] Ford CM. Laryngeal injection techniques. In: Ford CM, Bles DM, editors. Phonosurgery: assessment and management of voice disorders. New York: Raven Press; 1991. p. 123–41.

[23] Habashi S, Croft CB. Intracordal Teflon injection: a question of timing. J Laryngol Otol 1991;105:128–9.
[24] Hirano M, Mori K, Tanaka S, et al. Vocal function in patients with unilateral vocal fold paralysis before and after silicone injection. Acta Otolaryngol 1995;115:553–9.
[25] Remacle M, Dujardin JM, Lawson G. Treatment of vocal fold immobility by glutaraldehyde cross-linked collagen injection: long term results. Ann Otol Rhinol Laryngol 1995;104: 437–41.
[26] Shaw GY, Szewczyk MA, Searle J, et al. Autologous fat injection into the vocal folds: technical considerations and long-term follow-up. Laryngoscope 1997;107:177–86.
[27] Rihkanen H. Vocal fold augmentation by injection of autologous fascia. Laryngoscope 1998;108:51–4.
[28] Hallen L, Testad P, Sederholm E, et al. DiHA (dextranomers in hyaluronan) injections for treatment of insufficient closure of the vocal folds: early clinical experiences. Laryngoscope 2001;111:1063–7.
[29] Kasperbauer JL, Slavit DH, Maragos NE. Teflon granulomas and overinjection of Teflon: a therapeutic challenge for the otorhinolaryngologist. Ann Otol Rhinol Laryngol 1993;102: 748–51.
[30] Nakayama M, Ford CN, Bless DM. Teflon vocal fold augmentation: failures and management in 28 cases. Otolaryngol Head Neck Surg 1993;109:493–8.
[31] Anderson TD, Sataloff RT. Complications of collagen injection of the vocal fold: report of several unusual cases and review of the literature. J Voice 2004;18:392–7.
[32] Isshiki N, Yamamoto I, Fukagai S. Type 2 thyroplasty for spasmodic dysphonia: fixation using a titanium bridge. Acta Otolaryngol 2004;124(3):309–12.
[33] Blitzer A, Brin MF, Stewart CF. *Botulinum*, toxin management of spasmodic dysphonia (laryngeal dystonia): a 12-year experience in more than 900 patients. Laryngoscope 1998;108: 1435–41.
[34] Mahieu HF, Norbart T, Snel F. Laryngeal framework surgery for voice improvement. Rev Laryngol Otol Rhinol (Bord) 1996;177:189–97.

ELSEVIER
SAUNDERS

Otolaryngol Clin N Am
39 (2006) 77–86

OTOLARYNGOLOGIC
CLINICS
OF NORTH AMERICA

Phonosurgery for Pitch Alteration: Feminization and Masculinization of the Voice

Jeffrey H. Spiegel, MD, FACS

Department of Otolaryngology–Head and Neck Surgery, Boston University School of Medicine, 88 East Newton Street, Boston, MA 02118, USA

Transsexuality is a complex, difficult problem in which individuals of unambiguous genotype and phenotype for gender assignment feel that they belong to the opposite gender. It has been estimated that 1 in 54,000 individuals are transsexuals; 75% of whom desire reassignment from male to female (MTF), and the remainder are woman who desire to be men (female to male; FTM) [1]. There are several presumed contributing factors to transsexualism, but a specific cause has not been identified. There are specific organic differences in transsexual individuals, however (eg, a large nucleus suprachiasmaticus may be identified in the hypothalamus of these persons) [2].

A multitude of changes is necessary for the individual who desires to change his/her perceived gender. Hairstyle, mannerisms, gait, and clothing are just some of the characteristics that must be altered to permit these individuals to be identified rapidly by others as being the gender that they feel they are; however, voice often is of particular importance. The importance of voice was illustrated nicely by an analysis of a group of 14 MTF transsexuals. When impartial observers were asked to determine whether subjects were male or female, subjects were judged more often as female when only visual clues were presented. When audio and visual cues were given, fewer subjects were judged as feminine; with just audio cues, fewer still were judged as women. As the investigators noted, clearly "physical appearance positively influences the perception of femaleness while the voice tends to negatively influence the perception of femaleness. Of course, a female voice in the absence of a female appearance will be less helpful in 'passing' as

E-mail address: jeffrey.spiegel@bmc.org

a woman than when consistent with a feminine appearance, but the negative impact of masculine voice on those who look like women is evident" [3].

Once identified as being transsexual, individuals often initiate hormone therapy to assist in the development of phenotypic characteristics of their desired gender. It is generally presumed that hormone therapy is beneficial in "masculinizing" the voice of FTM transsexuals, but that the corresponding application of estrogen and other female hormones to men does not result in an acceptable change [3]. For FTM transsexuals, the results are good. In one larger series, after initiation of hormone therapy, 12 of 16 (75%) individuals believed that they had a voice that always would be considered masculine, whereas 4 of 16 (25%) believed that their voice definitely had become more male than female. In addition, 12 of 16 always were addressed as men when on the telephone. Fourteen of 16 patients believed that successful alteration in voice was of equivalent importance to them as sexual reassignment surgery (surgical modification of the sexual organs) [4].

For the 75% of transsexuals who are MTF, the matter is more difficult. These individuals have lower fundamental frequencies than women, different resonance characteristics, and significantly different speech characteristics, including phrasing, speed, volume, and presentation. The fundamental frequency of an individual should be at least 150 to 160 Hz to be perceived as female, although many other vocal characteristics come into play [5].

Is it possible to make a cello sound like a violin? Certainly one can try to play the cello with the same phrasing and tempo that are heard commonly from a violin, but the size of the instrument, length and weight of the strings, resonance, and tones clearly will be those of a cello. To raise the sound one could replace the cello strings with lighter wires applied at greater tension; however, other characteristics of the instrument will, of necessity, remain the same and the resulting sound is unpredictable. Will it sound like a violin or like a cello with different strings?

Similar questions exist when considering surgical alteration of the vocal cords to feminize the voice. Several inventive surgeons have designed procedures to achieve this goal, and the author presents many of them in this article, together with a review of the degree to which they were successful.

Women speak with phrasing, intonation, resonance, and pitch that are different from men. Of these, only pitch (and perhaps resonance) is amenable to possible surgical alteration. The choice of words and the way in which they are said only can be altered by speech therapy and behavioral modifications. Certainly, the goal is to achieve a mean fundamental frequency that is within the range of typical adult females (196–224 Hz). Typically, men have a much lower fundamental frequency (107–146 Hz) [6]. In general, there are four factors that control the pitch. These include the tension, mass, and length of the cords, as well as the subglottal pressure that is applied. Pitch is increased when the vocal cords are lengthened, which increases their tension and slightly decreases the vibrating mass [7]. Men have larger larynges than do women, so the cord is longer and has increased mass (similar to the difference between a cello and a violin). Lengthening the cords further is akin to tightening the string of an instrument, and increases the pitch.

In 1979, Kitajima and colleagues [8] reported on their experimental studies at raising vocal pitch. They specifically attempted to address how to restore the pitch of women with low voices, and had proposed a procedure that they called "cricothyroid approximation" between 1974 and 1975 [9,10]. They found a near linear relationship between vocal pitch and cricothyroid distance, and noted that pitch increment per unit of shortening is greater for female larynges than for male larynges. This may be due to the overall lower mass of the female vocal cord. Specifically, they found that 1 mm of approximation between the cricoid and thyroid cartilages resulted in a pitch elevation of 0.15 to 0.90 semitones [8].

Isshiki and colleagues [7] examined procedures to raise and lower the vocal pitch. For lowering the pitch, they suggested shortening of the antero-posterior length of the thyroid cartilage. This procedure reduces the tension, reduces the length, and increases the vibratory mass of the cord, and thus, should lower the voice pitch substantially. The investigators recommended removing a 2-mm wide strip of cartilage on one side, under local anesthesia, and then checking the results. If not adequate, additional cartilage can be removed on one or both sides (Fig. 1). The results of this operation, which they called "thyroplasty type III," can be significant. They reported a pitch reduction of 38 to 178 Hz in nine male patients.

To elevate the pitch, Isshiki and colleagues [7] suggested three options: (1) cricothyroid approximation to increase the tension on the cords, (2) scarring of the vocal cord to increase stiffness by longitudinal incision along the vocal

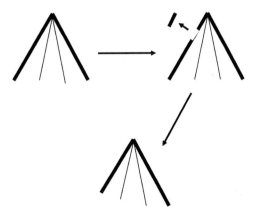

Fig. 1. Pitch reduction by shortening the length of true vocal cord (thyroplasty type III). A segment of cartilage is removed, preserving the inner perichondrium. The procedure can be repeated on the other side to increase effect.

cord, and (3) decreasing the mass of the cord by way of injection of steroids or destruction of tissue with CO_2 laser.

Cricothyroid approximation probably has been used most commonly to elevate the vocal pitch. In this technique, the cricoid and thyroid cartilages are exposed and sutured together with permanent sutures (Fig. 2). Small pieces of silicone may be needed underneath the sutures to distribute tension, and prevent the sutures from tearing through the soft cartilage. Cricothyroid approximation results in a lengthening of the cords, but with a corresponding anteroinferior rotation of the larynx. This rotation commonly causes the thyroid prominence ("Adam's apple") to become more visible beneath the skin of the anterior neck. In women, the thyroid prominence is less evident; MTF transsexuals consider the Adam's apple to be a significant problem in their struggle to present themselves as women. Chondrolaryngoplasty (in which those parts of the thyroid cartilage that project anteriorly superior to the insertion of the vocal cords are excised) is among the more common feminizing procedures that are requested by MTF transsexuals (Fig. 3) [11]. In nine female patients who had cricothyroid approximation, Isshiki and colleagues [7] achieved pitch elevation that ranged from 24 to 158 Hz. In one MTF transsexual, the combination of CT approximation and longitudinal incisions achieved elevation from 110 to 164 Hz; however, these short-term results were not long-lasting [12].

Yang and colleagues [13] reviewed the results of 73 patients who underwent cricothyroid approximation between June 1995 and June 2000; 20 patients had complete preoperative and postoperative acoustic voice data (at least 12 months postoperatively; mean, 22 months) for inclusion in their report. They found a mean change of 57 Hz (from 145 preoperatively to 202 postoperatively) in fundamental pitch. Whereas cricothyroid approximation has been criticized for reducing the pitch range, these investigators found no variation after surgery. Overall, 58% of the patients demonstrated satisfaction with their postoperative voice and 33% expressed dissatisfaction; 42%

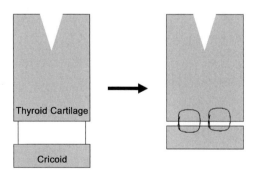

Fig. 2. Cricothyroid approximation (thyroplasty type IV). Sutures are placed between the thyroid cartilage and cricoid cartilage to pull the cartilages together. This effectively lengthens the vocal cords.

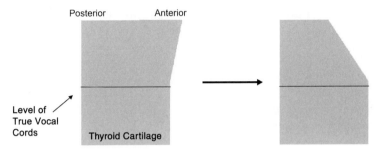

Fig. 3. Sagittal view of the larynx demonstrates the segment of cartilage that is removed to reduce the appearance of the Adam's apple. Preservation of structure at the anterior attachment of the true vocal cords is important to protect the voice. Disruption can result in undesirable lowering of pitch.

of subjects overall described their voices as "rough or hoarse." Only 31% reported that their voices were never considered masculine on the telephone, 47% noted that they were considered to have a masculine voice occasionally, and 22% noted that they frequently were considered to have a masculine voice. At follow-up (>1 year after surgery), 29% of subjects noted dysphagia with liquids.

Another study examined the pitch change in 14 MTF patients who had received speech therapy, and wanted pitch elevation—by way of cricothyroid approximation—along with chondroplasty to reduce the prominence of the Adam's apple [14]. Mean frequency did not change before or after surgery. They noted a preoperative mean of 152 Hz, a postoperative mean of 155 Hz, and a 6-month postoperative mean of 157 Hz. When considering the modal pitch (the pitch most commonly used during speech), however, the results were good. Subjects started at 142 Hz, had immediate postoperative results of 175 Hz, and 6 months postoperatively had a modal frequency of 186 Hz. These investigators believed that the modal pitch correlated significantly with the perceived gender of the speaker, as evidenced by listeners correctly judging the gender of 8 of the 14 patients. The degree to which conscious effort plays a role in modal frequency may be different than at fundamental frequency (ie, perhaps the subjects put more effort into sounding female postoperatively, but could not change their fundamental frequency). Conversely, cricothyroid approximation may have permitted the subjects to speak more easily at feminine modal frequency. The necessary randomized trial that will answer these questions has not been done.

More recently, two other groups reported their results with cricothyroid approximation. In 2004, Neumann and Welzel [2] of Germany described 67 MTF patients who underwent cricothyroidopexy (ie, their version of the Isshiki type IV thyroplasty [cricothyroid approximation]) using a combination of miniplates and wires. Nearly all patients had temporary hoarseness for up to 4 weeks. Two patients (3%) had a lowering of the fundamental frequency, and only 28% of patients had a postoperative fundamental frequency in the female range. Furthermore, nearly all patients had difficulty speaking loudly, and had a loss of dynamic range from 40 dB to 29 dB. These investigators noted that after 1 year follow-up, although volume had improved, preoperative vocal performance was not achieved. They suggested that vocal pitch elevation occurs when vocal fold length is increased by at least 2 mm.

More recently, a group from London reported their modification of the cricothyroid approximation operation with results in 21 MTF transsexuals [15]. These investigators used horizontal mattress sutures to approximate the cricoid and thyroid cartilages, but further, to sublux the inferior edge of the thyroid cartilage over the cricoid. Theoretically, this can achieve further lengthening of the vocal cords with subsequent increase in tension and voice elevation. The investigators reported an average modal frequency increase of 71 Hz in free speech, but did not report fundamental frequency changes. They noted that a significant number of patients had voice "irregularities" that improved with speech therapy, although many patients had voice irregularities before surgery. This is to be expected in a group of MTF transsexuals who have been straining their voices to speak in a near falsetto feminine voice over a prolonged period of time. Patients who had fewer vocal problems before surgery did better with surgery.

An additional method to increase the length of the vocal cords is advancement of the anterior commissure, as described in 1983 by Lejeune and colleagues [16] and in 1985 by Tucker [17]. A wedge of cartilage that contains the anterior commissure is advanced and secured in place with a splint of metal or silicone block. A modification of this technique was used by Wagner and colleagues [18], who advanced just a rectangular segment of cartilage that contained the attachment of the anterior commissure of the vocal folds. This was secured in an advanced position with clits of cartilage. They reported on 14 patients who underwent pitch elevation, 5 with anterior commissure advancement (1 with chondroplasty for appearance, 1 with chondroplasty for appearance and reversal of a previous attempt at cricothyroid approximation, and 3 with anterior commissure advancement coupled with cricothyroid approximation [1 of whom also had chondroplasty for appearance]). Their remaining patients had cricothyroid advancement with or without chondroplasty for appearance. Four of their 14 patients had postoperative fundamental frequency of less than 125 Hz; the median gain was 11 Hz overall (range, 0–113 Hz).

Isshiki and colleagues [7] also noted that pitch elevation can be achieved by anterior–posterior expansion of the thyroid ala. They performed this in one patient in their 1983 report, in addition to cricothyroid approximation with an elevation of pitch from 215 to 315 Hz. Injection of triamcinolone was attempted in five patients to induce atrophy (mass reduction) in the vocal fold, but the specific effect was not clear and the investigators concluded that further refinement is necessary, although the procedure remains theoretically sound.

Longitudinal incision of the vocal cord to increase the pitch was proposed in two different papers (Saito and Kokawa) in 1977 [7]. Scarring of
the vocal cord could result in stiffness and increased pitch, but the investigators proposed that reduced contraction of the vocalis muscle resulted in
the beneficial effect. In the two case reports, changes of 37 Hz and 36 Hz
were achieved after 3 months. A similar technique involves partial evapora-
tion of the vocal cord by CO_2 laser. Isshiki and colleagues [7] noted that one
patient achieved an elevation of 30 Hz with this technique, because of reduction in mass and increased stiffness from superficial scarring.

Two investigators have recognized that pitch elevation could perhaps be
achieved by shortening the cords, and attempted to do this by creation of an
anterior web. In 1982, Donald [19] reported three patients in whom a laryngofissure approach was used to denude and approximate the anterior third of
the vocal cords (Fig. 4). Donald noted that one patient had an elevation in
pitch of more than one octave, a second patient (described as noncompliant
with the recommended care regimen) had "some improvement" with a raspy
voice postoperatively, and a third patient had "excellent improvement in
voice pitch but some slight breathiness" [19].

A similar method was used by Gross [20], although with an endoscopic
approach rather than by way of laryngofissure. Gross reported on the first
10 patients (of 20 he operated on) in whom a laryngoscope was used to expose the vocal cords, and the anterior aspect was de-epithelialized and then
sutured together. Gross obtained postoperative change in habitual frequency of 39 to 125 Hz. He noted that deep voice pitch was not produced
even in "uncontrolled situations," such as laughter or surprise. After 3
months, most patients continued to show a reduction in loudness of voice,
but only 3 of 10 expressed concern about this.

An aggressive approach was taken by the Thai group of Kunachak and
colleagues [21]. They reported reducing the size of the vocal cords and the
overall size of the larynx to change from a masculine toward a feminine
structure. The anterior 4 mm of thyroid cartilage was removed from the larynx on both sides (including the attachment of the anterior commissure). Six
millimeters of vocal cord were removed from the anterior aspect of the vocal
cords. The vocal cords were sutured together in the midline, and pulled forward to the leading edge of the thyroid cartilage on each side which were
then reapproximated in the midline (Fig. 5). In six patients, fundamental

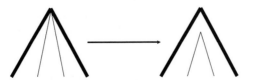

Fig. 4. Elevation of pitch achieved by shortening length of true vocal cord. This can be done by
way of laryngofissure or endoscopic approach.

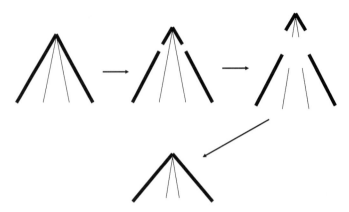

Fig. 5. Laryngoplasty and pitch elevation as per Kunachak and colleagues [21]. Four milli-meters of anterior thyroid cartilage and approximately 6 mm of true vocal cord are removed bilaterally, and then are reapproximated carefully in the midline.

pitch changed from 102 Hz to 320 Hz. The first two patients had vocal cord granulomas, perhaps from overly superficial placement of the cord reap-proximation sutures. This technique may have the advantage of improving the external appearance of the larynx and the pitch, but requires general an-esthetic (which prevents "tuning" of the vocal pitch at the time of surgery) and uses an external incision.

The ideal procedure would be done endoscopically, could improve the appearance of the larynx, and would increase the pitch without altering vo-cal quality, range, or loudness. Until the time that such a procedure exists, speech therapy may be the best alternative for patients who desire pitch el-evation. Dacakis [6] reported on 10 MTF transsexuals who had a long-term maintenance of at least a 21-Hz increase in fundamental frequency during spontaneous speech. These same patients enjoyed a mean increase of 43 Hz in spontaneous speech at the time of discharge from speech therapy, but were able to retain the necessary skills for substantial improvement, even when outside of therapy. Dacakis noted a correlation between the number of sessions of speech therapy that a patient attended and the long-term maintenance of an increase in fundamental frequency.

Speech therapy also must focus on intonation, because it has been dem-onstrated that women's voices have greater variability in intonation than do men's. Thus, the stereotype of the monotone male voice is substantiated to some degree [22]. Vocal tract resonance also must be addressed because lis-teners can identify correctly the gender of speakers using an electrolarynx at fundamental frequency of 85 Hz [23]. These findings suggest that surgery alone is not likely to be adequate, because elevation of the vocal pitch alone does not always result in a voice that is perceived as female. Methods to ad-just vocal tract resonance have been reported, and should be incorporated into the speech therapy of patients who request vocal feminization [23].

In general, the goals of speech therapy for the MTF transsexual should be to increase head resonance over chest resonance, increase pitch to at least 155 Hz, increase intonation variability with more upward intonations, and to encourage a delicate articulation with decreased loudness [24]. Nonetheless, while speech therapy is important and can have long-lasting benefits, an effective voice-elevating surgical procedure would be welcome as voice therapy does not always provide the desired change, and patients with just speech therapy may still have lower pitched voice when surprised or speaking without conscious preparation and use of learned vocal techniques [25].

Summary

The most widely used and reported technique for pitch elevation, cricothyroid approximation, may not have long-lasting benefit, and has a real incidence of complications (eg, decreased range, loudness, vocal quality). One leading laryngologist has proposed that because no surgical technique of pitch elevation exists that is satisfactorily safe and effective, pitch elevation surgery should not be performed until a more effective technique is developed (J.A. Koufman, personal communication, 2005). The laryngologist is advised to understand the existing methods, so that patients who request pitch elevation can be counseled appropriately.

References

[1] Landen M, Walinder J, Lundstrom B. Prevalence, incidence and sex ration of transsexualism. Acta Psychiatr Scand 1996;3:221–3.
[2] Neumann K, Welzel C. The importance of voice in male-to-female transsexualism. J Voice 2004;18(1):153–67.
[3] Van Borsel JV, De Cuypere G, Van Den Berge H. Physical appearance and voice in male-to-female transsexuals. J Voice 2001;14(4):570–5.
[4] Van Borsel J, De Cuypere G, Rubens R, et al. Voice problems in female-to-male transsexuals. Int J Lang Comm Dis 2000;35(3):427–42.
[5] Wolfe V, Ratusnik DL, Smith FH, et al. Intonation and fundamental frequency in male-to-female transsexuals. J Speech Hear Disord 1990;55:43–50.
[6] Dacakis G. Long term maintenance of fundamental frequency increases in male-to-female transsexuals. J Voice 2000;14(4):549–56.
[7] Isshiki N, Taira T, Tanabe M. Surgical alteration of the vocal pitch. J Otolaryngol 1983; 12(5):335–40.
[8] Kitajima K, Tanabe M, Isshiki N. Cricothyroid distance and vocal Pitch. Experimental surgical study to elevate the vocal pitch. Ann Otol 1979;88:52–5.
[9] Isshiki N, Morita H, Okamura H, et al. Thyroplasty as a new phonological technique. Acta Otolaryngol (Stockh) 1974;78:451–7.
[10] Isshiki N, Okamura H, Ishikawa T. Thyroplasty type I (lateral compression) for dysphonia due to vocal cord paralysis or atrophy. Acta Otolaryngol (Stockh) 1975;80:465–73.
[11] Wolfort FG, Dejerine ES, Ramos DJ, et al. Chondrolaryngoplasty for appearance. Plast Reconstr Surg 1990;86(3):464–9.
[12] Koufman JA, Isaacson G. Laryngoplastic phonosurgery. Otolaryngol Clin North Am 1991; 24:1151–77.

[13] Yang CY, Palmer AD, Murray KD, et al. Cricothyroid approximation to elevate vocal pitch in male-to-female transsexuals: results of surgery. Ann Otol Rhinol Laryngol 2002;111(6): 477–85.

[14] Brown M, Perry A, Cheesman AD, et al. Pitch change in male-to-female transsexuals: has phonosurgery a role to play. Int J Lang Comm Dis 2000;35(1):129–36.

[15] Kanagalingam J, Georgalas C, Wood GR, et al. Cricothyroid approximation and subluxation in 21 male-to-female transsexuals. Laryngoscope 2005;115:611–8.

[16] Lejeune FE, Guice CE, Samuels PM. Early experiences with vocal ligament tightening. Ann Otol Rhinol Laryngol 1983;92:475–7.

[17] Tucker HM. Anterior commissure laryngoplasty for adjustment of vocal fold tension. Ann Otol Rhinol Laryngol 1985;94:547–9.

[18] Wagner I, Fugain C, Monneron-Girard L, et al. Pitch-raising surgery in fourteen male-to-female transsexuals. Laryngoscope 2003;113:1157–65.

[19] Donald PJ. Voice change surgery in the transsexual. Head Neck Surg 1982;4:433–7.

[20] Gross M. Pitch-raising surgery in male-to-female transsexuals. J Voice 1999;13(2):246–50.

[21] Kunachak S, Prakunhungsit S, Sujjalak K. Thyroid cartilage and vocal fold reduction: a new phonosurgical method for male-to-female transsexuals. Ann Otol Rhinol Laryngol 2000; 109:1082–6.

[22] Wolfe VI, Ratusnik DL, Smith FH, et al. Intonation and fundamental frequency in male-to-female transsexuals. J Speech Hear Disord 1990;55:43–50.

[23] Mount KH, Salmon SH. Changing the vocal characteristics of a postoperative transsexual patient: a longitudinal study. J Commun Disord 1988;21:229–38.

[24] deBruin MD, Coerts MJ, Greven AJ. Speech therapy in the management of male-to-female transsexuals. Folia Phoniatr Logop 2000;52:220–7.

[25] Soderpalm E, Larsson AK, Almquist SA. Evaluation of a consecutive group of transsexual individuals referred for vocal intervention in the west of Sweden. Logoped Phoniatr Vocol 2004;29:18–30.

ELSEVIER
SAUNDERS

Otolaryngol Clin N Am
39 (2006) 87–100

OTOLARYNGOLOGIC
CLINICS
OF NORTH AMERICA

Laryngeal Dystonia

Gregory A. Grillone, MD, FACS*, Teresa Chan, MD

*Department of Otolaryngology-Head and Neck Surgery, Boston University Medical Center,
88 East Newton Street, D-608, Boston, MA 02118, USA*

Dystonias are a group of movement disorders that are characterized by involuntary, action-induced counterproductive muscle contraction. They may be classified as primary (also called sporadic or idiopathic) or secondary (related to trauma, infection, medication, or underlying neuromuscular disorder). Dystonias may be classified further according to age of onset (early and late onset) and distribution of muscle involvement: focal, segmental, multifocal, or generalized. Laryngeal dystonia (LD) is an example of a focal, action-induced dystonia that affects laryngeal motor control. LD can be classified as adductor type, abductor type, mixed type, and adductor laryngeal breathing dystonia (ALBD).

LD also is referred to often as spasmodic dysphonia, and these terms often are used synonymously. Historically, it also has been referred to as spastic aphonia, spastic dysphonia, phonic laryngeal spasm, coordinated laryngeal spasms, mogiphonia, and laryngeal stuttering [1]. The name "spastic dysphonia" was first used in 1871 by Traube [2] to describe a patient who had "nervous hoarseness." The reference to spasticity is a misnomer because no consistent lesion in the pyramidal or extrapyramidal tract has been identified. Furthermore, studies by Blitzer and colleagues [3] showed that patients who have LD do not have findings on electromyography that are consistent with other true spastic disorders.

Patients who have LD suffer from hyperfunction of their laryngeal muscles with excessive closing or opening of the glottis during phonation or respiration. With the adductor type, extreme effort is exerted in an attempt to achieve fluent speech, and consequently, the patient's voice is wrought with irregular breaks. The abductor type is characterized by excessive intermittent breathiness, sometimes to the point of aphonia. Mixed LD exhibits characteristics of the adductor and abductor types. ALBD is characterized by persistent inspiratory stridor, usually normal voice, and

---

* Corresponding author.
E-mail address: gregory.grillone@bmc.org (G.A. Grillone).

0030-6665/06/$ - see front matter © 2005 Elsevier Inc. All rights reserved.
doi:10.1016/j.otc.2005.11.001

oto.theclinics.com

paroxysmal cough. Some patients who have ALBD find it difficult to breathe and swallow at the same time, which results in dysphagia. Except for ALBD, patients who have LD usually are asymptomatic at rest (not phonating). Other laryngeal functions, including singing, humming, and laughing, usually are not affected.

LD may be associated with other focal dystonias, such as blepharospasm, torticollis, or writer's cramp [4]. These usually manifest focally and progress over time. Involvement of multiple focal areas is seen more commonly in early-onset dystonias with presentation before age 26 [1]. Up to 16% of patients who present with initial laryngeal involvement develop symptoms in another part of the body [5]. Symptoms of LD also can be found in association with underlying neurologic disorders or environmental exposure, such as infection, trauma, medication (phenothiazines, metoclopramide), or a psychogenic stimulus.

The prevalence of LD is unknown. It may not be as rare as once believed, and often may be misdiagnosed. It seems to occur more frequently in women, with a male/female ratio of 1:3 to 1:8 [5,6]. The peak age of onset is 35 to 45 years, but onset can occur anywhere between 13 and 71 years of age [6,7]. Patients with a family history of dystonia usually present before the age of 25 [7]. Blitzer and colleagues [5] found a positive family history of dystonia in 12% of patients who had LD over a 12-year period. In general, primary dystonias carry a 20% likelihood of other dystonias within the family; many studies have begun to discover a genetic basis for this phenomenon [5,8,9]. Other risk factors include stress or antecedent viral infection [6].

Some investigators propose that LD is a continuum disorder with adductor and abductor components present in all patients, and symptoms are dependent on the predominant type [10]. Adductor LD is the most common form and represents about 80% of all LDs [5]. It is characterized by intermittent closure of the true vocal cords during speech, which results in phonatory breaks and a strained, strangled voice quality. Pitch is monotonal and projection is compromised. Irregular breaks occur in the middle of words, especially with vowels in connected speech, liquids (l and r), or semi-vowel sounds (w and y). Patients who have adductor LD often complain that it is a great effort to speak. Abductor LD is far less common; patients have a whisper-soft, breathy voice that sometimes progresses to aphonia when severe spasm occurs. Patients who have abductor LD have particular trouble with voiceless consonants (p, t, l, s, f, h, th). Sounds, such as "s," "h," or "k," preceding open vowels in words like "coffee" and "cake" usually are affected most. Both types of LD can have associated, irregular tremors that are distinct from essential tremor in up to 25% of cases [3].

Etiology

Classically, spasmodic dysphonia was believed to be psychogenic in origin. When Traube first described the disorder more than 100 years ago, he attributed it to nervous hoarseness. Typically, patients note onset or decline of symptoms when under new stress or prolonged duress. Anecdotally, sensory distractions or "gestes antagonistes," such as yawning, sneezing, yelling, humming, or singing, have been effective in "tricking the patient" and relieving symptoms momentarily. Improvement with alcohol, sedatives, and tranquilizers also have been cited as evidence of a psychogenic or functional etiology.

A newer school of thought proposes that faulty central neurologic processing accounts for these symptoms. Work by several investigators has demonstrated measurable neurologic abnormalities in brainstem auditory-evoked responses, gastric acid secretory response to sham feedings, blink reflexes, finger tapping and peg board tasks, and cardiac response to the Valsalva maneuver [11–14].

Evaluation of laryngeal dystonia

There is no single test or pathognomonic sign or symptom that confirms the diagnosis of LD. The signs and symptoms vary among patients and are not always classic.

Any patient who presents with signs and symptoms that are suggestive of LD warrants a thorough multidisciplinary evaluation. This includes full otolaryngologic and neurologic assessments, as well as evaluation by a speech language pathologist. Onset of symptoms following a stressful life event (emotional or physical), the use of sensory tricks (eg, humming), brief absence of symptoms upon first awakening, improvement in symptoms with alcohol or other tranquilizer, and worsening of symptoms in stressful situations (eg, public speaking, speaking on the telephone) support the diagnosis of dystonia. The presence of other dystonias (eg, writer's cramp), as well as a family history of dystonia also help to support the diagnosis. LD, in particular the adductor LD and ALBD, must be distinguished from functional voice disorders. LD differs from functional voice disorders in that dystonias usually are progressive rather than acute in onset, and typically do not respond well to voice therapy alone. In questionable cases of adductor LD, the authors often initiate a course of voice therapy before considering botox injection. If symptoms resolve completely with voice therapy, the diagnosis likely is functional. ALBD can be distinguished from hysterical or functional stridor in that stridor is persistent rather than intermittent, and it occurs with virtually every inspiration during waking hours, only to disappear completely during sleep. It is important to rule out underlying neurologic disorders, such as Wilson's disease, Huntington's disease, and Parkinson disease, which may cause secondary LD. A full voice evaluation should be performed, including videolaryngoscopy during connected speech, videolaryngostroboscopy, and acoustic and aerodynamic measures to evaluate for tremor, fundamental frequency, pitch and amplitude perturbation, harshness, fluency breaks, and breathiness. It is important to document voice quality objectively and with the patient's own assessment using a visual analog global rating scale. The latter is important for long-term follow-up and outcomes measures [15]. It also is essential to glean the severity of disability or handicap in daily professional and social life, and to determine the possible emotional impact of the dysphonia.

The gold standard of evaluation has been fiberoptic laryngoscopy. Patients who have LD may have findings that range from a normal examination to extrinsic muscle hyperfunction with true and false vocal cord hyperadduction during speech [16]. Some patients who have adductor LD have supraglottic narrowing with anterior rotation of the arytenoid cartilages on speech [16,21]. Also, tremor may be seen often. Stroboscopy adds to the ability to assess the rhythm and regularity of these associated tremors [17]. It also may be helpful in assessing the severity of dystonia. Patients who have ALBD show paradoxic vocal cord movement on inspiration [18].

Several other testing modalities are at the disposal of the otolaryngologist. Electromyography (EMG) can be helpful, but there are no findings that are pathognomonic of LD. Abnormally high activity levels are seen often in the thyroarytenoid and the cricothyroid muscles in adductor LD. In patients who have abductor LD, the posterior cricoarytenoid and thyroarytenoid muscles demonstrate an increase in activity. Blitzer and colleagues [3] demonstrated inappropriate bursts of activity at rest, large polyphasic motor unit potentials with phonation, and irregular tremor on EMG in patients who had LD. A delay from initiation of electrical signal to sound production also may be found [3,12].

Aerodynamic analysis of voice production measures airflow and air pressure and their relationships during phonation. In adductor LD, the patient often is straining against a tight glottis, and mean airflow rates with phonation range from normal to extremely low. In abductor LD, mean airflow rates generally are greater than normal, with bursts of airflow occurring during the abductor spasm [17]. Subglottic pressure measures are estimated to be higher than normal for patients who have adductor LD [19].

Acoustic analysis provides a quantifiable measure of voice quality and vocal function. The patient's voice is recorded and the microphone signal is analyzed mathematically using a computer. More than 33 aspects of a patient's voice can be analyzed, including fundamental frequency changes, jitter, shimmer, voice breaks, and signal-to-noise ratio. Higher mean values of jitter (frequency), shimmer (amplitude), and voice break factor were found in patients who had LD. Significantly lower mean values of signal-to-noise ratio also were found compared with controls [17,20]; however, these findings are not specific enough to be diagnostic. Rather, they are indicators of function, and help to document severity and monitor response to treatment [21].

In contrast to the quantitative physical data that are provided by acoustic measurements, perceptual analysis provides a psychophysical evaluation of voice signals and may provide more qualitative information that is pertinent to the patient's practical phonatory disability. Measures of grade, roughness, breathiness, aphonia, asthenia, strain, staccato, tremor, falsetto, and vocal fry are rated on an analog scale by expert listeners [15].

Finally, spectral analysis provides a physical printout of vibrations and resonances in the glottis and oropharynx during voice production. This can be particularly helpful in defining the tremor component that often is associated with LD. Spectral analysis also can be used, as demonstrated by Koufman [22], to differentiate other laryngeal disorders (eg, muscle tension dysphonia) from LD.

Clinical classification

Several attempts have been made to create a specific classification system to better customize treatment of patients and predict response to therapies, such as botulinum toxin. No one classification system is used universally.

Ludlow and Connor [23] first devised criteria for classification based on constant versus intermittent symptoms and the presence or absence of tremor. When applied to adductor LD, patients were grouped into the following categories: (1) constant harsh and tight voice, (2) intermittent pitch and voice breaks in the middle of words, or (3) glottal stops with tremor at 4 Hz to 5 Hz in the middle of words. When applied to abductor LD, the following categories were applied: (1) constant whispering, (2) intermittent breathiness with consonants at the beginnings of words, or (3) voice tremor with breathy breaks at 4 Hz to 5 Hz in the middle of words.

The classification that was proposed by Koufman [22] is based on independent visual and acoustic evaluation using fiberoptic laryngoscopy and extensive voice analysis. They include focal dystonias (LD) and nonfocal laryngeal dystonias that are associated with more involved entities, such as Meige syndrome and cerebral palsy. LDs are classified further by letter according to primary component, adductor (D) or abductor (B); presence of tremor (T), and location of overclosure (for adductor LD only), either primarily glottic (G) or glottic and supraglottic (S). There also is a subcategory for respiratory type (R) and mixed types: adductor compensatory (BD) and abductor compensatory (DB).

Blitzer and colleagues [5] used a variation of the Koufman [22] and Morrison and Rammage [24] classification systems. Type 1 hyperadduction is forceful overcontraction at the glottic level only with tight compression of the vocal processes and arytenoids. Type 2 is forceful contraction, including contraction of the false cords. In types 3 and 4, there is supraglottic narrowing in the anteroposterior direction. The thyroarytenoid muscle pulls the arytenoids anteriorly in type 3. In type 4, there is sphincteric closure, whereby the arytenoids are pulled so far anteriorly that they close tightly against the epiglottis. For patients who have adductor LD, the authors have found it useful to classify severity of disease to help guide botulinum toxin dosing. Patients with intelligible speech and normal stroboscopic findings are classified as mild, those with barely intelligible or unintelligible speech and normal stroboscopy are considered moderate, and patients with unintelligible speech who are unable to trigger the strobe are considered severe.

Treatment options

There is no known cure for LD. Multiple treatment modalities, including voice therapy, biofeedback, psychologic counseling, sensory distractions, acupuncture, chiropractic, pharmacotherapy, and surgery, have been reported in the literature with anecdotal success. Although voice therapy alone does not seem to be effective in treating adductor LD, the authors have found it useful as an adjunctive therapy in patients who receive botulinum toxin type A injections. The compensatory mechanisms that sometimes contribute to poor voice quality in patients who have adductor LD often reappear as the toxins muscle weakening effect wears off. Voice therapy seems to minimize the re-emergence of these compensatory mechanisms, and effectively gives patients a longer period of serviceable voice. Treatment of LD that is associated with generalized or multifocal disease often begins with pharmacotherapy, whereas focal disease is more amenable to focused treatment (eg, botulinum toxin injection).

Pharmacotherapeutic options for the treatment of dystonias include anticholinergics (trihexyphenidyl, benztropine), benzodiazepines (clonazepam, lorazepam, diazepam), dopamine-depleting agents (tetravenzine, clozapine), or baclofen. The use of anticholinergics is effective in approximately 50% of children and 40% of adults who have dystonia [1]. Major side effects, such as dry mouth, blurred vision, difficulty with concentration, and cognitive impairment, limit patient compliance and the use of these medications. Use of anticholinesterases in conjunction with anticholinergics sometimes help to alleviate untoward side effects [1].

Classical surgical options in the treatment of LD include resection of the recurrent laryngeal nerve (RLN) unilaterally and lidocaine injection around the RLN. Dedo, who initially described RLN resection in the 1970s [25], reported wide successes and only a 15% failure rate over time [26]. In a review series of RLN resection by other investigators, failure rates were as high as 64% at 3 years; many subjects had worsening of their voice after surgery [27]. Accordingly, RLN resection largely has fallen out of favor among most otolaryngologists. Rescue operations and alternative procedures, such as laser thinning of the vocal cord, avulsion of the remaining RLN, RLN crush, resection of the superior laryngeal nerve alone, transection of the adductor branch only, and anterior thyroplasty with lateral or posterior displacement of the vocal ligaments, have been proposed [28–30]. These have not been shown to be consistently effective over time. Most recent alternative therapies include laser removal of one thyroarytenoid muscle, selective adductor denervation–reinnervation with ansa cervicalis, implantable nerve stimulator devices, and bipolar radiofrequency-induced thermotherapy [31–33]. The long-term effectiveness of these treatment modalities remains to be seen.

Since the mid 1980s, botulinum toxin injections into the affected laryngeal musculature have been the mainstay of treatment for most patients who have LD. In 1980, Alan Scott, an ophthalmologist, first described the use of botulinum toxin in the extraocular muscles for the treatment of strabismus [34]. Since that time, botulinum toxin has been used to treat focal dystonias as well as many other disorders (eg, myoclonus, tremors, bruxism, spasticity, dystonic tics, hemifacial spasm, facial wrinkles). Blitzer and colleagues [35] first reported using botulinum toxin for LD in 1986.

Botulinum toxin

Eight distinct types of botulinum toxin exist: A, B, C1, C2, D, E, F, and G [36]. Types A and B have been studied the most extensively studied and are used most widely. Botulinum A toxin is marketed in the United States under the trade name Botox (Allergan, Inc., Irvine, California) and in Europe as Dysport (Speywood, UK). It was approved by the U.S. Food and Drug Administration (FDA) in December 1989 for use in strabismus and certain focal dystonias, including blepharospasm and hemifacial spasm. These indications remain the only FDA-approved uses for Botox, but many well-founded "off label" clinical uses have been approved by the American Academy of Otolaryngology-Head and Neck Surgery, the American Academy of Neurology, and a 1990 National Institutes of Health consensus conference [36]. Botulinum toxin B, also known as Myobloc (Solstice Neurosciences, San Francisco, California) in the United States and Neurobloc (Elan Pharmaceuticals, Munich, Germany) in Europe, was approved by the FDA in December 2000 for treatment of cervical dystonia.

Botulinum toxin works at the level of the neuromuscular junction. By binding presynaptically, it blocks release of the neurotransmitter acetylcholine, and thereby, arrests muscle contraction to the innervated area. The weakness or paralysis that is induced is temporary and is overcome in two ways: production of new accessory axon terminals and production of new proteins by the cell. The blockade also can be overcome by nonphysiologic means [36,37]. Because LDs often result from poorly coordinated muscle movement, weakening one side of the agonist and antagonist muscle groups results in functional movement.

Structure and preparation of botulinum toxin

Botox is prepared as a single-chain polypeptide that is inactive as a neuromuscular blocking agent. To achieve potency, the single chain is converted into a double chain that consists of a heavy chain and a light chain. The toxin is extracted from fermented culture media, precipitated, purified, and crystallized with ammonium sulfate. Botox should be diluted in preservative-free saline (usually 1–4 mL of saline for a concentration of 2.5–10 U/0.1 mL), and ideally, should be used within 4 hours of reconstitution. To ensure stability, the pH should be kept between 4.2 and 6.8, the resuspended solution should be stored at less than 20°C, and it should not be shaken because this may inactivate the toxin. Use of preservatives, freezing, and physical agitation may denature the toxin and decrease overall potency [36]. The effects of Botox are seen within 24 to 72 hours with a maximal effect at about 2 weeks. The duration of beneficial effects lasts from 3 to 6 months [36].

Botox is dosed in mouse units. One mouse unit is equal to the median lethal dose to kill 50% of a group of female Swiss-Webster mice [37]. The relative potencies of the different preparations (Botox, Dysport, Myobloc, and Eurobloc) differ considerably. For example, the relative potency of Botox compared with Dysport is 1:4. Botox is dispensed in 100 U vials, whereas Dysport is dispensed in 500 U bottles. Furthermore, the potency of different batches of Botox may differ [36].

Mechanism of action

Acetylcholine is manufactured intracellularly and stored in vesicles. To exert its neuronal effects, it must bind to the axonal terminal membrane and be released into the postsynaptic cleft. This process is dependent on several proteins, including vesicle-associated membrane protein (VAMP) synaptobrevin, soluble NSF attachment protein (SNAP)-25, and syntaxin. The botulinum toxins are believed to be zinc endopeptidases that disrupt this process at several toxin-specific sites [36]. First, the toxin binds to the presynaptic terminal and is internalized. Different components from the various toxin subtypes exhibit specific proteolysis of the proteins that are involved in transport and binding of acetylcholine vesicles to the presynaptic membrane. Botox, in its active form, is composed of a heavy chain and a light chain. The light chain is the location of all protease activity, whereas the heavy chain is needed for initial binding and trafficking into the cell. The light chain from botulinum A and E cleave SNAP-25; the light chain from botulinum B, D, F, and G cleave VAMP/synaptobrevin; and the light chain from botulinum C cleaves syntaxin [36]. The structure, synthesis, and storage of acetylcholine are not disrupted by the toxin, and the cell can be made to fire by alternative nonphysiologic interventions.

According to studies by Borodic and colleagues [38], in which 10 U of botulinum toxin was injected into the longissimus dorsi muscle of rabbits, it diffused 4.5 cm from the site of a single injection. Because the extent of denervation is determined by dose and volume, multiple injection points may help to optimize toxin denervation effects to a given area, with fewer complications than a single, high-volume injection [39].

Fillippi and colleagues [40] discovered that botulinum toxin in rat models decreased the afferent discharge from muscle spindles. They proposed that decreased reflex muscle tone, as well as denervation of focal motor areas, may be responsible, in part, for relief of dystonic muscle spasm.

Side effects and contraindications of botulinum toxin

Possible minor side effects include transient breathy hypophonia (35%); hoarseness (50%); swallowing difficulties (15–60%), including clinically insignificant aspiration; and pain at the injection site (1%). Typically, these resolve over 1 to 2 weeks [5]. Local injections are believed to enter the systemic circulation in only minute amounts, if at all. Systemic side effects are rare and may manifest as flulike symptoms that can last from 24 hours to a few weeks. Serious side effects include dysphagia, airway compromise, or generalized weakness from intravascular injection. No deaths have been associated with botulinum toxin use in humans. The lethal dose is unknown, but is estimated to be approximately 2800 U to 3000 U for a 70-kg human [41].

No absolute contraindications exist for the use of Botox; however, a few patient populations warrant caution. Given the unknown potential for teratogenicity and adverse effects of even minute amounts of systemic Botox on neonates and infants, use in pregnant and lactating women is not advised. Botox has been used safely in children who have cerebral palsy, and the side effect profile parallels that seen in the adult population [42,43]. Patients who have associated motor neuron disease or neuromuscular disorders, such as myasthenia gravis and Eaton-Lambert syndrome, have been treated successfully with Botox; however, there are scattered reports of untoward local or systemic effects [44–46]. Given an already compromised neuromuscular status in these patients, additional insult from systemic effects of toxin could be devastating; use in these patients should be considered carefully on a case-by-case basis. Aminoglycosides may potentiate the effects of the toxin and combined use is not recommended. Patients who have known gastroesophageal reflux disease should be treated with antireflux therapy before administration of botulinum toxin. Theoretically, slowed vocal fold closure after injection may predispose them to aspiration.

When given in large or repeated doses, some patients have developed resistance to the toxin. This is believed to occur by development of antibodies and is estimated to happen in 3% to 10% of patients [46]. These antibodies bind to toxin when it is administered, and thereby, limit a patient's response. Risk factors for developing immunogenicity to botulinum toxin include use of higher doses, shorter intervals between injections (<3 months), booster doses, and young age [47]. There is no consistent assay to test for the presence of antibodies. Some centers confirm resistance by injecting 15 U of Botox into one side of the frontalis muscle. Retained symmetric function is indicative of resistance [35]. Patients who have developed resistance sometimes can be treated with other serotypes, such as botulinum toxin B. With the doses of botulinum toxin that are used to treat LD, the authors have not found resistance to be a significant factor.

Injection techniques

Although there are several techniques for injecting botulinum toxin into the larynx, the authors prefer the EMG-guided percutaneous technique. A tuberculin syringe with a 27-gauge, monopolar, hollow, Teflon-coated needle is used for injection. Botox in its crystalline, freeze-dried form is mixed with 4 mL of preservative-free normal saline to create a base dilution of 25 U/mL. Typically, patients who have adductor LD and ALBD are treated with injections into one or both thyroarytenoid muscles. The dose used ranges from 0.625 to 4 U per thyroarytenoid muscle, but each injection is tailored according to severity of disease and response to previous injections. A record of response to each injection is kept by the patient. Under EMG guidance, the needle is passed through the cricothyroid membrane in the midline, and is angled superiorly and laterally in the direction of the thyroarytenoid muscle. Intramuscular location is confirmed by muscle interference pattern on EMG and a change in the audible signal to a sound that is similar to "hard rain on a metal roof." Having the patient phonate while the needle is in the muscle can augment the EMG response. Injection is made after confirmation of the needle location within the muscle. During the procedure, the patient is asked not to cough or swallow. The authors have found that intra-tracheal injection of 1 to 2 mL of 1% lidocaine before toxin injection suppresses cough and swallow in problematic patients. Although this may reduce the EMG signal, the advantages of suppressing these reflexes seem to outweigh the decrease in signal. Sheppert and colleagues [48], in a study of cadaveric larynges, found that the concentration of neuromuscular junctions is highest in the middle third of the thyroarytenoid muscle. In accordance with their results, they advocate injecting into this high concentration area to optimize results. In practice, it is difficult to know the exact location of the needle tip within the muscle.

An indirect laryngoscopic approach for injection was advocated by Ford and colleagues [49] in 1990. Injection in this manner is perpendicular to the long axis of the muscle and does not require EMG guidance. The degree of benefit and duration of treatment seem to be clinically comparable to the more traditional percutaneous techniques.

Botox also can be used in patients who have persistent adductor LD after RLN section [50–52]; however, Sulica and colleagues [50] reported that patient perception of therapeutic effect was lower, despite comparable voice improvement, time to onset of initial and peak effects, and duration of effects. Which thyroarytenoid to inject after surgery remains controversial. Blitzer and colleagues [51] reported an 81% improvement with injection into the functional cord versus 60% improvement with injection into paralyzed cord. Conversely, Ludlow and colleagues [52] reported good results with injection of the paralyzed cord.

Injection for abductor LD requires access to the posterior cricoarytenoid (PCA). The patient's larynx is rotated manually away from the side of injection. The needle is passed just posterior to the posterior edge of the thyroid cartilage at the level of the cricoid. The needle is advanced toward the posterior plate of the cricoid cartilage, and is positioned in the PCA under EMG guidance. The patient is asked to sniff to contract the PCA maximally and verify the EMG signal. A sufficient response was noted in 20% to 25% of patients who had abductor spasmodic dysphonia by weakening just one posterior cricoarytenoid. If significant improvement is not seen with unilateral injection, smaller doses (0.675–2.5 U in 0.1 mL) are given in the contralateral side several weeks after the first injection. If stridor or significant narrowing of the glottic chink have occurred, then no further injections are performed. If breathiness is persistent after both posterior arytenoids have been weakened and the glottic chink has been narrowed, or if significant tremor is present, injection of the cricothyroid muscles is effective [53].

Outcomes

In a report of their 12-year experience with more than 900 patients who had spasmodic dysphonia, Blitzer and colleagues [5] noted that nearly 90% of patients who had adductor LD and 66.7% of patients who had abductor LD achieved a normal voice after injection. On average, this effect was seen at 2.4 days with a peak in effect at 9.0 days in patients who had adductor spasmodic dysphonia. The duration of benefit for the entire group was 15.1 weeks. Injection after nerve-section failure in this subset of patients showed up to 81% improvement; however, these patients never did as well as those who had never undergone surgery, and their perception of improvement was lower on average. Of the 154 patients who had abductor LD in their study, 20% developed a good voice with unilateral injection. After reinjection of the remainder of the group contralaterally, the patients, as a whole, achieved 54.8% of normal function initially; over time, this improved to 66.7%. The average onset of improvement was 4.1 days with a peak effect at 10.0 days. The duration of benefit was 10.5 weeks.

Grillone and colleagues [18] treated seven patients who had ALBD with botulinum toxin injections into both thyroarytenoid muscles. All patients had relief of stridor and coughing for an average of 13.8 weeks.

Studies by Cannito and colleagues [54] showed that patients who had more severe disease were more likely to show objective improvement and note subjective improvement by visual analog global rating scale after injection. In addition, older patients exhibited less improvement than did younger patients when differences in severity were controlled. In a meta-analysis of 27 studies, the average patient who had LD and who was treated with Botox obtained an 84% improvement in voice [55].

Patients who had combined dystonic abnormalities faired poorly (only 30% improvement). Poorest outcomes with botulinum toxin therapy were seen in patients who had tremor, with an average of 43% improvement. Occasionally, improving phonatory ability unmasks an unvoiced tremor to the detriment of voice quality. Consistent with this finding, Langeveld and colleagues [15] studied voice quality before and after Botox treatment using several modalities, including self-evaluation, perceptual voice ratings, and acoustic analysis. In all areas, postinjection ratings showed that voice characteristics were improved significantly, but were not perceived as normal, which indicated the persistence of pathology or unmasking of other vocal dysfunction (eg, voice tremor).

There are few studies on the long-term effects of botulinum toxin in humans. Denervation atrophy, fibrosis, and EMG changes may occur after long-term exposure [56–58].

Summary

Because no cure for LDs exists, the ultimate goal of current treatment modalities is functional symptomatic relief without airway compromise. Botulinum toxin has proven to be a safe and effective treatment for relief of the symptoms of spasmodic dysphonia. Its effects are localized, transient, and nondestructive, and its side effects are few. Outcomes may be improved with the universal use of classification schemes. New surgical approaches await the crucial test of time. Surgery is best reserved for the rare patient who does not benefit from, or cannot tolerate, botulinum toxin injections.

References

[1] Blitzer A, Brin M. Spasmodic dysphonia: evaluation and management. In: Fried MP, editor. The larynx: a multidisciplinary approach. 2nd edition. Salem (MA): Mosby-Year Book Inc; 1996. p. 187–98.

[2] Traube L. Spastische form der Nervösen Heiserkeit. Gesammelte Beitr Pathol Physiol 1871; 2:677.

[3] Blitzer A, Lovelace RE, Brin MF, et al. Electromyographic findings in focal laryngeal dystonia (spasmodic dysphonia). Ann Otol Rhinol Larngol 1985;94:591–4.

[4] Brin MF, Fahn S, Blitzer A, et al. Movement disorders of the larynx. In: Blitzer A, Brin MF, Sasaki CT, et al, editors. Neurological disorders of the larynx. New York: Thieme Medical Publishers; 1992. p. 240–8.

[5] Blitzer A, Brin MF, Stewart C. Botulinum toxin management of spasmodic dysphonia (laryngeal dystonia): a 12-year experience in more than 900 patients. Laryngoscope 1998; 108(10):1435–41.

[6] Schweinfurth JM, Billante M, Courey M. Risk factors and demographics in patients with spasmodic dysphonia. Laryngoscope 2002;112:220–3.

[7] Miller RH, Woodson GE. Treatment options in spasmodic dysphonia. Otolaryngol Clin North Am 1991;24(5):1227–37.

[8] Ozelius L, Kramer PL, Moskowitz CB, et al. Human gene for torsion dystonia located on chromosome 9q32–34. Ann Neurol 1990;27:114–20.

[9] Kramer PL, de Leon D, Ozelius L, et al. Dystonia gene in Ashkenazi Jewish population is located on chromosome 9q32–34. Ann Neurol 1990;27:114–20.

[10] Cannito MP, Johnson P. Spastic dysphonia: a continuum disorder. J Commun Disord 1981; 14:215.

[11] Feldman M, Nixon JV, Finitzo-Hieber T, et al. Abnormal parasympathetic vagal functions in patients with spastic dysphonia. Ann Intern Med 1984;100:491.

[12] Schafer SD, Roark RM, Watson BC, et al. Vocal tract electromyographic abnormalities in spasmodic dysphonia: preliminary report. Trans Am Laryngol Assoc 1987;108:187.

[13] Cohen LG, Ludlow CL, Warden M, et al. Blink reflex excitability recover curves in patients with spasmodic dysphonia. Neurology 1979;39:572.

[14] Cannito MP, Kondraske GV. Rapid manual abilities in spasmodic dysphonia and normal female subjects. J Speech Hear Res 1990;33:123.

[15] Langeveld T, Houtman E, Briaire J, et al. Evaluation of voice quality in adductor spasmodic dysphonia before and after botulinum toxin treatment. Ann Otol Rhinol Laryngol 2001;110:627–34.

[16] Woodson G. Use of flexible fiberoptic laryngoscopy to assess patients with spasmodic dysphonia. J Voice 1991;5:85.

[17] Zwirner P, Murry T, Swenson M, et al. Effects of botulinum toxin therapy in patients with adductor spasmodic dysphonia: acoustic, aerodynamic and videoendoscopic findings. Laryngoscope 1992;102:400–6.

[18] Grillone GA, Blitzer A, Brin MF, et al. Treatment of adductor laryngeal breathing dystonia with botulinum toxin. Laryngoscope 1994;104(1):30–2.

[19] Shipp T, Izdebski K, Schutte HK, et al. Subglottal air pressure in spastic dysphonia speech. Folia Phoniatr (Basel) 1988;40(3):105–10.

[20] Zwirner P. Acoustic changes in spasmodic dysphonia after botulinum toxin injection. J Voice 1991;5:78.

[21] Woodson GE, Zwirner P, Murry T, et al. Functional assessment of patients with spasmodic dysphonia. J Voice 1992;6:338–43.

[22] Koufman JA. New classification of laryngeal dystonias. The Visible Voice 1992;1:1–5.

[23] Ludlow CL, Connor NP. Dynamic aspects of phonatory control in spasmodic dysphonia. J Speech Hear Res 1987;30(2):197–206.

[24] Morrison M, Rammage L. Musculoskeletal approach to the classification of dysphonias. In: The management of voice disorders. San Diego (CA): Singular Publishing Group; 1994. p. 53–63.

[25] Dedo HH. Recurrent laryngeal nerve section for spastic dysphonia. Ann Otol Rhinol Laryngol 1976;85:451.

[26] Dedo H, Behlau MS. Recurrent laryngeal nerve section for spastic dysphonia: 5- to 14-year preliminary results in the first 300 patients. Ann Otol Rhinol Laryngol 1991;100:274.

[27] Aronson AE, Desanto LW. Adductor spastic dysphonia: three years after laryngeal nerve section. Laryngoscope 1983;93:1.

[28] Biller HF, Som M, Lawson W. Laryngeal nerve crush for spastic dysphonia. Ann Otol Rhinol Laryngol 1983;92:469.

[29] Tucker H. Laryngeal framework surgery in the management of spasmodic dysphonia: preliminary report. Ann Otol Rhinol Laryngol 1989;98:52–4.

[30] Isshiki N, Tsuji DH, Yamamoto Y, et al. Midline lateralization thyroplasty for adductor spasmodic dysphonia. Ann Otol Rhin Laryngol 2000;109:187–93.

[31] Friedman M, Toriumi DM, Grybauskas V. Treatment of spastic dysphonia without nerve section. Ann Otol Rhinol Laryngol 1987;96(5):590–6.

[32] Berke GS, Blackwell KE, Gerratt BR, et al. Selective laryngeal adductor denervation-reinnervation: a new surgical treatment for adductor spasmodic dysphonia. Ann Otol Rhinol Laryngol 1999;108(3):227–31.

[33] Remacle M, Plouin-Gaudon I, Lawson G, et al. Bipolar radiofrequency-induced thermotherapy (rfitt) for the treatment of spasmodic dysphonia. A report of three cases. Eur Arch Otorhinolaryngol 2005.

[34] Scott AB. Botulinum toxin injection into extraocular muscles as an alternative to strabismus surgery. Opthalmology 1980;87:1044–9.

[35] Blitzer A, Brin MF, Fahn S, et al. Botulinum toxin (BOTOX) for the treatment of "spastic dysphonia" as part of a trial of toxin injections for the treatment of other cranial dystonias. Laryngoscope 1986;96(11):1300–1.

[36] Blitzer A, Sulica L. Botulinum toxin: basic science and clinical uses in otolaryngology. La-ryngoscope 2001;111(2):218–26.

[37] Brin MF. Botulinum toxin therapy: basic science and overview of other therapeutic applications. In: Blitzer A, Binder WJ, Boyd JB, et al, editors. Management of facial lines and wrinkes. Philadelphia: Lippincott Williams & Wilkins; 2000. p. 279–302.

[38] Borodic GE, Pearce LB, Smith K, et al. Botulinum A toxin for spasmodic torticollis: multiple vs. single injection points per muscle. Head Neck 1992;14:33.

[39] Shaari CM, Sanders I. Quantifying how location and dose of botulinum toxin injections affect muscle paralysis. Muscle Nerve 1993;16:964–9.

[40] Fillipi GM, Errico P, Santarelli R, et al. Botulinum A toxin effect on rat jaw muscles spindles. Acta Otolaryngol (Stockh) 1993;113:400.

[41] Scott AB, Suzuki D. Systemic toxicity of botulinum toxin by intramuscular injection in the money. Mov Disor 1988;3:333–5.

[42] Pidcock FS. The emerging role of therapeutic botulinum toxin in the treatment of cerebral palsy. J Pediatr 2004;145(2 Suppl):S33–5.

[43] Koman LA, Brashear A, Rosenfeld S, et al. Botulinum toxin type a neuromuscular blockade in the treatment of equinus foot deformity in cerebral palsy: a multicenter, open-label clinical trial. Pediatrics 2001;108(5):1062–71.

[44] Mezaki T, Kaji R, Kohara N, et al. Development of general weakness in a patient with amyotrophic lateral sclerosis after focal botulinum toxin injection. Neurology 1996;46:845–6.

[45] Tuite PJ, Lang AE. Severe and prolonged dysphagia complicating botulinum toxin A injections for dysponia in Machado-Joseph disease. Neurology 1996;46:846.

[46] Brin MF. Botulinum toxin: chemistry, pharmacology, toxicity, and immunology. Muscle Nerve Suppl 1997;6:S146–68.

[47] Green P, Fahn S, Diamond B. Development of resistance to botulinum toxin type A in patients with torticollis. Mov Disor 1994;9:213–7.

[48] Sheppert AD, Spirou GA, Berrebi AS, et al. Three-dimensional reconstruction of immuno-labeled neuromuscular junctions in the human thyroarytenoid muscle. Laryngoscope 2003; 113(11):1973–6.

[49] Ford CN, Bless DM, Lowery JD. Indirect laryngoscopic approach for injection of botulinum toxin in spasmodic dysphonia. Otolaryngl Head Neck Surg 1990;103:752.

[50] Sulica L, Blitzer A, Brin MF, et al. Botulinum toxin management of adductor spasmodic dysphonia after failed recurrent laryngeal nerve section. Ann Otol Rhinol Laryngol 2003; 112(6):499–505.

[51] Blizter A, Brin MF, Fahn S. Botulinum toxin therapy for recurrent laryngeal nerve section failure for adductor laryngeal dystonia. Trans Am Laryngol Assoc 1989;110:206.

[52] Ludlow CL, Naunton RF, Fujita M, et al. Spasmodic dysphonia: botulinum toxin injection after recurrent laryngeal nerve surgery. Otol Head Neck Surg 1990;102:122.

[53] Ludlow CL, Naunton RF, Terada S, et al. Successful treatment of selected cases of abductor spasmodic dysphonia using botulinum toxin injection. Otolaryngol Head Neck Surg 1991; 104:840.

[54] Cannito MP. Perceptual analysis of spasmodic dysphonia before and after treatment. Arch Otolaryngol Head Neck Surg 2004;130(12):1393–9.

[55] Available at: http://www.cochrane.org/colloquia/abstracts/capetown/capetownPB30.html. Accessed July 1, 2005.

[56] Borodic GE, Ferrante R. Effects of repeated botulinum toxin injections on orbicularis oculi muscle. J Clin Neuro-Ophthalmol 1992;12:121–7.

[57] Ansved T, Odergren T, Brog K. Muscle fiber atrophy in leg muscles after botulinum toxin type A treatment of cervical dystonia. Neurology 1997;48:1440–2.

[58] Sanders DB, Massey EW, Buckley EG. Botulinum toxin for blepharospasm: single fiber EMG studies. Neurology 1986;36:544–7.

ELSEVIER
SAUNDERS

Otolaryngol Clin N Am
39 (2006) 101–109

OTOLARYNGOLOGIC
CLINICS
OF NORTH AMERICA

Treatment of Adductor Spasmodic Dysphonia with Selective Laryngeal Adductor Denervation and Reinnervation Surgery

Dinesh K. Chhetri, MD*, Gerald S. Berke, MD

*Division of Head and Neck Surgery, 62-132 CHS, Head and Neck Surgery,
UCLA Medical Center, 10833 Le Conte Avenue, Los Angeles, CA 90095, USA*

Spasmodic dysphonia (SD) is a voice disorder characterized by abnormal intermittent spasms of intralaryngeal muscles that result in voice breaks during speech. In the adductor variant of spasmodic dysphonia (ADSD), spasms of the adductor muscles cause strangled voice breaks and a strained-strangled voice quality. In the abductor variant (ABSD), spasms of the posterior cricoarytenoid muscle (PCA) cause breathy voice breaks and a breathy voice quality. Patients with SD typically have no other associated chronic medical problems or handicaps and are highly functioning individuals. The voice breaks lead to a significant difficulty in daily communication. Therefore individuals with SD perceive their voice significantly limits them functionally, physically, and emotionally. Successful treatment of vocal spasms thus leads to a dramatic improvement in the patient's perception of health and social functioning.

The ideal treatment for any disease is a single noninvasive therapy that results in a permanent cure without associated complications. Such ideal treatment does not exist for most medical disorders, and SD is no exception. One main hurdle toward achieving a cure for SD is that the cause and pathophysiology of SD remain unclear. There are no animal models for this disorder. What we know from laryngoscopic and electromyographic exams is that voice breaks in SD are associated with abnormal electrical activity of the laryngeal nerves, resulting in increased muscle movements [1]. SD is thus classified as a focal dystonia that affects the larynx. However, we do

---

* Corresponding author.
E-mail address: dchhetri@mednet.ucla.edu (D.K. Chhetri).

0030-6665/06/$ - see front matter
doi:10.1016/j.otc.2005.10.005 *oto.theclinics.com*

not know what triggers the onset of SD or how the abnormal neural activities in the recurrent laryngeal nerves (RLN) are generated. Chhetri and colleagues [2] performed a histochemical examination of the lateral cricoarytenoid muscle (LCA) and a morphologic analysis of the adductor branch of the recurrent laryngeal nerve in patients with ADSD and found no obvious neuromuscular abnormalities. Type-II fiber predominance was seen in muscle samples, but this could also be induced by the increased neural activity seen in the pathophysiology of ADSD. Therefore it is likely that the pathophysiologic changes in ADSD are at the level of the central nervous system, and the technological resolution to examine them is unavailable at present.

The voice breaks of ADSD can be understood biomechanically as a mismatch between laryngeal resistance and subglottic pressure, leading to cessation of airflow. The sudden, strong adduction of the vocal folds in ADSD dramatically increases laryngeal resistance that requires matching high subglottic pressure levels for uninterrupted phonation. The lung-thorax system is unable to instantaneously and smoothly generate the increased subglottic pressure required to overcome the sudden increase in laryngeal resistance, and phonatory break ensues until relaxation of the vocal folds leads to decreased resistance and the resumption of airflow. When airflow cessation is not complete but severely reduced, the strained vocal quality is produced.

Selective adductor denervation reinnervation surgery

This article focuses on the surgical management of ADSD by selective laryngeal adductor denervation and reinnervation (SLAD-R). All current treatments for ADSD are designed to reduce the intraglottic adductory force of the larynx. Chemodenervation of the thyroarytenoid (TA) muscles with botulinum toxin (botox) was initiated in the 1980s by Blitzer and colleagues [3] and is now considered the standard of care by many laryngologists. Although this therapy is effective, there are significant disadvantages, including the need for repeated injections, a period of undesirable breathiness after the injection, and the lack of uniform dose-response relationship with this medication. Many patients with ADSD are young and find it difficult to adjust to the potential for lifelong laryngeal injection therapy. However, before the introduction of botulinum toxin, SD was treated mostly with psychotherapy and speech therapy, which were ineffective for this condition. Although Dedo [4] had introduced unilateral recurrent laryngeal nerve section for this disorder in 1976, laryngologists did not embrace this technique because it creates an iatrogenic unilateral vocal cord paralysis and because of studies, for example, by Aronson and Desanto [5], that showed a symptom recurrence rate of up to 64% within 3 years. It was believed that the recurrence of symptoms was the result of a persistent abnormality in the untreated side and the regrowth of axons into the larynx from the cut nerve stump. Therefore, some otolaryngologists caution against surgery for SD that involves irreversible steps such as the division of the RLN or its branches [6].

SLAD-R surgery for ADSD was developed to avoid the failures of the Dedo operation. Several in vivo canine studies performed at the University of California Los Angeles in the late 1980s established the potential for long-term treatment of spasmodic dysphonia symptoms by selective adductor denervation and reinnervation. Green and Berke [7] measured the intra- and subglottic pressures as the RLN was stimulated from low to high, while keeping the superior laryngeal nerve (SLN) stimulation constant from low to high. They noted that RLN stimulation led to a linear increase in both pressures. Interestingly, SLN stimulation resulted in the attenuation of RLN effects on pressure. The RLN was thus established as the correct target for surgery. Bilateral laryngeal denervation was necessary to effectively treat abnormal signals coming to both vocal cords, and reinnervation was added to prevent the regrowth of axons back into the larynx. It was clear that the nerve section had to be performed distal to the PCA branches to avoid bilateral vocal cord paralysis. However, the effect of bilateral adductor denervation on laryngeal biomechanics was unclear. This was studied by Sercarz and colleagues [8] in a canine model, using photoglottography and electroglottography. After bilateral adductor denervation, high levels of subglottic pressure could not be generated even with high levels of RLN stimulation. More importantly, the geometry of glottic vibration was maintained. In the same study, the laryngeal vibration and vocal-fold histopathology were studied 4 months after surgery in two animals that underwent selective reinnervation of the distal TA nerve stump with the ansa cervicalis nerve and were compared with two animals that did not undergo reinnervation. Non-reinnervated vocal cords were characterized by asymmetric and aperiodic vibration. The vocal-fold bulk and tension were maintained in the reinnervated vocal folds. Thus, the importance of laryngeal reinnervation is to maintain glottal bulk and geometry as well as to prevent reinnervation of the laryngeal muscles by axons from the cut adductor nerve stump.

SLAD-R surgery initially targeted the TA muscle alone. As experience was gained with this operation and intralaryngeal microanatomy was further understood, the LCA branch was also routinely observed coming off the distal adductor branch. The LCA branch was then divided routinely. However, the LCA branch is too short and small for reinnervation, and therefore LCA myotomy was added in the late 1990s to prevent reinnervation of the LCA muscle from the proximal adductor nerve stump. LCA myotomy improved the long-term success of the procedure but also lengthened the period of breathiness after surgery. A few patients (usually male) developed permanent breathiness resulting from incomplete posterior commisure closure. Presently, partial LCA myotomy is performed, and no cases of severe or permanent breathiness have occurred with this modification in technique.

Preoperative evaluation for SLAD-R surgery

The most important consideration for the long-term success of SLAD-R surgery is that ADSD be accurately diagnosed preoperatively. There are no objective diagnostic tests for ADSD. However, experienced clinicians can diagnose it by its typical voice breaks during connected speech and by normal voice qualities during emotional vocalizations such as laughing, crying, and other instances. Botox therapy can be both diagnostic and therapeutic, and the authors often suggest that patients try botox and experience the "botox lifestyle" before surgery. Patients with concomitant tremor are advised that surgery may control the SD symptoms but not the tremor. The patient should be medically cleared by colleagues in internal medicine to undergo a 3-hour procedure under general anesthesia. The main reasons given by patients for seeking surgery are listed in Table 1.

Surgical technique

The operation proceeds in steps and is repeated on each side of the neck. An endotracheal tube that allows electromyographic monitoring of the recurrent laryngeal nerves (NIM-Response System, Medtronic Xomed, Inc., Jacksonville, FL) is used for intubation. The bed is turned 90° away from the anesthesiologist so that the surgeon can stand at the head of the bed as needed. A shoulder roll is placed to extend the neck. A 10-mg dose of dexamethasone and prophylactic antibiotics are given intravenously before the skin incision is made.

The skin incision is placed on a skin crease along the inferior border of the thyroid lamina. The incisions should extend bilaterally to the midpoint of the carotid triangle, which is bordered by the sternocleidomastoid and the omohyoid muscles, to obtain adequate exposure for identification of the ansa cervicalis nerves. Subplatysmal flaps are elevated superiorly, approximately to the hyoid bone and inferiorly just below the cricoid cartilage.

Table 1
Reasons for seeking surgery for ADSD

Reasons for seeking surgical intervention	Percentage of patients
Just wanted to cure SD for good	94
Ups and downs of botox	71
Prolonged voice difficulties after botox	52
Botox stopped working	32
Cost of botox	30
Swallowing difficulties after botox	16
Botox never worked	16
Difficulty with traveling to obtain botox	15

Identification of the ansa cervicalis nerves

The ansa cervicalis nerve is an excellent choice for use in laryngeal reinnervation because of its proximity to the larynx and because it is quite active during phonation. Its anatomy has been reviewed elsewhere [9]. It is a cervical motor nerve formed by the junction of two main nerve roots derived entirely from the ventral cervical rami and innervates the infrahyoid strap muscles. The superior (anterior) root is derived from C1, which joins the hypoglossal nerve for a short distance before branching off from this nerve at the level of the origin of the occipital artery, and descends on the lateral surface of the internal jugular vein. The inferior (posterior) root usually arises from the junction of two primary ventral cervical rami, most commonly C2 and C3, and travels posteriorly and deep to the internal jugular vein. A loop is formed at the point of anastomosis of the superior and inferior roots, usually on the lateral surface of the internal jugular vein.

The carotid artery and internal jugular vein lie immediately beneath the fascial tissue filling the carotid triangle. The fascial tissue is dissected in a superior-to-inferior manner and divided. Dissection proceeds until the internal jugular vein is identified. The superior root of the ansa cervicalis nerve can be identified typically at this time running along the lateral wall of the vein. Occasionally this branch is located more anteriorly under the anterior belly of the omohyoid muscle as it courses inferiorly. Retraction of the sternocleidomastoid muscle laterally and the omohyoid muscle medially often further exposes the ansa cervicalis. The ansa cervicalis nerve is exposed from the level of the superior border of the thyroid lamina and is followed distally until a length needed for easy rotation into the larynx is exposed. Dissection often proceeds under the omohyoid muscle to achieve this length. The nerve is then tagged for later use in reinnervation.

Laryngotomy

The strap muscles are divided in the midline from the hyoid bone to the cricoid cartilage. The thyrohyoid muscle is elevated from the thyroid ala using a freer elevator. The attachment of the thyrohyoid and sternothyroid muscles to the inferior border of the thyroid lamina is bovied with bipolar electrocautery and then divided sharply. Attention is given to preserve the external branch of the superior laryngeal nerve, which runs along the superior border of the cricothyroid muscle. When the oblique line is reached, its superior and inferior attachments to the thyroid lamina are divided. The posterior border of the thyroid lamina can then be palpated, and a single pronged hook is placed on the posterior lamina to rotate the larynx medially, thus fully exposing the thyroid lamina.

An inferiorly based rectangular, cartilaginous laryngotomy window is cut into the thyroid lamina (Fig. 1). A sagittal saw is used to make the cartilage cuts, although in younger patients this can be accomplished with a knife blade. The posterior cut is made just anterior to the inferior cornu. The

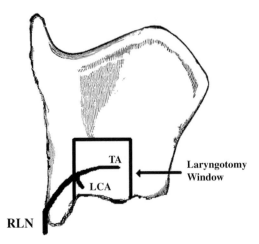

Fig. 1. Normal laryngeal anatomy showing the intralaryngeal course of the adductor branch of the recurrent laryngeal nerve and its relationship to the laryngotomy window.

superior cut is parallel to the inferior border of the thyroid lamina and is placed approximately halfway between the upper and the lower borders of the lamina. The anterior cut is made just anterior to the inferior thyroid tubercle. The cuts can be made through to the inner thyroid perichondrium but not deeper. The cartilaginous window is mobilized with an elevator and rotated inferiorly.

Adductor denervation and lateral cricoarytenoid muscle myotomy

The intralaryngeal portion of the operation is performed with microinstruments and magnification. The adductor branch runs typically in an oblique course from the posteroinferior corner of the window toward the midbelly of the TA muscle anterosuperiorly (see Fig. 1). Small blood vessels and adipose tissue often surround the nerve along its course to the muscle. Occasionally, the nerve lies deeper in the surgical bed, between the bellies of the TA and the LCA. A 3-0 silk suture is used to tie the nerve close to its insertion into the TA muscle. It is important to leave an adequate distal stump to allow unencumbered neural anastomosis to the ansa cervicalis nerve. The nerve is divided distal to the suture, and the nerve is retracted posteriorly with the suture and freed from its attachments all the way to the posterior border of the laryngotomy window. The branch to the LCA is seen typically during this maneuver and is divided. The suture is then threaded through a French-eye needle, and the nerve is sutured outside the larynx to the posterior lamina (Fig. 2). Partial LCA myotomy is then performed at the midbelly using microscissors. The present authors typically cut less than 50% of the thickness of the LCA muscle.

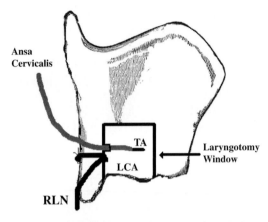

Fig. 2. Neural anatomy after selective adductor denervation and reinnervation. The adductor branches to the TA and the LCA are cut and exteriorized. The ansa cervicalis nerve is anastomosed to the distal adductor nerve stump.

Adductor reinnervation

The previously tagged ansa cervicalis nerve is cut distally, passed under the strap muscles, and brought to the laryngotomy window. The inferior root usually requires division for adequate rotation of the nerve. Typically, the nerve to the sternohyoid or sternothyroid is used. Epineurial anastomosis is performed using 8-0 nonabsorbable sutures between the ansa cervicalis and the distal stump of the adductor nerve branch (see Fig. 2). The laryngotomy window is replaced after a 2 × 2-mm piece of thyroid cartilage is removed from the posterior border to make an entryway for the ansa cervicalis nerve to enter the larynx. The skin incision is closed over a Penrose drain.

Postoperative course and surgical outcome

Intravenous dexamethasone and antibiotics are continued while the patient recovers in the surgical ward. The Penrose drain is removed the next day. Dysphagia is common during the first postoperative day, with most difficulty experienced with swallowing liquids. A dysphagic diet is given, and the patient is taught to thicken liquids as needed. Most patients' swallowing improves by postoperative day 2, and they are discharged on a medrol dose pack and antibiotics. The voice is typically breathy, similar to the voice after a large dose of bilateral TA injection.

The postoperative laryngoscopic examination should reveal normal abduction and nearly complete adduction at the vocal processes but a large midcord glottal gap. Breathiness lasts between 3 and 6 months, at which time the glottal closure is complete, and reinnervation presumably occurs. Further improvement in vocal strength occurs between 9 and 12 months.

The long-term results of SLAD-R have been very good. The initial surgical update on 21 patients was published in 1999 [10]. Nineteen of 21 patients had absent to mild voice breaks postoperatively. A recent long-term follow-up study of 81 patients at an average follow-up 49 months showed that 83% of the patients had significantly improved Vocal Handicap Index 10 scores, and 91% of patients indicated that their voice after surgery was more fluent than after botox therapy [11].

Patients who have suboptimal results after SLAD-R can be divided into two groups. The first group consists of patients with a recurrence of dystonia, a true failure of the operation. This has occurred in approximately 11% of the present authors' patients. When symptoms recur, they recur in approximately 12 months. These authors have not witnessed any recurrence of symptoms more than 24 months after surgery. Recurrent symptoms do respond to repeat botox injections. The second group consists of patients who have permanent breathiness, a complication of the operation. In the latest follow-up voice evaluation, the rate of moderate breathiness was approximately 14%, with approximately 6% of patients experiencing severe breathiness caused by vocal cord paresis. Severe breathiness appears to be related to the degree of LCA myotomy and resultant posterior glottal chink. Males seem to tolerate posterior glottal chinks much less than women. However, with conservative LCA myotomy, no cases of permanent vocal-fold paresis have occurred.

The voice after SLAD-R surgery is normal in over 75% of patients, with the rest having some degree of dysphonia [11]. The latter group includes some limitation in the upper and lower limits of pitch and loudness. Some patients continue to exhibit abnormal compensatory behaviors, although their voice is fluent. Professional singers will not be able to return to a singing career. To maintain long-term voice quality, excellent vocal hygiene and control of laryngopharyngeal reflux are mandatory. In the present authors' experience, the symptoms of ADSD are generally so disabling and disruptive to patients' daily communication that most find their fluent voice after surgery much more useful and preferable to the "roller coaster" ride with botulinum toxin therapy, despite the vocal limitations described above. SLAD-R is the only surgical treatment for ADSD with demonstrated long-term control of symptoms, and therefore it continues to play an important role in our management of ADSD.

Summary

SLAD-R is an alternative therapeutic modality in the treatment of ADSD. It provides long-lasting control of symptoms, and patient satisfaction is very high. The majority of patients achieve a fluent voice, with a range of breathiness from none to minimal. Patients should be counseled about the possibility of recurrent symptoms and permanent postoperative breathiness. The latter complication has been minimized by conservative LCA myotomy. A prospective study is underway to further understand this surgery.

References

[1] Hillel AD. The study of laryngeal muscle activity in normal human subjects and in patients with laryngeal dystonia using multiple fine-wire electromyography. Laryngoscope 2001; 111(Suppl 97):S1–47.

[2] Chhetri DK, Blumin JH, Vinters HV, et al. Histology of nerves and muscles in adductor spasmodic dysphonia. Ann Otol Rhinol Laryngol 2003;112(4):334–41.

[3] Blitzer A, Brin MF, Fahn S, et al. Botulinum toxin (BOTOX) for the treatment of "spastic dysphonia" as part of a trial of toxin injections for the treatment of other cranial dystonias. Laryngoscope 1986;96(11):1300–1.

[4] Dedo HH. Recurrent laryngeal nerve section for spastic dysphonia. Ann Otol Rhinol Laryngol 1976;85(4 Pt 1):451–9.

[5] Aronson AE, Desanto LW. Adductor spastic dysphonia: three years after recurrent laryngeal nerve resection. Laryngoscope 1983;93:1–8.

[6] Sulica L, Blitzer A, Brin MF, et al. Botulinum toxin management of adductor spasmodic dysphonia after failed recurrent laryngeal nerve section. Ann Otol Rhinol Laryngol 2003; 112(6):499–505.

[7] Green DC, Berke GS. An in vivo canine model for testing treatment effects in laryngeal hyperadduction disorders. Laryngoscope 1990;100(11):1229–35.

[8] Sercarz JA, Berke GS, Ming Y, Rothschiller J, et al. Biilateral thyroarytenoid denervation: a new treatment for laryngeal hyperadduction disorders studied in the canine. Otolaryngol Head Neck Surg 1992;107(5):657–68.

[9] Chhetri DK, Berke GS. Ansa cervicalis nerve: review of the topographic anatomy and morphology. Laryngoscope 1997;107(10):1366–72.

[10] Berke GS, Blackwell KE, Gerratt BR, et al. Selective laryngeal adductor denervation-reinnervation: a new surgical treatment for adductor spasmodic dysphonia. Ann Otol Rhinol Laryngol 1999;108(3):227–31.

[11] Chhetri DK, Mendelsohn BA, Berke GS. Long term follow-up results of selective adductor denervation reinnervation surgery for adductor spasmodic dysphonia. Presented at the 126th Annual Meeting of the American Laryngological Association (ALA). Boca Raton, FL, May 11–12, 2005 [abstract].

ELSEVIER
SAUNDERS

Otolaryngol Clin N Am
39 (2006) 111–133

OTOLARYNGOLOGIC
CLINICS
OF NORTH AMERICA

Office-Based Laryngeal Procedures

Peak Woo, MD, FACS

Department of Otolaryngology, Mount Sinai School of Medicine, The Grabscheid Voice Center, Mount Sinai Medical Center, 5 East 98th Street, Box 1653, First Floor, New York NY 10029-6574, USA

Office-based interventional laryngology for voice and swallow disorders will increase steadily. Some of the office-based procedures scarcely would have been done even 10 years ago; these include biopsies, injections, and lesion removals.

Why would office-based procedures be on the upswing when such procedures have been known and written about since the nineteenth century [1]? Some of the factors are related to economics, others are due to demographics, and still others are due to technology. This article outlines treatments that can be performed under local anesthesia in the general otolaryngologist's office. These procedures can be performed without a lot of expensive equipment and can be done with existing diagnostic equipment that is supplemented by a few simple instruments. This article gives details about the technique of office anesthesia, and the necessary office equipment and instruments. The procedures and their indications follow.

The major reason why office procedures will increase in popularity is based on patient acceptance. This is because an office-based procedure, when compared with a procedure that is performed under general anesthesia, is always deemed less invasive by patients and physicians. When given the option of an office-based laryngeal biopsy or a trip to the operating room, most patients will opt for a brief procedure under local anesthesia. This is especially true in elective surgery or procedures. Where voice enhancement for quality of life improvement is being discussed, an office procedure is accepted more readily than the same procedure that necessitates a trip to the operating room. The ability to offer the patient a safe and quality experience under local anesthesia increases the otolaryngologists' options for delivery of care [2].

E-mail address: peak.woo@mssm.edu

0030-6665/06/$ - see front matter © 2005 Elsevier Inc. All rights reserved.
doi:10.1016/j.otc.2005.11.008

A second reason why office procedures will increase is patient demographics. As the aging of America continues, it is anticipated that the elderly and their need for better voice and swallow function will parallel the disease processes that are due to aging and development. Increasing numbers of patients who come to the otolaryngologist with voice and swallow complaints that are due to laryngitis sicca, presbyphonia, Parkinson's disease, and nonspecific pharyngitis and laryngitis are elderly. Other disease processes that are limited to the larynx and result in voice loss that is related to aging and increased life span are acquired conditions, such as sulcus vocalis, intubation trauma, and phonotrauma. As patients demand better voice, the reply by the otolaryngologist that the patient's voice condition is a natural effect of aging will be not tolerated. The search by the patient for better function will drive additional procedures. Procedures that are safe, effective, and can be offered in an office environment will have an increasing role.

A third reason why office procedures will increase is economics. For most otolaryngologists who participate in health care insurance plans, the trip to the operating room for a laryngeal biopsy or laryngeal injection is laborious and is not compensated adequately. The office sits empty with its overhead while the physician must make the trip to the operating room, wait to do the procedure, wait for the induction and extubation, and check the patient after surgery before leaving. Often, preoperative, operative, and postoperative time that is involved in a procedure far exceeds the relative value units that are assigned by Health Care Finance Administration for endoscopy procedures. Even efficient operating rooms cannot compensate for the need for anesthesia induction and recovery time that often take longer than the operation itself. This means that the surgeon may take all day to do only a few cases with fixed codes that limit the amount of reimbursement. If the surgeon could use the office setting to do the procedures, and use other rooms for other patients while the patient is being anesthetized, this would be a more efficient use of time and resources.

As technology becomes ever more sophisticated, office delivery of drugs, lasers, and instrumentation will improve. Already, new laser fibers offer the clinician different laser wavelengths [3,4]. With different delivery systems, it is now possible to offer CO_2 laser, pulsed dye laser, and the Nd-YAG laser in a fiberoptic configuration that can be delivered through the channel of a therapeutic laryngoscope, bronchoscope, or esophagoscope. Sensory testing of the larynx is available in an office setting [5]. Brush biopsies that are obtained in the office can be scanned by supercomputers to evaluate all of the cells that were sampled by the surgeon [6]. The use of chips in a scope technology is superior enough that stroboscopy can be accomplished through a flexible laryngoscope. Such technology was not available until recently.

The reason that otolaryngologists give for not doing more office procedures is the false notion that excess time and technical expertise are required to master these procedures. These reasons will become moot with simple guidelines for training. With experience from practice, simple laryngeal procedures are done daily in our practice.

The history of office laryngology is replete with colorful characters and descriptions. In his seminal book on laryngology, Mackenzie [1] demonstrated many tools, sprays, and medicated treatments for office-based procedures. Even in one of the first textbooks on operative laryngoscopy, Brünnings [7] illustrated the role of operative laryngoscopy under local anesthesia. Jackson [8], in a textbook on laryngology and bronchoesophagology, illustrated many operative procedures under local anesthesia with a separate role for endoscopist and a role for the operator. A revisit of the procedures that were mastered so well by our predecessors is worth a review in light of today's technology.

Anesthesia

Selecting appropriate patients for office-based procedures should be mentioned first. Some insight by the patient as to the procedure being done is helpful. An informed consent that describes the local anesthesia process. It is helpful to describe to the patient what it will feel like to have local anesthesia of the larynx and pharynx. The loss of sensation may feel like difficulty with swallowing. The duration of the procedure and how it will feel afterward will help to allay the fears that surround the prospect of having instruments in the mouth and nose. At the end of the informed consent process, some patients will decline the procedure. It is better to err on the side of caution and not start the local procedure, than to expend a long period of time in an anxiety-ridden patient only to have the procedure fail because of patient reluctance to undergo the procedure. Thorough trust in the surgeon's ability will reduce the patient's fear. If the surgeon is confident, calm, and has good expectations for the patient to do well, it will set the tone for the procedure to go well. Topical anesthesia procedures for the upper airway have become popular because flexible endoscopy allows the endoscopist to perform routine investigations of the upper aerodigestive tract in the office without sedation [9].

The largest obstacle to doing an easy interventional laryngoscopy is the failure to obtain adequate local anesthesia of the larynx and pharynx. A well-done local anesthesia allows the surgeon to obtain reliable results with little variability. The duration of local anesthetic application is 15 minutes and cannot be hurried.

The local anesthetic is applied topically by spray into the oropharynx and the hypopharynx. A medical assistant may do the spraying process but the author insists on doing the direct topical application. An assistant physician also may do the local anesthesia, but he or she must be rigorous and consistent in his/her results. At the end of the process of applying local anesthesia, the expected result is a calm patient who can tolerate touching and manipulation of the vocal folds, larynx, and base of the tongue. If the procedure is to include subglottis visualization or tracheal manipulation, these areas also must be addressed systematically during the local anesthesia process.

The topical medication that is used may be 4% topical lidocaine or 2% Pontocaine (Cetacaine). Lidocaine's half-life is shorter than that of Cetacaine. The use of flavors or additives is to be avoided because it causes more coughs in some patients. Cocaine has some theoretic advantages in terms of secretion and vasoconstriction, but is not used because of fear of central excitation. For vasoconstriction of the nasal cavity, 25% neosynephrine spray is used. In some cases, a topical pledget in the nose to obtain adequate decongestion may be needed to pass the therapeutic scopes. Fig. 1 shows the typical local laryngotracheal anesthetic set-up. This consists of the air pump–powered directional spray, the cotton ball with carrier to paint the larynx with topical anesthesia, 4 × 4 cotton sponges, tongue blades, and tissues for the patient. Nasal speculum, kidney basin, and a medication cup are added occasionally. Cotton tip applicators or cottonoid strips are used if vasoconstriction of the nose is necessary. If the procedure is to involve the local injection of anesthesia, then 1% lidocaine with epinephrine is drawn up separately in a 27-gauge, 1.5-inch needle with a 5-mL syringe.

To get adequate anesthesia of the larynx by local application, divide the local anesthesia into three parts. First, spray the oropharynx with a 2-second spray of 2% Pontocaine with the nozzle directed posteriorly. Second, spray the larynx and hypopharynx with a 2-second spray of 2% Pontocaine with the nozzle directed inferiorly. Third, perform direct application of the larynx and the base of tongue with a cotton pledget or cotton ball.

The protocol for flexible endoscopic laryngotracheal anesthesia is as follows. Each nostril is sprayed with two 0.5-second sprays while the patient is asked to sniff quickly. Follow-up sniffs may be necessary to anesthetize the nasopharynx. Direct the nozzle of the spray straight while the tongue is depressed downward with the tongue depressor. Spray the oral cavity and each tonsil area. The patient is asked to hold his own tongue, roll the tongue down, and sit forward in a chin forward position. This trains the patient

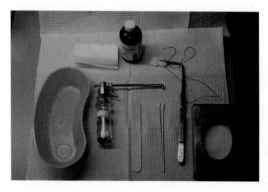

Fig. 1. Topical anesthesia tray.

to put his or her head and neck into an endoscopy position for rigid interventional endoscopy. The spray is directed downward 90°. When asking the patient to take a deep breath, the spray nebulizer is turned in a slow circle to spray the larynx and hypopharynx liberally. It is important to spray during inhalation. This is done twice. If the patient coughs, it must be repeated, because it means that no anesthesia was delivered to the larynx and trachea. The patient is observed for 10 minutes. If there is no further cough, the topical application continues by cotton ball application of the pharynx and the larynx.

The curved cannula with cotton is dipped in the topical 2% Pontocaine. The cotton ball should be 1.5 cm and have a slight tail so it will trail the anesthesia into the mucosal surfaces of the larynx and pharynx. The cotton ball will be used to paint each tonsil and the vallecula, and then is directed into each piriform sinus along the lateral border of the hypopharynx. This anesthetizes the lingual, glossopharyngeal, and the internal branch of the superior laryngeal nerve. It is difficult to direct the cannula into the depth of the piriform sinus to block the recurrent laryngeal nerve, and direct application of the laryngeal introitus is preferred. To do this, the refreshed cotton ball is held in the operator's right hand and the cotton ball is directed into the introitus of the larynx by 2 to 3 cm. Visualization is provided by the left hand holding the videolaryngoscope. Fig. 2 is an endoscopy view of the larynx being painted by the cotton swab. The rigid technique is performed with the patient holding the tongue while assuming the head forward, neck flexed, and head extended position. When the cotton ball is inserted deeply into the larynx, it will occlude the airway partially. The patient is instructed to cough with the cotton ball within the introitus of the larynx. This assures an even topical application to the entire supraglottic and glottic larynx. If additional anesthesia is required in the trachea for fiberoptic tracheoscopy or bronchoscopy, the therapeutic bronchoscope is placed deep into the trachea and

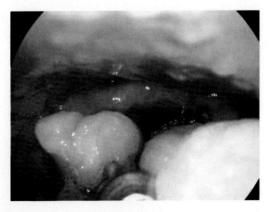

Fig. 2. Cottonball with potocaine used to swab the larynx.

additional anesthesia is instilled. Alternatively, transtracheal block may be used by cricotracheal puncture.

After 5 to 10 minutes, the patient should be ready for the local procedure. A test palpation of the larynx can be done using a blunt probe or the biopsy forceps. Tolerance to passive palpation should be confirmed before invasive procedures that may require suction, biopsy, or injection.

The total time that is necessary to anesthetize the larynx is approximately 15 minutes and cannot be rushed. Therefore, it is best to have blocked time for this when there are not other demands for the room. While the patient is undergoing the anesthetic process, the physician should be available for any complications. Smelling salts and the ability to lay the patient flat are helpful if the patient feels faint. Familiarity with the crash cart and the rudimentary basics of oxygen administration and CPR are advisable, but has not been necessary.

Using this protocol, one can expect good nasal, oral, oropharyngeal, and laryngeal anesthesia for most rigid and flexible interventional laryngeal procedures. Additional supplementation of anesthesia by nerve block or oral medication may be needed, but is not usual.

Equipment used for injection and office procedures

The physician can find many laryngeal instruments from many vendors (eg, fine scissors, directionally active cups, punch forceps). The basic instruments are needle injection of medications, punch forceps for biopsy, and alligator or cup forceps for holding brush biopsies. The basic set-up is shown in Fig. 3. The four basic instruments are needle injector gun, cotton ball holder, needles for injection, and biopsy forceps. There are variations in terms of disposable needles, their size, and holders; these depend on the personal preference of the operator and their availability.

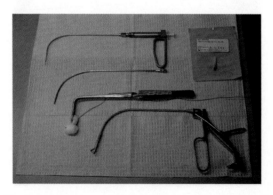

Fig. 3. Instruments used for laryngeal injection and biopsy.

Mitomycin injection, scar lysis, and laryngeal dilation

After open or endoscopic laryngeal surgery, scarring, synechia, and web formation may impede progress toward satisfactory outcome. One option for treatment is repeated trips to the operating room for granulation and scar management. Office-based procedures for granulation and web management offer an alternative. Several investigators showed that the application of mitomycin after wound creation can reduce the incidence of restenosis [10,11]. In selected cases, mitomycin can be applied to the wound as an office procedure. In patients who have early web formation, web lysis during the acute healing phase can break the synechia that is forming, and allow good healing without a web and a repeat trip to the operating room [12]. The author has used office-based scar lysis to good effect after surgery to maintain a sharp anterior commissure in patients who had laryngeal papilloma with bilateral vocal fold involvement.

Scar lysis and mitomycin application are done best using an office-based indirect rigid endoscopy technique. This is because direct pressure against the area of interest is necessary. When scar lysis is done for early anterior webs, a rigid blunt instrument, such as a curved biopsy forceps, is used. Telescopic endoscopy allows the surgeon to use one hand for the telescope with documentation and the other hand for the instrument or the pledget with mitomycin. Such an approach is difficult to do using flexible laryngoscopy.

Mitomycin is ordered from the pharmacy in a concentration of 0.4 mg/mL. Typically, 2 mL is adequate for each application. A cotton pledget with an attached string is used to apply the mitomycin directly to the raw surface. The pledget used is 1 cm × 2 cm and should be small enough not to occlude the airway, but large enough to cover the raw surface where topical mitomycin is desired.

The patient is prepared for topical application of mitomycin using laryngeal local anesthesia. One should pay particular attention to the direct application using the cotton ball deep into the throat, because total anesthesia of the sensory afferent of the larynx is necessary to do the procedure. Three minutes is a long time to hold a topical pledget against the mucosa, and only the most well-anesthetized larynges can tolerate topical applications of 3 minutes.

Scar lysis is far easier to perform than is mitomycin application. The indication for the procedure is early synechia formation at the anterior commissure after microlaryngeal surgery for bilateral vocal fold involvement with papilloma or after bilateral polypoid corditis surgery. Fig. 4 shows a patient who had anterior synechiae after laser surgery who was treated by scar lysis in the office. Two applications were done at 4-week intervals starting at 4 weeks after surgery. Fig. 5 shows a much improved anterior commissure. After laser cordectomy for T1B cancer of the larynx, anterior web may form. Lysis of the anterior web may be performed. After laryngeal stent

118   WOO

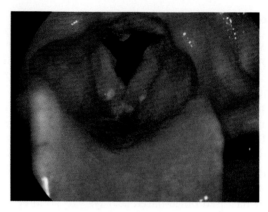

Fig. 4. Before office lysis of scar.

removal for laryngeal stenosis, residual granulation and web formation may be "touched up" by careful removal of granulation or by lysis of the granulation tissue.

To perform the scar lysis, the larynx is anesthetized by local spray. The patient may be given Valium, 5 or 10 mg, 1 hour before the procedure. After the larynx is anesthetized, the curved cannula is inserted into the larynx by endoscopic control. The blunt tip of the instrument is placed below the vocal folds and pushes against the inner, anterior border of the thyroid cartilage. With a firm anterior pressure of the blunt tip of the instrument against the patient's larynx, the instrument is pulled, firmly and steadily, out across the web. This action must be done quickly, but firmly, to break the web. A small amount of blood-tinged mucus will be expectorated. The area is inspected to see that the web has been lysed. A second application may be necessary.

The wound may be reinspected at 2 to 4 weeks and the procedure may be repeated if necessary. Repeated mitomycin application and repeated

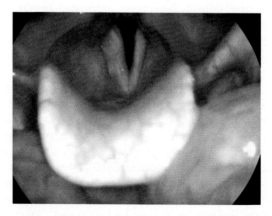

Fig. 5. Post scar lysis and mitomycin application.

laryngeal dilation may be necessary; this is performed at 3- or 4-week intervals. Repeat laryngeal endoscopy confirms if the larynx has healed enough to avoid a repeat procedure. Using this approach, scar and granuloma often can be treated without a return to the operating room. This protocol of examination and treatment is done until the area has epithelialized fully or the benefits of the dilation and lysis are exhausted.

After lysis of the synechia, mitomycin or steroid may be applied. Mitomycin is applied topically to the wound. It may not be possible to hold the pledget for the entire time; if so, several set interrupted applications are necessary. The total duration of application should be approximately 3 minutes. After the application is complete, the area is washed by nebulized saline or by wiping the site of mitomycin application with a cotton ball that has been soaked in saline.

Office-based injection laryngoplasty

Office-based injection laryngoplasty can be done by a transcervical or a transoral technique. A local injection technique gives great latitude to the surgeon who performs rehabilitation procedures for patients who have glottal incompetence. Even if the surgeon is adept at operative laryngoplasty, office-based injection laryngoplasty procedures give the laryngologist greater options in treatment. Laryngoplasty as an office procedure will transform the office from a diagnostic arena into a therapeutic arena. It is possible to consider office injection for the immediate relief of glottal incompetence. Ford and colleagues [13] initially championed the office injection of collagen for treatment of glottic insufficiency, and showed the ease which collagen can be placed into the medial edge of the vocal folds. The transcervical approach was described first as an alternative by Strasnick and colleagues [14], and has gained popularity.

Selection of patients for office injection should be individualized. A relative indication for office injection is the patient who is high risk for general anesthesia. Relative contraindications for office-based procedures are bleeding coagulopathy, a patient who has a high level of anxiety, and the professional voice user in whom precise injection is necessary.

The difference between transoral and transcervical injection is a matter of preference. The transcervical route uses less volume to fill the syringe and needle. In general, the transoral approach allows placement of the injectable to the edge of the vocal fold margin. The transoral route also allows the surgeon to inject multiple sites along the vocal margin; however, it is limited by the amount of material that can be injected. If a large volume needs to be injected in the lateral paraglottic space, the transcervical approach is preferred.

Trans-cervical approach may be done by way of a transthyroid cartilage injection, through the thyroid hyoid membrane, through cricothyroid membrane, or by the sub thyroid cartilage approach. The author prefers to insert the needle on the thyroid cartilage and inject the space just inferior to the thyroid cartilage on the side of the affected vocal cord. By staying just underneath the thyroid cartilage and aiming cephalad, the needle is placed at the level of the inferior lip of the vocal fold. Furthermore, by carefully avoiding entrance of the needle into lumen of the larynx, the injection of a greater volume may be able to be achieved.

The indirect trans-oral approach done by using a curved cannula. Usually a disposable needle such as available (Medtronic/Xomed; see Fig. 3), the needle can be used for finer particles, such as collagen or hydroxyapatite cement. Larger bore needle of 20 g or greater will be necessary for fat, micronized dermis or gel foam. A gun such as the Brunning syringe or its variation may be necessary. The trans-oral approach can further be divided into a one team or a two-team approach. The single team approach uses indirect laryngoscopy with a 70-degree telescope. A two-team approach uses flexible laryngoscopy with a mediastinal needle. By working off the television monitor, the endoscopist is responsible for visualization of larynx while the surgeon places the needle into position and performs the injection.

Materials that are available for augmentation depend on the viscoelastic properties. An ideal office injection of material should be made readily available product. It should have sufficient volume to permit injection by a transoral or transcervical approach. Current materials are saline or glycerin, collagen, micronized dermis, hydroxylapatite, and hyaluronic acid.

Micronized dermis (Cymetra Lifecell, Branchburg, New Jersey) is the particulated form of Alloderm. It is immunogenically inert and has been used in many other applications (eg, burns, reconstruction). Mixing 325 mg of micronized dermis with 1.5 mL of 1% lidocaine makes 2.0 mL of injectable material. The material should be mixed evenly to avoid clumping. It takes practice to achieve a smooth, thick, toothpaste-like consistency. It is important not to overdo the mixing because it may result in lower yields. The 3-mL syringe is coupled to a 19- or 20-gauge 1.5-inch needle for transcervical injection. A 19-gauge needle is used because the manufacturer does not recommend too fine a needle because it will disrupt the micronized particles and make it less stable. With the dilution as described, the material should flow smoothly through the syringe.

There continues to be controversy regarding whether the Alloderm implant is a temporary or a permanent implant. There is no doubt that initial experience with the injection showed absorption of 40% after the initial 3 months. In the author's experience, the permanent nature of the result probably is related to the amount of material that is injected. If only 0.5 mL to 0.8 mL of material is injected, the injection results in good correction to just across the midline; however, this is unlikely to be enough for all but the smallest of glottal gaps. Because the material is well tolerated by the patient who has little tissue reaction, the amount injected has increased steadily over the years; a typical injection volume for vocal fold paralysis is 1.4 mL to 1.8 mL. This amount of injection results in gross overcorrection with filling of the paraglottic space. Mandatory overinjection and avoidance of injection or extravasation of the Alloderm into the airway is necessary to avoid problems of undercorrection or absorption over time. The ability to inject more volume is the reason why transcervical injections have become preferred over transoral injections.

The site of vocal fold injection for micronized dermis is just deep to the vocal ligament. This area is different from the plane for Teflon injection, and is different for collagen injection for vocal fold scars as described by Ford and colleagues [13]. This "intermediate" zone of injection is aimed at bulking up the mass of the vocal fold lip. In addition, intermediate zone injection helps to correct the thin vocal fold lip that is characteristic of atrophied vocal folds. By re-establishing the thickness of the vocal folds, they will be able to oscillate with the upper and lower lip phase difference. This increases the closed phase of the vocal fold vibratory cycle and improves loudness. Direct subepithelial injection is performed in only limited cases (ie, vocal fold scar, sulcus, after partial laryngectomy). This is done best under anesthesia, because the reliability of placement into the superficial layer of the lamina propria cannot be certain using an office-based technique.

Indications for office-based injection laryngoplasty are the same as for operative injection laryngoplasty. The most common indication is the rehabilitation of acute vocal fold paralysis. Indications for injection laryngoplasty in non-recurrent laryngeal nerve paralytic dysphonias that result in glottal incompetence include physiologic sulcus, bowing and vocal atrophy, superior laryngeal paralysis, and scar.

To perform transcervical injection with fiberoptic monitoring, a two-team approach is necessary. The endoscopy team is responsible for the anesthesia and the exposure, whereas the surgeon determines the external landmarks and the needle placement. Both teams work off a high-quality TV monitor to verify completion of the procedure.

Indications for transcervical injection laryngoplasty are the same as for operative laryngoscopy or office-based laryngoscopy. Relative contraindications for injection laryngoplasty are posterior laryngeal gap or large interarytenoid defects. Some relative contraindications are patients who have poor pulmonary reserve. Injection is not indicated for severe scar tissue, because the site will not accept the intended soft tissue implant. The best indications are patients who have soft vocal folds with glottal incompetence. Because of airway concerns, injection laryngoplasty for patients who have bilateral paresis should be performed one side at a time. Bilateral injections for patients who have bowing and atrophy can be performed without concern for the airway. Patients who have nonparalytic dysphonia that may benefit from the injection laryngoplasty approach include those who have physiologic sulcus, bowing and atrophy, superior laryngeal nerve paresis, or small segmental scar. If the defect is in the membranous larynx and the tissue is supple, the injection will have a good chance of success. The size of the glottal defect also predicts whether the injection will be a success. Small midcourt

gaps that are smaller than 2 mm in size do better than do large glottal caps
that are irregular or have an associated posterior gap. When stroboscopy reveals an opened phase pattern, injection laryngoplasty has the ability to reduce the open-phase abnormality. Injections for patients who have bilateral
scar should be performed with caution, because office-based injections are
not precise enough to place the intended material exactly into the defect.
Unintended injection into sites that are pliable may cause a further deterioration in the voice.

Transcervical injection is done by a two-person approach. One person is
the endoscopist and the other is the operator. The procedure is done best
with the patient seated in the examination chair, and the surgeon and the
endoscopist work off a high-quality video monitor. The videoendoscope
with a distal chip technology are superior in image quality to a standard fiberoptic laryngoscope. The endoscopist passes the laryngoscope into the
nose contralateral to the affected side, and visualizes the vocal fold so
that the injection needle can be identified before entrance into the airway lumen. Premature entrance of the needle into the airway is not desirable, because it portends a high likelihood of leakage of the injectable material into
the airway. By keeping the tip of the endoscope just above the vocal fold, the
subglottis and the affected vocal fold can be seen.

After the endoscope has been positioned, the surgeon identifies the landmarks for injection by a mapping out the midline, the notch of the thyroid
cartilage, the inferior border of the thyroid cartilage, and the top of the cricoid cartilage. The neck is prepped and draped, and 1 mL of lidocaine 1%
with 1:100,000 epinephrine is injected into the skin and down to the thyroid
cartilage. The thyroid hyoid membrane is palpated; this palpation usually
can be verified on the endoscopy as a depression in the cricothyroid membrane. Furthermore, there should be some transillumination of the cricothyroid membrane by the light that is transmitted from the airway onto the
skin. Using the transilluminated light as a guide, the operator places his index finger onto the lower border of the thyroid cartilage. The needle is
pushed down onto the thyroid cartilage approximately 5 mm from the midline and 5 mm above the lower border of the thyroid cartilage. Fig. 6 is
a schematic of the injection trajectory. After solid cartilage is reached, the
needle is stepped down the thyroid cartilage until the inferior border of
the thyroid cartilage is reached. The needle is angled perpendicular to the
thyroid cartilage and slightly cephalad. After the inferior border of the thyroid cartilage is reached, the needle traverses this the cricothyroid membrane. The operator wiggles the needle gently and carefully advances it
while locating needle placement on the television monitor. For patients
who have soft cartilage, it is possible to traverse the cartilage directly.
This approach may be complicated by a cartilage plug that makes injection
difficult. By going below the inferior border of the thyroid cartilage, this
complication is avoided. When the needle placement has been a localized,
the needle is moved to a midmembranous portion and injection is begun.

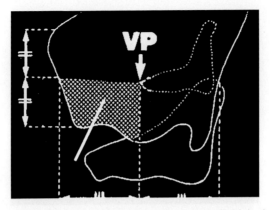

Fig. 6. Schematic of needle trajectory for transcervical injection.

Approximately 0.8 to 1.5 mL of minimized dermis is given. A good injection start by medializing the membranous vocal fold and followed by injection into the paraglottic space.

With experience, the author has determined that overinjection by 50% is necessary. The appearance of overinjection by expansion of the paraglottic space and false vocal fold seems to be necessary to have a good result. If the injection medializes only the membranous vocal fold, the effect is temporary. Fig. 7 is an endoscopic view of a patient who had a sizable left vocal fold gap that was treated by office-based injections. Fig. 8 is the view of the larynx 3 months after office-based injection.

With this much volume of injection, the patient may experience ear pain or transient stridor. After injection, the patient is observed in the waiting room for 20 minutes. The patient is cautioned about the possibility of transient stridor and postoperative pain. Cough and excessive phlegm or mucus keeps the patient in the recovery area until all local anesthesia is gone. If the

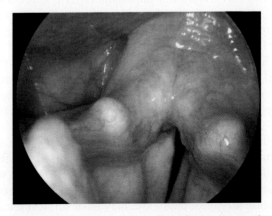

Fig. 7. Vocal fold paralysis before office injection laryngoplasty.

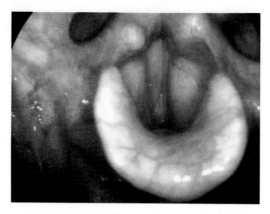

Fig. 8. Complete closure 6 months after office injection laryngoplasty.

airway was traversed inadvertently, a slight amount of blood-tinged mucus may be present. Rarely, paradoxical vocal fold breathing or laryngeal spasm may require a prolonged observation period. Reassurance, deep slow breathing, and rarely, oxygen, are used to treat laryngeal spasm or vocal fold dysfunction. Instruction is given to the patient and family to call if there is persistent stridor or shortness of breath after 24 hours.

Injection of cidofovir for papilloma management

Snoeck and colleagues popularized intralesional injection of the antiviral agent, cidofovir, as an adjunctive procedure in the management of laryngeal papilloma [15]. Bielamowicz and colleagues [16] reported good responses to intraoperative injections of cidofovir into the papilloma site. Response rates have been as high as 50%. Usually, the procedure is done for patients who have rapidly recurrent respiratory papilloma (RRP). Under the protocol of injection, the cidofovir is injected by monthly injections of cidofovir. The dosing and concentration have been variable. Some investigators reported using 4 mg/mL to oral communications from physicians of concentration used as high as 75 mg/mL. The procedures required repeated endoscopy under general anesthesia, with its inherent risks. In adults who are tolerant of laryngoscopy and who can give consent, office-based cidofovir may be a good option [17]. This can be given to the patient using serial injections.

The indications for injection are adult patients who have RRP that has a recurrence rate that results in significant symptoms at less than 1-year intervals. Other indications are patients who have RRP and in whom surgery may result in significant web and complications. Thus, a patient who has anterior commissure laryngeal papilloma may have surgical removal followed by serial injection.

The author prefers to perform the first injection under general anesthesia after gross disease debulking. This is followed by office-based serial injections of cidofovir. Injection without surgical debridement also is considered if there is a reasonable chance that adequate injections may be accomplished in the office. The sites at which good injection may be accomplished include the right and left true vocal folds, the superior surface of the vocal folds, the right and left false vocal folds, the aryepiglottic folds, and the petiole of the epiglottis. The areas that are difficult to gain access to include subglottic sites of laryngeal papilloma, deep in the ventricle and saccule of the larynx, and the interarytenoid area. Areas, such as the vocal process and the laryngeal surface of the epiglottis, also are challenging because there is not much soft tissue to hold the injectate without spillage.

Equipment for injection includes a 70° endoscope and an injector needle. Injector needles may be a reusable curved needle or a disposable injection cannula system. Cidofovir is dispensed in a 75 mg/mL concentration in 5-mL vials. The patient to has a stock bottle of 5 mL of cidofovir for injection. The usual sequence is three injections in 3 months, with approximately 75 mg of cidofovir injected at each setting. After trials in the office, the author uses a concentration of 20 mg/mL. The drug is prepared by drawing up 75 mg of cidofovir and diluting it one third to make a 20 mg/mL concentration of injectable solution. The amount that can be injected comfortably into the vocal folds is 0.5 mL into the right and left true vocal folds, 0.5 mL into the right and left false vocal folds, and 0.5 mL into the arytenoid mucosa and the aryepiglottic folds. Thus, the total amount is 3 mL of injection of 20 mg/mL injection. Using such volumes, airway distress that is due to large volume injection has not been a problem.

The injections may be tailored to the site of papilloma. For example, in patients in whom there is extensive involvement of the true and false cords, more is given to the true cords and the lateral ventricles than to the epiglottis; in patients in whom there is more involvement of the supraglottic larynx, more is injected in the supraglottic sites of involvement. For best results, one should work distally and then proximally. It is not necessary to be intralesional when the injection is given. More importantly, it seems that if there is adequate tissue diffusion and tissue elevation can be accomplished, the results will be better. Complications from injections have been minor. The author has not noted any side effects with kidney function. With the low dosing, prehydration has not been done. In some patients, the volume injected may result in mild inspiratory stridor for the first few minutes. Office observation is performed until the patient is stable. The patients are discharged with instructions to call if they have pain, stridor, or dysphagia. With doses that are greater than 20 mg/mL, pain at the injection site and prolonged hoarseness may be a side effect. These anecdotal experiences have kept the injection concentration at less than 20 mg/mL.

Office-based steroid injection

Office-based intralesional steroid injections give the otolaryngologist the added therapeutic option of intervening with the scar and healing process, without the need for general anesthesia. Corticosteroid injections are used in three main ways: reduce granulation tissue and promote primary healing, reduce hypertrophic scar formation and soften scar, and reduce acute inflammation and chronic inflammation before surgery. Steroid reduces the duration of inflammatory response after vocal fold surgery. Therefore, the granulation phase of healing is blunted. Steroid injection into local tissue has good effect for patients who have excessive granulation tissue response after surgery. This is the treatment of granulomas from contact or intubation. In cases of postoperative granuloma that is due to large secondary healing deficits, it also can be treated by removal of granulation and intralesional steroid injection.

The treatment of recurrent granuloma of the vocal process can be challenging. The granuloma often is recurrent after repeated removal. To improve the outcome, local steroid injections into the granuloma site reduces the inflammatory response that causes the patient to cough and perpetuate the granuloma formation. To perform the procedure in the office, the granuloma is injected with 40 mg/mL of Depo-Medrol around the lesion; this is followed by careful removal of the exophytic granulation tissue with a cup forceps. This procedure—combined with aggressive use of proton pump inhibitor and voice therapy—is effective for some patients who have recurrent granuloma. The reduced deep granuloma reaction allows the surface epithelium to heal and promotes wound closure.

Steroids may be used in the postoperative period to soften the scarred vocal fold. Increased vascularity, thicker vocal cords, and a reduced vibratory capability characterize the vocal fold scar. Much as we would treat any hypertrophic scar of the skin with steroid injections every 6 weeks, repeat injections of steroid in the office can be done to soften the stiff vocal fold margin.

To treat patients who have hypertrophic scar, it should be deemed that the vocal pathology is related directly to the excessive scar and thickening from the surgery. The patient may have reported initial improvements in the voice that were followed by worsening roughness and voice loss. Stroboscopy shows the patient to have a unilateral stiffness with hyperemia.

Injection is done best with a small needle. The Xomed Oral-Tracheal Injection Needle (Xomed-Medtronic, Jacksonville, Florida) is especially helpful, because the needle is small and disposable.

In selected patients in whom local inflammation and reaction is part of phonotrauma, preoperative management with local steroid injection can be used with good effect in two situations. The first is to avoid or delay the surgery. In a patient who has vocal fold edema or traumatic laryngitis, inflammation responds to steroid injection (eg, a singer who cannot go on voice rest). Fig. 9 is the endoscopic view of the vocal fold injection in a singer who has a left vocal fold fibrovascular lesion. Fig. 10 is the end result after the left vocal fold was injected with less than 0.1 mL of Depo-Medrol. The injection is placed into the superficial layer of the lamina propria and not deep to the vocal ligament. This is important to avoid vocal muscle atrophy. Local injection of steroid has a greater effect than does systemic steroid administration. Office injections may be used in lieu of systemic steroids to relieve persistent edema of the vocal folds. Fusiform polyps, acute hemorrhagic polyps, and polypoid corditis respond well to steroid injection. The treatment of fibrous polyps or cysts with steroid injection is less effective.

The method of injection is by curved cannula using indirect laryngoscopy, because the injection technique with a transbronchial needle uses a needle that is too thick for the vocal fold edge. Wastage of material in the long needle is unacceptable. Kenalog, 10 mg; Kenalog, 40 mg; Depo-Medrol (aqueous methylprednisolone, 40 mg/mL); or Depo-Medrol, 80 mg/mL may be used. Depo-Medrol, 40 mg/mL, has a longer duration than does Kenalog. Usually, 0.1 mL to 0.2 mL of Depo-Medrol is used per site. Fig. 10 is a videophotograph of a singer being given steroid injections in the vocal fold margin for small intracordal swelling and hemorrhage.

The site of injection also is important. Patients who have granuloma should have the area of the contact ulcer and the rim of the granuloma injected. This includes the arytenoid near the vocal process and the granuloma. For patients in whom vocal scar is being treated, the site of injection is the vocal ligament and in the flap of mucosa superficial to the vocal ligament. Care should be taken to keep the injection site superficial and to avoid deep intramuscular injections. Although deep intramuscular injections of small amounts of steroid probably are safe, muscle atrophy and bowing that are due to repeated injections is a concern. For patients who have vocal fold edge edema, polypoid corditis, or vocal fold nodules steroids should be

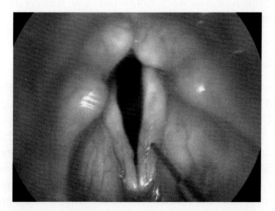

Fig. 9. Endoscopic view of injection into left vocal fold.

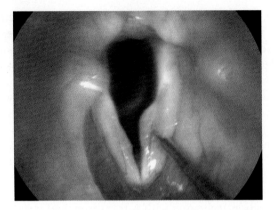

Fig. 10. Swelling of lamina after injection into left vocal fold.

injected in the superficial layer of the lamina propria. Going parallel to the vocal fold edge, depressing the mucosa laterally and dimpling the mucosa best enters the superficial layer. After the needle is in the mucosa, the needle is slipped deeper into the edge of the vocal fold margin. The steroid will disseminate along the length of the vocal fold parallel to the vocal ligament. Because the pocket that is defined by the lamina propria is limited, a small pumping action on the syringe is necessary so that a sudden bleb of material is not injected into the superficial lamina propria. If there is inadvertent overinjection, the vocal fold may be massaged with the closed tip of a cup forceps to even out the amount of material that was injected into the vocal fold.

Complications from the injection in the office are infrequent. Steroid injection may be repeated at 6- to 12-week intervals for the scar. Follow-up injections are dictated by the degree of scar improvement. It is unrealistic to expect the scarred vocal fold to be restored to full vibratory capability with normal mucosal wave. Comparison studies with serial stroboscopy should show improved vibratory amplitude and relative improvement in the pressure phonatory threshold.

Office brush biopsy and biopsy

Office brush biopsy of the larynx is not new. Surface exfoliative cytology has been used extensively. What is new is the sampling technique using transepithelial brush biopsy and the technique of the analysis. Laryngeal brush biopsy, using the endo-CDx system, differs from traditional surface exfoliative cytology in two ways. First, the brush biopsy is meant to obtain a transepithelial brush sampling down to the basal layer. This requires the operator to be vigorous in sampling the area by going back and forth until a small amount of blood is noted. This assures that a transepithelial biopsy has been sampled Fig. 11 shows the concept of a transepithelial biopsy

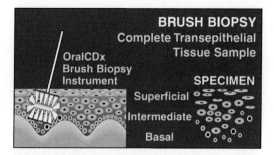

Fig. 11. Schematic of brush biopsy using transepithelial tissue sampling brush.

compared with surface cytology. Second, a sample is prepared for examination by traditional smear and by cellblock, using a proprietary computerized sampling technique that classifies each cell. The cells are read by a trained cytopathologist. Brush biopsies have been an excellent surveillance tool for the detection of premalignant and malignant lesions of the oral cavity. In the larynx, such an approach is used to follow, diagnose, and treat red and white lesions of uncertain behavior. Fig. 12 shows a brush biopsy specimen, and Fig. 13 shows the same specimen sampled by traditional operative laryngeal biopsy. The cells are well samples and are comparable with some absent tissue architecture. Nevertheless, the cells may be interpreted as normal, atypia or frank dysplasia, or carcinoma.

In the larynx, white or red lesions of the vocal fold and their surrounding structures are common. Repeated biopsies or excision may compromise the patient's voice if unwanted scarring follows the biopsy. These problems are

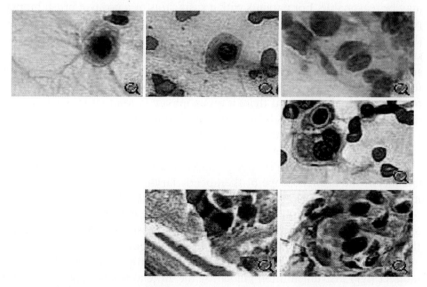

Fig. 12. Brush biopsy specimen of a patient with laryngeal cancer.

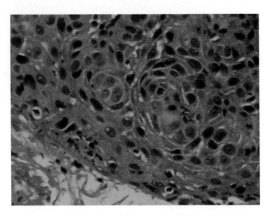

Fig. 13. Histology biopsy of same patient in Fig. 12. Note the similarity in cell type.

especially troublesome in preneoplastic lesions or lesions of uncertain behavior that arise from the membranous vocal folds. Repeated excisional biopsies for benign keratosis and mild reactive atypia may be avoided if these
lesions can be separated from the more aggressive lesions, such as intraepithelial neoplasia or invasive carcinoma.

Brush biopsy offers the advantage of an office-based sampling of tissue,
without the need for general anesthesia. The screening procedure of transepithelial biopsy may help the surgeon to decide whether to proceed with
a more formal biopsy. The positive and negative predictive value of a brush
biopsy of the larynx can help to guide therapy choice. For patients with
a negative brush biopsy, observation that is based on clinical grounds alone
may be reasonable. For patients with a suspicious or a positive brush biopsy
result, a full thickness biopsy is necessary. In a small series of 24 patients
that was collected at the author's institution in whom brush biopsy and
standard biopsies were done, positive predictive value of brush biopsy results compared to standard biopsy result was 87%. Brush biopsy is easier
to do than is standard cup force biopsy of the larynx. Cup forceps biopsies
of the vocal fold are easy if there is an exophytic lesion that is suggestive of
carcinoma. If the biopsy is being done on a red patch or a white patch of the
vocal fold, the lack of control using cup forceps through a fiberoptic endoscope makes biopsies through the endoscope undesirable.

The technique of brush biopsy is simple; the brush is passed through the
channel of the bronchoscope or therapeutic laryngoscope to obtain a specimen, much as a cup biopsy is done through a flexible bronchoscope. An al-
ternate method for brush biopsy is by rigid endoscope control. This uses an
alligator or cup forceps to hold the brush and brush the lesion, while using
the 70° rigid endoscope to control the brush placement.

Brush biopsy of the larynx may be done by fiberoptic laryngoscopy or by
indirect rigid instrumentation guided by the 70° endoscope. The rigid scope
is preferred because of the magnification and the possibility of palpation.

The rigid technique requires a cooperative patient who can hold his tongue and maintain a steady position. The flexible endoscopy technique requires an assistant to open and close the brush, and to twirl the brush against the lesion. In some areas, such as the petiole of the epiglottis and the area below the vocal fold, flexible endoscopy has an advantage.

Some technical details about performing the brush biopsy procedure will help the operator to get the best possible result.

The brush must be rotated or brushed vigorously in an up-and-down direction against the lesion. The end point is the finding of a small amount of red or pink material mixed with sputa. This assures the operator that the brush has traveled beyond the basal layer and has reached the small capillaries below the basement membrane. This reduces the possibility that "inadequate sampling" will appear on the brush biopsy report.

Avoid contamination by withdrawing the sample without touching other sites. The brush can be withdrawn safely after it has been retracted into the sheath.

Prepare the specimen by following the instructions for preparing the smear and cellblock according to the manufacturer's instructions.

Office-based laryngoscopy and biopsy and office-based laryngoscopy and removal of lesions

Office-based laryngoscopy and biopsy and office-based laryngoscopy and removal of lesions should be considered only if the benefits outweigh the risks. With the excellent operative and magnification instruments, office-based procedures are performed on only a small fraction of patients who are being considered for microlaryngoscopy and biopsy or excision.

This primary reason for considering office-based biopsy is the wish to avoid repeated general anesthesia. Not all lesions are amenable to office-based procedures. The following are suitable for consideration for office-based procedures.

Recurrent granuloma of the larynx. Exophytic granulomas of the larynx may be amenable to office-based removal and steroid injection, instead of repeated microlaryngoscopy.

Removal of polyps that are pedunculated, and can be excised with little risk of extension by mucosal stripping.

Removal of polypoid corditis to improve the airway for patients who have large polypoid corditis.

Biopsy of a malignant lesion before radiation or chemotherapy in a patient who is poor candidate for general anesthesia.

Biopsy of a malignant or benign lesion before definitive surgery, when the phonosurgery results from the biopsy are not a consideration.

Biopsy in the office is done with a minimum of instrumentation. Although a variety of instrumentation is available, the expense and the specialized nature of the instruments makes useful only in the most dedicated laryngologist's office. In the author's clinic, only the forward or straight grasping forceps or the cup forceps is necessary. A 3-mm round cup forceps serves a variety of purposes. The cup in the closed position is used as a blunt probe for palpation. The open cup forceps is used to apply topical anesthesia by way of the cotton ball. This same instrument is used to obtain biopsy, and remove exophytic lesions of the vocal fold. Although smaller biopsy instruments are available, often they are too small to be useful without stabilization. The cup forceps that are used are directionally changeable. This allows the surgeon to use the same instrument in the larynx by adjusting the direction of the cups for directed biopsy.

To do the laryngeal biopsy using the indirect technique, the operator instructs the patient to hold the tongue with his or her index finger and thumb. The operator holds the rigid laryngoscope in one hand and the curved biopsy forceps in the other hand. The surgeon may attach the rigid laryngoscope to a video camera and work off the video monitor. This approach allows the surgeon to be further away from the patient and allows for greater freedom with the operator's hand. The patient is asked to breathe quietly in a constant to-and-fro manner. Quiet breathing keeps the larynx from adducting and abducting in an unpredictable manner. As the patient breathes quietly, the surgeon puts the cup forceps onto the lesion. After the lesion is within the jaws of the forceps, removal of the lesion must be done rapidly and decisively. The motion necessary is a downward displacement that is followed quickly by an upward avulsion action. This rapid motion separates the lesion cleanly from the tissue below. If this is not done quickly, the patient will wince and cough, and unwanted tissue trauma may occur.

There is a temptation to take a biopsy that is too small, or sample just the surface of the lesion. If this is done, the remaining lesion will be difficult to remove. Invariably, bleeding becomes problematic as the operator tries to remove the remainder of the lesion. If the lesion appears vascular, the author does not perform the procedure in the office. A small amount of bleeding is expected; the patient is asked to expectorate the blood and sputum into a kidney basin repeatedly to avoid aspiration. After the expectoration is clear, the patient may be discharged. If bleeding does not stop, local pressure using a cotton pledget soaked in 1:10,000 epinephrine may be necessary. Surgical control of bleeding for simple biopsies is a possibility, but it has not been encountered.

Summary

Office-based procedures, such as biopsies, injection laryngoplasty, and cidofovir injections, give the laryngologist new options in the management of laryngeal lesions. Lysis of scar, management of vocal fold paralysis, treatment of granuloma, and biopsy of laryngeal cancer are some of the procedures that may be considered. These techniques represent a small sampling of possibilities that will become more common. New injectable materials and technologic advancements will become available. With the changing demographics of the U.S. population and the factors that favor healthcare cost containment, office-based procedures will become more popular.

References

[1] Mackenzie M. Diseases of the pharynx, larynx, and trachea. Wood's library of standard medical authors, vol. 77. New York: William Wood; 1880.
[2] Simpson CB, Amin MR. Office-based procedures for the voice. Ear Nose Throat J 2004; 83(7, Suppl 2):6–9.
[3] Zeitels SM, Franco RA, Dailey SH, et al. Office-based treatment of glottal dysplasia and papillomatosis with the 585-nm pulsed dye laser and local anesthesia. Ann Otol Rhinol Laryngol 2004;113(4):265–76.
[4] Devaiah AK, et al. Surgical utility of a new carbon dioxide laser fiber: functional and histological study. Laryngoscope 2005;115(8):1463–8.
[5] Aviv JE, et al. Laryngopharyngeal sensory deficits in patients with laryngopharyngeal reflux and dysphagia. Ann Otol Rhinol Laryngol 2000;109(11):1000–6.
[6] Svirsky JA, Burns JC, Carpenter WM, et al. Comparison of computer-assisted brush biopsy results with follow-up scalpel biopsy and histology. Gen Dent 2002;50:500.
[7] Brünnings W. Direct laryngoscopy, bronchoscopy and oesophagoscopy, vol. xiv. London: Bailliere, Tindall and Cox; 1912.
[8] Jackson C. Diseases and injuries of the larynx, a textbook for students and practitioners. 2nd edition. New York: Macmillan; 1942.
[9] Simpson CB, Amin MR, Postma GN. Topical anesthesia of the airway and esophagus. Ear Nose Throat J 2004;83 (7)(Suppl 2):2–5.
[10] Roh JL, Yoon YH. Prevention of anterior glottic stenosis after transoral microresection of glottic lesions involving the anterior commissure with mitomycin C. Laryngoscope 2005; 115(6):1055–9.
[11] Rahbar R, Shapshay SM, Healy GB. Mitomycin: effects on laryngeal and tracheal stenosis, benefits, and complications. Ann Otol Rhinol Laryngol 2001;110(1):1–6.
[12] Shapshay SM, et al. Endoscopic treatment of subglottic and tracheal stenosis by radial laser incision and dilation. Ann Otol Rhinol Laryngol 1987;96(6):661–4.
[13] Ford CN, Bless DM, Loftus JM. Role of injectable collagen in the treatment of glottic insufficiency: a study of 119 patients. Ann Otol Rhinol Laryngol 1992;101(3):237–47.
[14] Strasnick B, Berke GS, Ward PH. Transcutaneous Teflon injection for unilateral vocal cord paralysis: an update. Laryngoscope 1991;101(7 Pt 1):785–7.
[15] Snoeck R, et al. Treatment of severe laryngeal papillomatosis with intralesional injections of cidofovir. [(S)-1-(3-hydroxy-2-phosphonylmethoxypropyl)cytosine]. J Med Virol 1998;54(3): 219–25.
[16] Bielamowicz S, et al. Intralesional cidofovir therapy for laryngeal papilloma in an adult cohort. Laryngoscope 2002;112(4):696–9.
[17] Chhetri DK, et al. Office-based treatment of laryngeal papillomatosis with percutaneous injection of cidofovir. Otolaryngol Head Neck Surg 2002;126(6):642–8.

ELSEVIER
SAUNDERS

Otolaryngol Clin N Am
39 (2006) 135–158

OTOLARYNGOLOGIC
CLINICS
OF NORTH AMERICA

Contemporary Management of Laryngeal Papilloma in Adults and Children

Jennifer G. Andrus, MD[a],*,
Stanley M. Shapshay, MD, FACS[b]

[a]Department of Otolaryngology – Head & Neck Surgery, Boston Medical Center,
88 East Newton Street, Suite D-610, Boston, MA 02118, USA
[b]Department of Otolaryngology – Head & Neck Surgery Mount Sinai
School of Medicine, New York, NY

Occurring in children and adults, recurrent respiratory papillomatosis (RRP) is the most common neoplasm in humans. Although benign, malignant transformation of these human papillomavirus (HPV)-associated lesions is well documented, but rare. More commonly, RRP can be life threatening because of airway obstruction from growth and proliferation of the papilloma lesions.

RRP typically presents as hoarseness, although more advanced cases manifest with stridor and respiratory distress. The disease most commonly occurs on the true vocal folds. Treatment has focused on removal of obstructing lesions, with additional ablation of the root of the papilloma in hope of preventing regrowth. Since the popularization of the carbon dioxide (CO_2) laser for laryngeal surgery in the 1970s, repeated laser ablation has been the mainstay of therapy; some pediatric patients have undergone suspension microlaryngoscopy with laser treatment monthly or even more frequently. There is a high rate of recidivism because lesions regrow at the sites of ablation, and others develop in previously seemingly uninvolved areas. Thus, although some investigators have had limited success at keeping the lesions controlled through regular repeat surgeries, it is generally accepted that laser treatment, along with other surgical techniques (cold excision, use of a microdebrider), usually is not curative [1–9]. In the last 30 years, more attention has been directed toward adjuvant treatments, which range

* Corresponding author.
E-mail address: jennifer.andrus@bmc.org (J.G. Andrus).

0030-6665/06/$ - see front matter © 2005 Elsevier Inc. All rights reserved.
doi:10.1016/j.otc.2005.10.009   *oto.theclinics.com*

from systemic immune modulators to locally injected antivirals, in patients who have localized or disseminated disease. Successful long-term eradication of RRP lesions is unreliable, but there has been some improvement in reducing the number and frequency of procedures that require general anesthesia through the use of adjuvant treatments and in-office procedures.

Epidemiology

The true incidence and prevalence of RRP are unknown, most likely because of the lag between the onset of hoarseness or voice change and definitive diagnosis. In 1995, based on a survey of otolaryngologists in the United States, the Task Force on RRP reported a projected total of 3623 new cases and 9015 active cases of adult RRP, and a projected total of 2354 new cases and 5970 active cases of pediatric RRP [10]. Significantly more surgical procedures were performed on the pediatric population than on adults (16,597 versus 9284), at more than twice the cost ($109 million versus $42 million). The Task Force data were extrapolated to estimate an RRP prevalence of 4.3 per 100,000 children and 1.8 per 100,000 adults in the United States [10]. This was comparable to studies that were conducted in the state of Virginia (4 per 100,000 children and 1 per 100,000 adults) [10], and in Denmark (3.84 per 100,000 population) [11].

There are two clinically distinct forms of RRP: juvenile onset and adult onset [12]. Juvenile-onset RRP (JORRP) is diagnosed most commonly between 2 and 4 years of age [13] (1 day is the youngest documented age at diagnosis [10]); 75% of diagnoses are made before the fifth birthday [14]. JORRP is equally common in boys and girls who are younger than 12 years of age, and is generally more aggressive than adult-onset RRP (AORRP). Similarly, within the pediatric population, JORRP tends to be more aggressive the earlier it presents. Children who were diagnosed with RRP before the age of 3 years had 3.56 times the chance of undergoing more than four surgeries, and were at twice the risk for having more than two anatomic sites involved with lesions, when compared with children who were diagnosed with JORRP after 3 years of age [11]. AORRP is diagnosed most commonly between the ages of 20 and 40 years (84 years is the oldest documented age at diagnosis [10]), has a slight male predilection, and is overall less common than JORRP. Although the aggressive form of RRP is more common in children, it can occur in adults [12].

Human papillomavirus

With more than 90 subtypes identified, and after decades as the suspected etiology behind RRP, HPV-6 and -11 were confirmed as the causative agents for RRP in the 1990s using viral probes. The virus is a small, nonenveloped, icosohedral capsid virus that contains a 7900–base pair–long, double-stranded circular DNA. HPV enters cells at the basal layer of epithelium and elaborates RNA to produce viral proteins. HPV has been found consistently in the epithelium of papilloma lesions and adjacent normal appearing tissue; this explains the ability of the virus to cause recurrent disease, despite apparent surgical eradication of lesions. Viral subtype also seems to predict severity of disease; children who are infected with HPV-11 frequently have more aggressive airway obstruction and greater need for tracheotomy [15]. Forty-five percent of respondents to a 2002 survey of the American Society of Pediatric Otolaryngologists (ASPO) reported routinely obtaining HPV subtyping at initial biopsy [16]. This number may be high compared with the overall percentage of otolaryngologists who subtype for HPV when evaluating airway lesions that are suspicious for RRP, given the cost of subtyping. A better understanding of the epidemiology and relationship of HPV subtype to disease severity would result from routine HPV subtyping; however, the direct benefit to individual patients has not been established.

Risk factors

HPV-6 and -11 also are the most common subtypes in cervical condylomata acuminata, and multiple investigators noted an association between mothers who had genital HPV infection and the incidence of RRP [17–21]. In different series, from 50% to 70% of patients who had JORRP were born to mothers who had genital warts during pregnancy or childbirth. Kashima and colleagues [22] found that 72% of 26 patients who had JORRP versus 36% of 33 patients who had AORRP had the clinical triad of: (1) being the firstborn, (2) being delivered vaginally, and (3) being born to a teenaged mother; this triad has been observed by other investigators. Patients who had AORRP also were more likely than controls to have more lifetime sexual partners and a higher frequency of oral sex. The presence of HPV in the genital tract of women of child-bearing age is believed to be at least 25% worldwide; clinical infection of pregnant women in the United States is between 1.5% and 5% [10,14,23,24]. These data predict a much higher incidence of RRP than that which has been found. Shah and colleagues [23] estimated that only 1 in 400 children who are born to mothers who have active condylomata contracts RRP. HLA class I and II genotyping on 56 white and 14 black patients who had RRP showed an increased frequency of HLA-DRB1*0102 in white patients; this suggested that this allele predisposes patients to RRP [25]. In the same study, other HLA alleles were enriched in the patients who had RRP, which suggested their possible role in determining disease severity. Other risk factors, which have yet to be elucidated, must account for an individual's susceptibility to RRP. Finally, although the numbers are small, RRP has been identified in children and adults who have HIV or congenital immunodeficiencies, or who are medically immunosuppressed after organ transplantation [10]. These risk factors may be anecdotal; however, they could be important in elucidating the pathophysiology of RRP because the host–immune response obviously is decreased in these cases.

Clinical presentation and evaluation

Because of the variable aggressiveness of RRP, as well as the diverse number of airway sites that can be involved, patients present with a range of symptoms and physical examination findings. Subtle voice changes over long periods of time may go unnoticed by many adult patients, and never progress to frank hoarseness, dysphonia, or dyspnea. Children who have RRP may be misdiagnosed. They often present with symptoms of hoarseness, stridor, and respiratory distress after diagnosis and treatment of recurrent croup, worsening asthma, or severe bronchitis have been unsuccessful. RRP should be considered in any patient of any age who presents with hoarseness, voice change, and shortness of breath, and especially in young children who have feeding difficulties, failure to thrive, recurrent pneumonia, or dysphagia. Careful history taking can help "place" RRP in a differential diagnosis for other laryngeal lesions. Slowly progressive hoarseness without risk factors for other airway lesions, especially in patients who have parental histories of genital condylomata, should raise suspicion for RRP [12].

Contemporary evaluation of patients begins with physical examination, with the utmost attention being paid to general appearance and the overall integrity of the patient's airway. If the patient's airway is stable, the examination should include flexible nasopharyngolaryngoscopy or rigid videostroboscopy to define, if any, the nature, extent, and severity of airway pathology. This will be achievable in most patients, with some challenge posed by young, school-aged children ($\sim$4–9 years old) who may require general anesthesia and direct laryngoscopy for laryngeal evaluation. Conversely, patients who have noisy breathing (stridor), who appear anxious or air hungry, with or without the use of accessory breathing muscles, require immediate attention in a "safe" setting where support staff and airway equipment are available. Most often, this is an operating room setting with a full complement of laryngoscopes, bronchoscopes, endotracheal tubes, a tracheotomy set, and a team of anesthesiologists, nurses, and operating room staff that is familiar with complex airway cases. In the hospital setting, an acute airway may need to be evaluated in the ICU setting, in which case the aforementioned equipment and personnel should be available.

Diagnosis

Generally, the diagnosis of RRP is a clinical one that is based on the gross appearance of the airway lesions, and is confirmed by histopathology. Lesions of the anterior nasal passages, oral cavity, and oropharynx can be seen readily on examination. Indirect mirror laryngoscopy can be used to identify supraglottic and glottic lesions, but clinicians rely heavily on flexible nasopharyngolaryngoscopy for identification and description of most lesions. Most patients who have an upper airway lesion require suspension microlaryngoscopy under general anesthesia to evaluate fully the extent of the lesion and obtain a biopsy; however, select adult patients may tolerate biopsy in the office setting with local anesthesia.

RRP has a predilection for anatomic sites that are junctions between squamous and ciliated epithelium, and thus, follow a predictable pattern of distribution. The growth pattern of papillomas, the recurrence rate, and the remission rate, however, are unpredictable. In general, papillomas occur most commonly on the limen vestibuli, the nasopharyngeal surface of the soft palate, the midzone of the laryngeal surface of the epiglottis, the upper and lower margins of the ventricle, the under surface of the vocal folds, the carina, and at bronchial spurs [12,26]. Grossly, papillomas are pink or white, sessile or exophytic lesions, pedunculated or broad based, with small, frondlike projections (Fig. 1). Multiple clusters of papilloma can be seen at one or more sites in the airway; RRP also can manifest as a carpet of papillomatous epithelium over a wide distribution (Fig. 2). Under magnification, as in suspension microlaryngoscopy, punctate vasculature is evident over the surface of papillomas. Histologically, RRP is composed of multiple fingerlike projections of nonkeratinized stratified squamous epithelium overlying a vascularized core of connective tissue stroma (Fig. 3) [12,14]. The basal epithelium can be normal to hyperplastic, and cellular differentiation can be normal or abnormal with variable expression and production of keratins [14]. Generally, mitotic figures are limited to the basal layer. Lesions rarely undergo malignant degeneration; however, the papilloma virus is oncogenic and varying degrees of atypia are common.

Treatment

The goal of treating RRP is to remove as much disease as possible to improve or maintain respiratory function, while preserving laryngeal function.

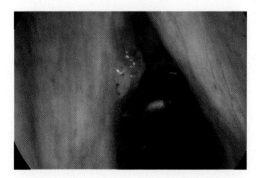

Fig. 1. Isolated papilloma of the left anterior true vocal fold.

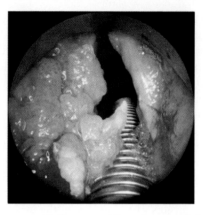

Fig. 2. Diffuse papillomatous epithelium over bilateral true and false vocal folds and left ventricle.

This is particularly important in approaching RRP of the glottis and subglottis, because overaggressive ablation of disease can result in severe scarring. Historically, the mainstay of RRP treatment has been primary resection of lesions under general anesthesia. Some patients who have mild to moderately aggressive disease are treated adequately with only a few procedures; however, many pediatric patients require multiple procedures in their lifetime, often on the order of 8 to 12 per year. With the risk of general anesthesia, most clinicians work closely with patients to maximize the time between procedures, using either respiratory or phonatory compromise as a barometer by which to gauge the timing of procedures. In recent years, with the development of other

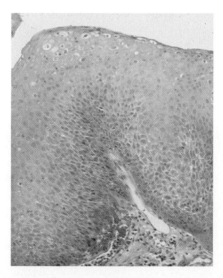

Fig. 3. Central fibrovascular core with overlying fingerlike projection of nonkeratinized stratified squamous epithelium (hematoxylin-eosin preparation).

primary and adjuvant treatments, many laryngologists are treating their adult patients at shorter intervals in the office under local anesthesia, and thus avoiding frequent general anesthetics.

Treatment modalities available to the modern otolaryngologist and discussed below include: cold excision, CO_2 laser ablation, pulsed dye laser (PDL) ablation, cidofovir, α-interferon, indole-3-carbinol (I3C), and photodynamic therapy (PDT).

Primary treatment modalities

Techniques of RRP surgical resection have evolved remarkably in the last 30 years. Likewise, as new modalities have emerged, otolaryngologists' preferences for, and use of, various options have changed; however, no mode of primary treatment for RRP has been able to eradicate the disease. Thus, even with the use of combined techniques, patients generally undergo multiple procedures to control disease, because a cure has not been found. RRP has proven to be a chronic disease.

Cold excision and carbon dioxide laser ablation

Before the 1970s and the implementation of the CO_2 laser, cold excision of papillomas to debulk disease was the mainstay of treatment. Phonomicrosurgical techniques that place more emphasis on preservation of normal tissue are used today, and have been enhanced by the development of microflap and subepithelial injection techniques, and by the use of larger binocular laryngoscopes. Generally, these techniques are best applied to localized, minor disease and are not indicated for diffuse laryngeal disease.

The development of the CO_2 laser in the 1970s was an important milestone for the treatment of RRP. Used with suspension microlaryngoscopy, the CO_2 laser permits precise ablation of lesions and excellent hemostasis. With a wavelength of 10,600 nm, the CO_2 laser converts light into thermal energy, and targets water in treated tissues, which results in tissue destruction by vaporization. The laser can be used in a defocused mode to debulk massive RRP, and then switched to a focused spot size to ablate residual RRP in areas in which minimal damage to laryngeal structures is desired (ie, the phonatory producing areas, the commissures, and the subglottis) [12]. CO_2 laser operative technique is described at length in the literature [12,14,27]. A particularly effective technique for the laser removal of sessile papillomatous growth has been our "laser brush technique." The laser is used at the lowest wattage setting to permit vaporization of tissue, usually 2 to 3 W. The time exposure is 1 second and the spot size diameter is 300 μm (0.3 mm). The laser is applied in "brush strokes" in an anterior to posterior direction to the broad surface of the papillomas, which causes some superficial vaporization and carbonization of the surface. The depth of penetration is superficial. The carbonization is removed with open microsuctions or with the use of a small, saline-soaked neurosurgical patty ("the brush") and suction. Under the operating microscope at 16× magnification, the depth of removal can be detected easily. The laser is used in brush strokes to remove the next layer of papillomas in a similar manner until the uninvolved submucosa is identified. Because papillomas only involve the mucosa, this layered approach with microhemostasis from the laser and occasional use of topical adrenaline is effective and safe. In 1995, the Task Force on RRP reported that 92% of respondents to their survey preferred the CO_2 laser for initial treatment of RRP; the remaining 8% favored suspension microlaryngoscopy with cold excision [10].

Despite the excellent results that are obtained with the CO_2 laser, its drawbacks are significant. Inappropriate choice of power settings and time exposure or overaggressive use of the laser can result in thermal damage to tissues that are deep or adjacent to the papilloma. Consequences in the endolarynx can be severe, and include acute and chronic glottic edema with airway compromise, vocal fold scarring, and poor voice [12]. Damage to surrounding normal airway tissue also increases its susceptibility to viral particle implantation and subsequent mucosal seeding of RRP [12,26]. In order to balance the goals of obtaining adequate control of disease and minimizing tissue damage and scarring, many surgeons resort to performing frequent procedures on their patients. With this practice come the attendant risks of general anesthesia, and with operating theatre expenses, add to the overall high cost of caring for RRP patients.

585-nm Pulsed dye laser therapy

With concern for the significant cumulative risk of soft tissue complications from CO_2 laser ablation that patients who have RRP often face, in 1994, McMillan and colleagues [28] proposed 585-nm PDL treatment as a minimally traumatic alternative. Subsequent in vivo studies using a canine model demonstrated that PDL irradiation of normal laryngeal tissue produced vascular destruction without acute or delayed disruption of epithelium, laryngeal atrophy, or fibrosis [28,29]. Based on reports that PDL may cause regression of HPV-induced cutaneous lesions, and the safety of PDL in canine larynges, a pilot study was launched in patients who had RRP [30]; complete regression of lesions was demonstrated within 1 month of treatment without adverse consequences. Other studies have shown the PDL to be useful in minimizing RRP burden without the scarring that is associated with CO_2 laser ablation [31,32]. This advantage is attributed to the unique wavelength of the PDL, which causes photoablation of vasculature that nourishes the papillomata, with minimal thermal conductivity into surrounding tissues. The chromophore for the PDL is oxyhemoglobin in erythrocytes, which is targeted selectively during treatment, and, on irradiation, extravasates from the supporting vasculature into the papilloma stroma. This results in a dark purpura that is apparent during treatment, and is used as a treatment end point (Fig. 4). The oxyhemoglobin targeting is selective, and water is not vaporized as in treatment with CO_2 laser. Thus,

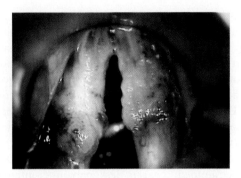

Fig. 4. Appearance of glottic papilloma after treatment with 585-nm PDL laser. Note the dark purpura which results from the extravasation of oxyhemoglobin from the fibrovascular core into the papilloma stroma.

the surface mucosa is preserved during PDL treatment; this prevents the development of raw surfaces that are vulnerable to metaplasia, scarring, and implantation of viral particles. If the PDL is used at higher power settings, there can be thermal damage to the surrounding tissues. The laser should be used at power settings that cause photovasculature ablation and not tissue destruction or vaporization. Franco and colleagues [32] used a Photogenica V 585-nm PDL (Cynosure Inc., Chelmsford, Massachusetts) at 450-μs pulse width, 5 J per pulse maximum output of 1 Hz, 1-mm fiber, 1- to 2-mm spot size, and 38 to 255 J/cm^2 fluence. We reported results using a Model SPTL-1A 585-nm PDL (Candela Corporation, Wayland, Massachusetts) at 300- to 500-μs pulse width, 1-mm fiber with 2.7-mm spot size or 600-μm silica fiber in a flexible nasolaryngoscope with 3-mm spot size, and 6 to 10 J/cm^2 fluences with one to five pulses per area treated [31]. The higher fluence of energy destroys the papilloma using thermal energy beyond the wavelength-selective approach on blood vessels. The surgeon needs to take care to limit thermal effects to avoid collateral tissue damage.

One drawback to PDL is that it is not effective on large, bulky lesions; best results have been seen on sessile lesions [31,32]. This implies that large lesions may be treated best initially with the CO_2 laser, cold excision, or microdebrider, before the base or anterior commissure is treated with PDL. This also implies that more frequent follow-up procedures may be necessary to control RRP with PDL; however, because it can be used under local anesthesia in an outpatient setting, the cost savings and anesthesia risk reduction are significant. The authors predict that PDL will be used more frequently in the outpatient setting, and possibly supplant CO_2 laser ablation as the primary mode for follow-up surgical management of adult patients who have RRP.

Microdebridement

In 1999, Myer and colleagues [33] reported the first experience with a laryngeal microresector system for treating RRP. Powered instrumentation for sinus surgery was adapted for use in the larynx (Xomed, Inc., Jackson-ville, Florida), and has evolved in the last 5 years to include longer, thinner, angled oscillating blades that incorporate suction and irrigation. This allows surgeons to resect papillomas with one hand, while manipulating lesions as needed with the other hand under suspension microlaryngoscopy. Other in-vestigators use the microdebrider and a hand-held telescope connected to a video monitor. By 2004, 53% of APSO member responders to a web-based survey on RRP management preferred the microdebrider for surgical re-moval of lesions (versus 42% who preferred the CO_2 laser) [16]. Proponents of the microdebrider cite several advantages over the CO_2 laser, including a less expensive equipment charge, less personnel-intensive, no thermal trauma, and less risk to operating room staff (ie, no exposure to laser plume, nor risk of ocular injury) [33]. There also is no risk of airway fire, which is ever present when using the CO_2 laser. In a retrospective review of 18 pa-tients who were younger than of 18 years of age who were treated at two institutions with CO_2 laser and microdebrider techniques, Patel and col-leagues [34] reported a significantly shorter operative time for the microde-brider (mean times 32.4 minutes versus 59.2 minutes). The microdebrider seems to be particularly effective for bulky exophytic disease; however, the device should be used with caution for the sessile growth pattern of papillo-mas. There is some danger of extending the depth of resection deep into the submucosa or muscle, and causing scarring and loss of phonatory function. In addition, there is no hemostasis with use of the debrider, which impairs visualization of the depth of resection.

Adjuvant treatments

Although surgery remains the mainstay of treatment for RRP, adjuvant treatments have an important place in patient management. Between 2001 and 2004, the reported use of adjuvant treatments in pediatric patients increased from 10% to 22% [14,16]. Clinical guidelines for instituting adjuvant therapy have not been developed; however, the most common criteria in the literature are patients who require more than four surgical procedures in 1 year, spread of disease to multiple distal sites, or rapid regrowth of lesions with airway compromise [14,16]. The most common adjuvant therapy was systemic α-interferon [14], until the emergence and adoption of intralesional cidofovir [16]. Other therapies that are used in ad-dition to surgery, and under study, are I3C and PDT. Acyclovir, isotreti-noin, methotrexate, and ribavirin have been used, but are not used widely today. Heat shock protein (Hsp) E7 is a novel adjuvant that showed prom-ising results in a phase II trial, and warranted a confirmatory phase III trial.

Cidofovir

Cidofovir [(S)-1-(3-hydroxy-2-phosphonylmethoxypropyl)cytosine] is a nucleoside analog (Gilead Sciences, Inc., Foster City, California) that is approved by the U.S. Food and Drug Administration for intravenous use to treat cytomegalovirus retinitis in patients who have AIDS [35]. Although not approved for topical or intralesional use, cidofovir has been used to treat several cutaneous and mucosal viral lesions [2–5,7–9,11–13,35–37]. The first report of successful intralesional use of cidofovir for RRP was by Van Cutsem and colleagues [7] in 1995. The investigators successfully treated a 69-year-old patient's hypopharyngeal and esophageal papillomas through direct injection of cidofovir into the papillomas. Three years later, in 1998, Snoeck and colleagues [2] reported the successful treatment of 16 of 17 patients who had severe laryngeal papillomatosis by intralesional injection of cidofovir in various volumes of 2.5 mg/mL at 2-week intervals. Following this report, in 1998 the authors began the use of cidofovir for recurrent respiratory papillomatosis through intralesional injections of the medication diluted to 2.5 mg/mL as reported by Snoeck and colleagues [2]. Our observed success was largely good, but not in all patients. Other surgeons were having the same clinical results, because reports began to emerge of combining cidofovir with other treatments, and of increasing the concentration of cidofovir in the injection. Cidofovir comes from the manufacturer at a concentration of 75 mg/mL; however, physicians typically have reported significant dilutions of the medication before intralesional injection. Following the literature, the authors have doubled the concentration of cidofovir that they use to 5.0 mg/mL, although other surgeons have begun to use higher concentrations (7.5–10 mg/mL). Co and Woo [38] reported their initial experience with serial office-based intralesional injections of cidofovir in awake patients using concentrations of 7.5 mg/mL concentrations. Woo now routinely uses concentrations of 20 mg/mL (personal communication, 2005).

The potential for renal toxicity of systemic (intravenous) cidofovir has been well documented [39], and Bienvenu and colleagues [36] reported a case of acute renal failure that was induced by topical cidofovir. Few prospective studies have been conducted on the local toxicity of intralaryngeal cidofovir [40]. Chhetri and colleagues [40] published the first report on local effects of intralaryngeal cidofovir injection in a canine model. The study found dose-dependent injury to the vocalis muscle after 12 injections at 2-week intervals. Endomysial edema resolved in the groups that received low dosages (0 and 2.5 mg), it resolved partially in the groups that received intermediate dosages (5 and 10 mg) with superficial residual damage; permanent, full-thickness necrosis, atrophy, and fibrosis was found in the groups that received high dosages (20 and 37.5 mg), after an additional 6-month observation period. Spiegel and colleagues [41] reported the first evaluation of the local effects of cidofovir injection on cartilage using a rabbit model. After evaluating the gross and histologic effects of local perichondrial injection of cidofovir into 96 1-cm^2 sections of rabbit auricles (24 each of 0 mg/mL, 5 mg/mL, 25 mg/mL, and undiluted 75 mg/mL), they concluded that delayed skin changes or histopathologic change in the cartilage may be expected at approximately one third of sites injected. Although there was a statistical likelihood for increased local change after cidofovir injection, there was no correlation of severity with injected dose.

Cidofovir has come to the forefront of adjuvant treatments for RRP in the last 10 years. Direct intralesional injection of cidofovir has found increasingly widespread use as a primary treatment for RRP in children and adults [2–8]. Multiple investigators have shown that cidofovir for RRP markedly decreases the frequency and severity of local disease recurrence. Ideally, the medication would work in a single setting to eliminate papillomatous lesions; however, clinical experience suggests that repeated injections are necessary. No prospective randomized study has been done on the effectiveness of dose and repetition. Most important, cidofovir does not offer a cure for RRP. Further research on its toxic effects and most effective dose likely will unfold in the next decade.

α-Interferon

In 1981, Haglund and colleagues [42] reported the first results of using human leukocyte interferon in seven patients who had RRP. This uncontrolled study was encouraging and led to multiple other studies that demonstrated positive early results with interferon therapy, primarily in the reduction of disease severity. Most series also showed recurrence of disease on continued treatment, as well as a rebound phenomenon—or increased severity of disease—on withdrawal of therapy [42–51]. At best, complete response rates vary from 30% to 60%. In 1988, Healy and colleagues [52], conducted a multicenter, randomized, clinical trial that recruited 123 patients. They were assigned to receive surgery or surgery and interferon over 1 year, and were followed for 1 year; the initial benefit of interferon therapy was not sustained over time.

Nonetheless, interferon therapy had an important place in the treatment of patients who have severe RRP that requires multiple surgeries. In 1995, the Task Force on RRP survey revealed that 9% of pediatric patients, and 1% of adult patients had been treated with interferon [10]. By 2004, the ASPO survey showed a marked decline of interferon use to 4% of pediatric patients who had RRP [16]. In this report, Schraff and colleagues [16] noted the availability and parallel increase in the use of other adjuvant treatments, especially cidofovir, as one possible reason for the decrease in interferon therapy. Additionally, the use of alternative adjuvants may reflect concern over the undesirable side effects of interferon, which include fever, nausea, vomiting, malaise, renal and hepatic dysfunction, growth retardation (even if temporary), and spastic diplegia. The authors have used interferon in occasional adult patients who had extremely aggressive disease with good results; however, the risks of interferon's side effects often outweigh the benefits of therapy.

Indole-3-carbinol

I3C is found in cruciferous vegetables (cabbage, cauliflower, broccoli, brussels sprouts), and is a potent inducer of the cytochrome P-450 metabolism of estrogen, which results in 2-hydroxylation of estradiol. Estrogen increases HPV gene expression. In the oxidation and hydroxylation of estrogen, different relative levels of 2-hydroxyestrone (2-OHE1) and 16alpha-hydroxyestrone (16α-OHE1) are associated with a higher or lower risk for developing hormone-dependent tumors and epithelial cell hyperproliferation. Higher 2-OHE1/:16α-OHE1 ratios, as increased by I3C, decrease the likelihood of papilloma formation because hyperproliferation of epithelial cells is not induced [53].

I3C inhibited the development of papillomas in HPV-infected laryngeal tissue that was transplanted into immunocompromised nude mice [53]. Based on their successful treatment of a 30-month-old girl who required nine surgeries in 6 months to control aggressive RRP with daily dietary supplementation with cabbage juice [54], Rosen and colleagues [55] conducted an open-label, phase I prospective trial of chemically pure I3C in 18 patients. I3C was well tolerated without major complications or severe side effects. A few patients experienced transient nausea and dysequilibrium. There was no adverse effect on pediatric growth patterns. None of the patients had accelerated growth of their papillomas. Mean follow-up was 14.6 months, during which time 6 patients had a complete response to I3C, with no growth of their papillomas; 6 had partial response, with significantly slowed growth; and 6 had no change in the growth rate of their RPP. Similar results of 33% complete responses, 30% partial responses, and 36% no response to I3C were reported by Rosen and Bryson [56] in a larger, long-term series of 33 patients who were followed over a mean of 5 years; in this study, adults had a better overall response to I3C than did children.

I3C is a promising adjunctive treatment for RRP that is easy to administer, has few side effects, and offers good results to at least one third of patients. Further clinical trials are warranted with larger numbers of patients, especially in the pediatric population.

Photodynamic therapy

Described in the early 1900s, PDT has been used to destroy neoplasms by light activation of a photosensitive dye that selectively concentrates in tumor cells. Vascular and tumor destruction result from the vascular stasis that occurs with the in situ generation of singlet oxygen by laser activation of the photosensitizer [57]. In 1986, Shikowitz and colleagues [58] reported the first effective use of PDT on virally induced cutaneous papillomas in an animal model. Abramson and colleagues [59,60] next established the safety parameters of PDT in the canine larynx—by demonstrating the effects of increasing light intensities at 630 nm—then began trials in human subjects [60]. Combined, studies by these investigators at Long-Island Jewish Medical Center demonstrated that PDT was an effective therapy for RRP when used with dihematoporphyrinether (DHE), which has a predilection for highly vascular tissue, and decreased RRP growth rates by 50% [57–61]. Light-dose effect studies did not show significant changes in response rates with increased light intensities [57]; however, a greater decrease in papilloma growth rate was seen in patients who received 4.25 mg/kg DHE (versus 3.25 mg/kg DHE) 48 to 72 hours before photoactivation with the optimal 50 J/cm^2 argon-pumped dye laser light. Despite good clinical response to this regimen at 3 years, HPV-DNA persisted in tissue biopsies [61].

The main side effect of using DHE for PDT is the 6- to 12-week increased photosensitivity; mild to severe sunburn results from exposure to natural UV and indoor fluorescent light if precautions are not taken. This prompted a search for alternative photosensitizers, and resulted in the study of PDT with meso-tetra (hydroxyphenyl) chlorin (m-THPC), because of its better tissue selectivity and shorter washout time [62]. The study showed a delayed response in most patients, and an initial transient increase in disease severity in many patients. Recurrences occurred in the patients who were followed for 3 to 5 years, but at rates that generally were less than the pretreatment recurrence rates. Latent HPV-DNA was not eliminated with m-THPC treatment. m-THPC was not compared with DHE in this study, so comparative conclusions cannot be made.

Heat shock protein E7: a novel therapy

HspE7 is a recombinant fusion protein that covalently links the C terminus of 638 amino acids from Hsp65 (derived from *Mycobacterium bovis* bacille Calmette-Guérin) with the E7 protein of HPV-16. Nonclinical studies demonstrate the activity of the fusion protein in vivo and in vitro, but also show that its individual components are not active when given alone or as mixtures. Goldstone and colleagues [63] showed that subcutaneous administration of HspE7 in an animal model generated an E7-specific, cell-mediated and humoral immune response. Chu and colleagues [64] showed that HspE7 induces dose-dependent regression of the epithelial cell–derived murine tumor, TC-1, which expresses HPV-16 E7. Based on these and other studies that suggest that HspE7 is cross-reactive for HPV types other than HPV-16, Derkay and colleagues [65] conducted an open-label, single-arm intervention study at eight medical centers on the clinical effects of subcutaneous HspE7. Fourteen female and thirteen male immune-competent patients between the ages of 2 and 18 years—all with histologically proven RRP that required at least four surgical procedures in the 12 months before enrollment, and 7 who had pulmonary disease—were recruited for the study. None of the participants had received adjuvant therapy for RRP within 30 days, nor had they received immunotherapy within 9 months of starting the study. After a baseline debulking surgery, each patient received three monthly subcutaneous injections of HspE7, 500 μg, over 60 days. The primary end point was the length of the interval between the initial debulking surgery and the first debulking surgery that was required in the posttreatment period. This was compared with the median intersurgical interval of the four surgeries before study enrollment. Study results showed a marked positive effect of HspE7 on the number of surgeries required. The first posttreatment intersurgical interval increased 93% over the pretreatment interval for the overall population. There also was a statistically significant increase in the median of all posttreatment intersurgical intervals over a 60-week follow-up, which indicated a sustained effect of HspE7. Incidentally, the effect was more pronounced in female patients than in male patients. Finally, based on the laryngoscopic staging and severity score that was developed for, and used in, the study, HspE7 also reduced the lesion growth rate. Generally, HspE7 was well tolerated. The study reported that a high proportion of participants experienced transient injection site reactions of mild to moderate severity.

HspE7 is being studied under the guidance of the U.S. Food and Drug Administration; a phase III pivotal trial seemed to be warranted by these results. HspE7 offers the benefit of a more systemic approach to RRP than does intralesional cidofovir, without the adverse side effects of interferon, and it can be administered in an outpatient setting. Although HspE7 is unlikely to offer a cure for RRP, it may reveal itself as the treatment that is most effective in keeping the disease in check.

Tracheotomy

The Task Force on RRP reported the need for tracheotomy in 6% of adult patients and 14% of pediatric patients [10]. Children who required a tracheotomy were diagnosed with RRP at a younger age than were those who did not require a tracheotomy (2.7 years versus 3.9 years) [66]. These rates are similar to those that were reported by Lindeberg and Elbrond [67] for Danish patients who had RRP (4% of adults and 14% of children). Cole and colleagues [68] reported that 21% of 58 pediatric patients who were treated over 10 years needed a tracheotomy. The need for tracheotomy arises when disease has progressed to the point of causing respiratory distress that is due to significant airway obstruction, above or below the glottis. Regardless of the incidence of tracheotomy, most investigators agree that the procedure should be avoided if possible, because of its association with distal tracheal spread, which is believed to be caused by the interruption that is made in respiratory epithelium and the creation of a new squamociliary epithelial junction. For the same reason, decannulation after tracheotomy should occur as soon as possible, with emphasis on achieving disease control by way of endoscopic procedures, and a goal of preventing extralaryngeal spread.

Prognostic factors and quality of life issues

As the basic science and clinical communities have continued to expand and evaluate treatment options for RRP in the last 20 years, new emphasis has been placed on identifying prognostic factors that might influence the aggressiveness of treatment that is warranted. Similarly, in the current era of economically oriented medical practice and patient-centered research, the cost of RRP to patients and society has gained more attention.

Age at onset is a well-established factor in predicting the severity of RRP. Epidemiologic studies in Denmark and the United States have shown that patients whose disease manifests before the age of 5 years require more surgical interventions, and undergo adjuvant therapy and tracheotomy more frequently than do patients whose disease occurs at older than 5 years, given the higher rate of tracheal and pulmonary extension in these younger patients [10–12,69].

HPV viral type has been of focal interest in evaluating the aggressiveness of RRP since its confirmation as the etiologic agent in RRP in the 1990s. With the establishment of HPV-6 and -11 as the most common types identified in airway lesions, several retrospective studies attempted to correlate viral type with disease aggressiveness. Early evidence was conflicting, and HPV-6 and -11 each was identified as the more aggressive viral type, or as equally aggressive [70–72]. More recently, Wiatriak and colleagues' [15] longitudinal prospective study of 73 patients who had JORRP demonstrated that patients who were infected with HPV-11 had more aggressive disease than did those who were infected with HPV-6, as evidenced by higher disease severity scores, need for more frequent surgical interventions, greater requirement for adjuvant therapy, higher incidence of tracheal and pulmonary disease, and greater need for tracheotomy. Gerein and colleagues [73] conducted a multicenter prospective study of 42 patients who had RRP who were treated with α-interferon. HPV-11 was associated with poorer response to therapy, and greater incidence of pulmonary spread and malignant transformation than was HPV-6. Taken with other retrospective studies, it seems that HPV-11 is the more aggressive viral subtype in RRP; however, the clinician's ability to perform viral typing, and the influence of identifying viral type on successful treatment is not well established.

In addition to predictors of severe disease, predictors of remission may help clinicians to counsel patients and their families during the course of RRP management. Few studies have addressed factors that may predict remission, and "remission" itself is not defined universally. Data on 165 new cases from the national registry for JORRP were analyzed by Ruparelia and colleagues [74] in search of factors that lead to remission—defined in that study as no surgical procedures needed for at least 1 year. The only factor that was predictive of remission was older age at diagnosis, with the maximum probability of remission being 44.2% at 3.6 years of age. The hazards of remission increased by 1.13 for every 1 year in age at diagnosis. Patients who underwent fewer than four procedures in the year after diagnosis also were more likely to experience remission than were those who required more than four surgical procedures in the year after diagnosis. Factors that were evaluated, but were not associated with remission, included adjuvant drug therapy in the first year of diagnosis, nonwhite race, and gender. Although patients who have AORRP can have an aggressive form of the disease, in general, they undergo fewer lifetime surgical procedures than do patients who have JORRP; this may imply a higher rate of remission in patients who have adult-onset disease. Again, however, there is a paucity of literature on remission rates in adult patients. Given that RRP is more likely to recur in respiratory mucosa that undergoes metaplasia or injury, recurrence may be more likely in smokers and patients who have reflux disease. Future research is required to establish control of reflux and smoking cessation/nonsmoking as predictors of remission.

In 1995, the Task Force on RRP estimated that the annual cost of surgical procedures for RRP was more than $150 million in the United States. With inflation alone, this figure must have grown over the last 10 years, and does not include the cost of adjuvant treatments and in-office procedures which are growing in popularity. The toll that RRP takes on patients and their families is well known among clinicians who care for them; however, studies on the cost to patients and caregivers in the way of time out of work and school, limitation of occupation/disability, transportation, and home care have not been published. Bishai and colleagues [75] assessed the medical costs and number of quality-adjusted life years (QALYs) for a statistical patient who had JORRP in 1997. Annual costs for this statistical case were nearly $58,000 (range, $32,000–$94,000), with a lifetime cost of $202,000 (range, $62,000–$474,000), and included the surgery-associated costs of hospital stay, physician fees, and outpatient visits. The burden of QALYs was estimated at 0.31 QALY per year of disease (range, 0.10–0.96 QALY per year of JORRP). This correlated to a lifetime loss of 2.01 QALY for a single case of JORRP (range, 1/28–4.61 total QALYs). The investigators speculated on the cost-effectiveness of offering women who had visible condylomata an elective cesarean section in an effort to attempt to prevent new cases of JORRP. There is not enough prospective evidence to support a policy that promotes this practice; however, analyzing the economics of such policies likely will play a greater role in the continued research on RRP prevention and treatment.

Several patient questionnaires were developed in the 1990s to assess the impact of various voice problems on the individual, including the voice-related quality of life instrument, and the voice handicap index, which addresses the social impact of dysphonia of any cause [76–78]. To monitor the burden of disease, Hill and colleagues [79] developed a questionnaire that is specific to RRP, and issued it with an established, generic multi-item health questionnaire (the United Kingdom Short Form–36; SF-36) to 36 patients who had RRP. Twenty-six patients responded; all had lower scores on the SF-36 than did controls, particularly in the domains of pain, physical limitation, and energy/vitality. Results from the RRP questionnaire identified 22 symptoms that patients who had RRP also were more likely to suffer than were controls (eg, difficulty speaking in noisy environments/for more than 15 minutes/on the phone, difficulty shouting/singing, or difficulty with depression/fatigue/sore throat). Responsiveness of the questionnaires to change in disease burden was not assessed. Despite its limitations and the lengthiness of the questionnaire, the study again reflects the increased interest in developing instruments that consistently measure the impact of RRP on patients' quality of life. Lindman and colleagues [80] similarly highlighted the need to develop means of longitudinally evaluating quality of life issues for children who have RRP. Identifying issues that are most important and burdensome to patients will direct clinicians in their treatment of, and research on, the disease.

New frontiers: updates in pathophysiology

Along with persistent efforts to improve RRP management, the last decade yielded a surge of interest and work in the realm of molecular biology that focused on defining the pathophysiology of RRP. Investigators questioned the roles of cellular immunity, cell cycle regulatory proteins, angiogenesis, and host–susceptibility factors in the development and persistence of RRP. Most studies are of small caliber—involving fewer than 25 patients—and most have not been reproduced. These numbers are not surprising given the small number of patients that is affected by RRP; but they do point to the need for large, multicenter efforts in the future.

Four areas of research are discussed below. All of them seek to identify specific molecular entities that are involved in RRP and that potentially can be targeted in novel treatments.

RRP is known to arise in immune-suppressed patients—including those who HIV, transplant recipients who are on immune suppressive drugs, and others who have congenital immune deficiencies—and in otherwise healthy patients. Because the defense against viral infections is mediated by T helper 1 (Th1) cells, and involves the interaction between Th1 cells and tissue antigen-presenting cells (APCs), which produces interleukin (IL)-2 as a critical messenger in the cytokine cascade that ensues, Snowden and colleagues [81] identified serum levels of IL-2 and the APC–Th1 cell upregulated IL-2 receptor (IL-2R) as plausible markers of immune activity to evaluate in patients who had RRP. Serum levels of IL-2 and IL-2R were determined by ELISA in samples from 15 children who had RRP and 10 control subjects. Serum IL-2 and IL-2R levels were significantly lower in patients who had papilloma. Among patients who had RRP, those who had more aggressive disease were significantly younger than were those who had less aggressive disease, and they had higher levels of serum IL-2 and IL-2R (although they were lower than in normal controls). The investigators concluded that these data support an aberrant cell-mediated immune response in children who have RRP, and they are undertaking a multicenter study to corroborate their findings in a larger population.

Given the apparent unregulated neoplastic growth of papillomas in RRP, Poetker and colleagues [82] looked at the possible role of apoptosis and its dysregulation in this disease process. The expression of several proapoptotic and antiapoptotic factors were studied. Particular attention was paid to survivin, a cell cycle–regulated antiapoptotic factor that is expressed in normally developing fetal tissues and many tumors and premalignant lesions, but rarely in normal differentiated tissues. The effects of HPV infection on apoptosis and the expression of apoptotic factors is unknown; however, this group found that the mean protein expression of survivin was nearly fivefold greater in RRP papillomas that were taken from 11 RRP specimens than in five normal laryngeal tissue specimens that were tested (14.2% ± 2.5% versus 3.0% ± 0.8% of normalized ribosomal protein L32, P = .003). Protein levels of survivin were completely absent by Western blot analysis in the normal laryngeal tissue, whereas survivin was found in the papilloma samples. This differential expression of survivin in RRP samples may represent the dysregulation of apoptosis by certain factors in patients who are infected with HPV, and could be targeted by novel treatments in the future.

Vascular endothelial growth factor (VEGF)-A exerts a variety of effects on vascular endothelium and is known to play a role, with its endothelial receptors, in several nonneoplastic processes that involve angiogenesis. Overexpression of VEGF-A also has been demonstrated in several neoplasms. Rahbar and colleagues [83] investigated whether VEGF-A could be a factor in the pathogenesis of RRP. In a retrospective study of 12 patients who had RRP, formalin-fixed papilloma specimens and samples of larynx tissue from five normal autopsy specimens were examined for the presence of mRNA for VEGF-A and vascular endothelial growth factor receptors (VEGFR)-1 and -2. VEGF-A mRNA was expressed strongly in the epithelium of papillomas of all 12 patients who had RRP, and VEGFR-1 and -2 mRNA were expressed strongly in the vascular endothelium of the fibrovascular cores of the papillomas. Conversely, the control samples showed no expression of VEGF-A mRNA or VEGFR-1 or -2 mRNA. With the knowledge that tumor growth was suppressed by the inhibition of VEGF-A or its receptors in several experimental models, Rahbar and colleagues [83] entertain the possibility of suppressing these factors to treat RRP.

Finally, perhaps the largest undertaking to understand the pathophysiology of RRP is described by Buchinsky and colleagues [84] as the Multicenter Initiative Seeking Critical Genes in Respiratory Papillomatosis. Twenty-one hospitals are aiming to recruit 400 patients and their parents through a collaboration between the RRP Task Force and the Center for Genomic Sciences at Allegheny-Singer Research Institute in Pittsburgh. The investigators postulate that susceptibility to RRP is encoded genetically, because millions of neonates are exposed to RRP during vaginal delivery, but few develop the disease. The objective is to determine the host genes that govern susceptibility to RRP by conducting a genome-wide association study on family triads of patients who have RRP and their parents. Data from the human genome project will be used to identify alleles that are over- and undertransmitted from parents to their offspring who are affected by RRP. Blood specimens will be collected from each person in the triad, the DNA will be extracted, each genotype will be determined, and that of the patient who has RRP will be compared with those of his/her parents. RRP biopsy specimens for each patient also will undergo HPV typing. It is hoped that defining the genes that govern host susceptibility to RRP will enhance our understanding of the disease and host–viral interactions in general.

Summary

As has been the case for decades, clinicians and scientists continue to struggle with the treatment of RRP. They are seeking new and better management strategies, while striving to identify the risk factors for acquiring RRP and predictors of disease severity and disease remission. RRP remains a "predictably unpredictable disease" with a varying natural history that makes the study of various effective therapies difficult. The surgeon remains charged to use the tools and techniques that work best for him or her in caring for patients who have RRP, to maximize disease control, and to minimize collateral damage to normal tissues and function. The creation of the RRP Task Force and the initiation of several multicenter studies reflect the increased collaborative nature of the work that is being done to understand RRP. New efforts in the last decade have focused on assessing the economic and social costs of RRP, and on eliciting the pathophysiology of the disease on a molecular level. These new areas of interest will blossom over the next half century. In time, novel treatments that target specific protein modulators of RRP will be developed as the genetics of host susceptibility to RRP are revealed.

References

[1] Dedo HH, Yu KCY. CO_2 laser treatment in 24 patients with respiratory papillomas. Laryngoscope 2001;111:1639–44.
[2] Snoeck R, Wellens W, Desloovere C, et al. Treatment of severe laryngeal papillomatosis with intralesional injections of cidofovir [of (S)-1-(3-hydroxy-2-phosphonylmethoxypropyl)cytosine]. J Med Virol 1998;54:219–25.
[3] Pransky SM, Magit AE, Kearns DB, et al. Intralesional cidofovir for recurrent respiratory papillomatosis in children. Arch Otolaryngol Head Neck Surg 1999;125:1143–8.
[4] Pransky SM, Brewster DF, Magit AE, et al. Clinical update on 10 children treated with intralesional cidofovir injections for recurrent respiratory papillomatosis. Arch Otolaryngol Head Neck Surg 2000;126:1239–43.
[5] Chhetri DK, Blumin JH, Shapiro NL, et al. Office-based treatment of laryngeal papillomatosis with percutaneous injection of cidofovir. Otolaryngol Head Neck Surg 2002;126(6):643–8.
[6] Van Valcke I, Wellens W, De Boeck K, et al. Systemic cidofovir in papillomatosis. Clin Infect Dis 2001;32:62–4.
[7] Van Cutsem E, Snoeck R, Van Ranst M, et al. Successful treatment of a squamous papilloma of the hypopharynx-esophagus by local injections of (S)-1-(3- hydroxy-2-phosphonylmethoxypropyl)cytosine. J Med Virol 1995;45:230–5.

[8] Snoeck R, Andrei G, De Clercq E. Cidofovir in the treatment of HPV-associated lesions. Verh K Acad Geneeskd Belg 2001;63(2):93–122.
[9] Bielamowicz S, Villagomez V, Stager S, et al. Intralesional cidofovir therapy for laryngeal papilloma in an adult cohort. Laryngoscope 2002;112:696–9.
[10] Derkay CS. Task force on recurrent respiratory papillomatosis: a preliminary report. Arch Otolaryngol Head Neck Surg 1995;121(12):1386–91.
[11] Reeves WC, Ruparelia SS, Swanson KI, et al. National registry for juvenile-onset recurrent respiratory papillomatosis. Arch Otolaryngol Head Neck Surg 2003;129(9):976–82.
[12] Derkay CS, Darrow DH. Recurrent respiratory papillomatosis of the larynx: current diagnosis and treatment. Otolaryngol Clin North Am 2000;33(5):1127–41.
[13] Derkay CS, Malis DJ, Zalzal G, et al. A staging system for assessing severity of disease and response to therapy in recurrent respiratory papillomatosis. Laryngoscope 1998;108(6):935–7.
[14] Derkay CS. Recurrent respiratory papillomatosis. Laryngoscope 2001;111(1):57–69.
[15] Wiatrek BJ, Wiatrek DW, Broker TR, et al. Recurrent respiratory papillomatosis: a longitudinal study comparing severity associated with human papilloma viral types 6 and 11 and other risk factors in a large pediatric population. Laryngoscope 2004;114:1–33.
[16] Schraff S, Derkay CS, Burke B, et al. American Society of Pediatric Otolaryngology members' experience with recurrent respiratory papillomatosis and the use of adjuvant therapy. Arch Otolaryngol Head Neck Surg 2004;130(9):1039–42.
[17] Cook TA, Brunchswig JP, Butel JS, et al. Laryngeal papilloma: etiologic and therapeutic considerations. Ann Otol Rhinol Laryngol 1973;82:649–55.
[18] Strong MS, Vaughan CW, Healy GD. Recurrent respiratory papillomatosis. In: Healy GB, editor. Laryngo-tracheo problems in the pediatric patient. Springfield (IL): Charles C. Thomas Publisher; 1979. p. 88–98.
[19] Quick CA, Kryzek RA, Watt SL, et al. Relationship between condylomata and laryngeal papillomata clinical and molecular virological evidence. Ann Otol Rhinol Laryngol 1980;89:467–71.
[20] Hallden C, Majmudar B. The relationship between juvenile laryngeal papillomatosis and maternal condylomata acuminata. J Reprod Med 1986;31:804–7.
[21] Quick CA, Farris A, Kryzek R. The etiology of laryngeal papillomatosis. Laryngoscope 1978;88:1789–95.
[22] Kashima HK, Shah F, Lyles A, et al. A comparison of risk factors in juvenile-onset and adult-onset recurrent respiratory papillomatosis. Laryngoscope 1992;102:9–13.
[23] Shah K, Kashima H, Polk BF, et al. Rarity of cesarean delivery in cases of juvenile onset respiratory papillomatosis. Obstet Gynecol 1986;68:795–9.
[24] Bennett RS, Powell KR. Human papillomavirus: association between laryngeal papillomas and genital warts. Pediatr Infect Dis J 1987;6:229–32.
[25] Bonagura VR, Vambutas A, DeVoti JA, et al. HLA alleles, IFN-gamma responses to HPV-11 E6, and disease severity in patients with recurrent respiratory papillomatosis. Hum Immunol 2004;65:773–82.
[26] Kashima H, Mounts P, Leventhal B, et al. Sites of predilection in recurrent respiratory papillomatosis. Ann Otol Rhinol Laryngol 1993;103:580–3.
[27] Vaughan CW, Healy GB, Cooperband SR, et al. Recurrent respiratory papillomatosis: management with the CO_2 laser. Ann Otol Rhinol Laryngol 1976;85:508–16.
[28] McMillan K, Pankratov MM, Wang Z, et al. Atraumatic laser treatment for laryngeal papillomatosis. Proceedings of the International Society of Optical Engineering (SPIE) 1994;2128:104–10.
[29] Woo P, Wang Z, Perrault DF Jr, et al. Pulsed dye laser application in ablation of vascular ectasias of the larynx: a preliminary animal study. Proceedings of the International Society of Optical Engineering (SPIE) 1995;2395:336–41.
[30] McMillan K, Shapshay SM, McGilligan JA, et al. A 585-nanometer pulsed dye laser treatment of laryngeal papillomas: preliminary report. Laryngoscope 1998;108:968–72.

[31] Valdez TA, McMillan K, Shapshay SM. A new laser treatment for vocal cord papilloma 585-nm pulsed dye. Otolaryngol Head Neck Surg 2001;124:421–5.
[32] Franco RA Jr, Zeitels SM, Farinelli WA, et al. 585-nm pulsed dye laser treatment of glottal papillomatosis. Ann Otol Rhinol Laryngol 2002;111:486–92.
[33] Myer CM, Willging JP, McMurray S, et al. Use of a laryngeal micro resector system. Laryngoscope 1999;109(7, Part 1):1165–6.
[34] Patel N, Rowe M, Tunkel D. Treatment of recurrent respiratory papillomatosis in children with the microdebrider. Ann Otol Rhinol Laryngol 2003;112:7–10.
[35] Safrin S, Cherrington J, Jaffe H. Cidofovir: review of current and potential clinical uses. Antiviral Chemo 1999;5:111–20.
[36] Bienvenu B, Martinez F, Devergie A, et al. Topical use of cidofovir induced acute renal failure. Transplantation 2002;73(4):661–2.
[37] Stragier I, Snoeck R, De Clercq E, et al. Local treatment of HPV-induced skin lesions by cidofovir. J Med Virol 2002;67:241–5.
[38] Co J, Woo P. Serial office-based intralesional injection of cidofivir in adult-onset recurrent respiratory papillomatosis. Ann Otol Rhinol Laryngol 2004;113:859–62.
[39] Cundy D, Bidgood AM, Lynck G, et al. Pharmacokinetics, bioavailability, metabolism, and tissue distribution of cidofovir (HPMC) and cyclic HPMC in rats. Drug Metab Dispos 1996; 24(7):745–52.
[40] Chhetri DK, Jahan-Parwar B, Hart SD, et al. Local and systemic effects of intralaryngeal injection of cidofovir in a canine model. Laryngoscope 2003;113(11):922–6.
[41] Spiegel JH, Andrus JA, Stefanato CM, et al. Histopathologic effects of cidofovir on cartilage. Otolaryngol Head Neck Surg 2005;133(5):666–71.
[42] Haglund S, Lundquist P, Cantell K, et al. Interferon therapy in juvenile laryngeal papillomatosis. Arch Otolaryngol Head Neck Surg 1981;107:327–32.
[43] Goepfert H, Sesions RB, Gutterman JU, et al. Leukocyte interferon in patients with juvenile laryngeal papillomatosis. Ann Otol Rhinol Laryngol 1982;91:431–6.
[44] Sessions RB, Goepfert H, Donovan DT, et al. Further observations on the treatment of recurrent respiratory papillomatosis with interferon; a comparison of sources. Ann Otol Rhinol Laryngol 1983;92:456–61.
[45] Lundquist PG, Haglund S, Carlsoo B, et al. Interferon therapy in juvenile laryngeal papillomatosis. Otolaryngol Head Neck Surg 1984;92(4):386–91.
[46] Kashima H, Levethal B, Dedo H, et al. Interferon alfa-n1 (Wellferon) in juvenile onset recurrent respiratory papillomatosis: results of a randomized study in twelve collaborative institutions. Laryngoscope 1988;98:334–40.
[47] McCabe BF, Clark KE. Interferon and laryngeal papillomatosis: the Iowa experience. Ann Otol Rhinol Laryngol 1983;92:2–7.
[48] Lusk RB, McCabe BF, Mixon JH. Three year-experience of treating recurrent respiratory papilloma with interferon. Ann Otol Rhinol Laryngol 1987;96:158–62.
[49] Bomholt A. Interferon therapy for laryngeal papillomatosis in adults. Arch Otolaryngol Head Neck Surg 1983;109:550–2.
[50] Sessions RB, Dichtel WS, Goepfert H. Treatment of recurrent respiratory papillomatosis with interferon. Ear Nose Throat J 1984;63:488–93.
[51] Zenner HP, Kley W, Claros P, et al. Recombinant interferon-alpha-2C in laryngeal papillomatosis: preliminary results of a prospective multicentre trial. Oncology 1985;42:15–28.
[52] Healy GB, Gelber RD, Trowbridge AL, et al. Treatment of recurrent respiratory papillomatosis with human leukocyte interferon: results of a multicenter randomized clinical trial. N Engl J Med 1988;319(7):401–7.
[53] Newfield L, Goldsmith A, Bradlow HL, et al. Estrogen metabolism and human papillomavirus-induced tumors of the larynx: chemoprophylaxis with indole-3-carbinol. Anticancer Res 1993;13:337–42.
[54] Coll DA, Rosen CA, Auborn K, et al. Treatment of recurrent respiratory papillomatosis with indole-3-carbinol. Am J Otolaryngol 1997;18(4):283–5.

[55] Rosen CA, Woodson GE, Thompson JW, et al. Preliminary result of the use of indole-3-carbinol for recurrent respiratory papillomatosis. Otolaryngol Head Neck Surg 1998;118: 810–5.

[56] Rosen CA, Bryson PC. Indole-3-carbinol for recurrent respiratory papillomatosis: long-term results. J Voice 2004;18(2):248–53.

[57] Abramson AL, Shikowitz MJ, Mullooly VM, et al. Variable light-dose effect on photodynamic therapy for laryngeal papillomas. Arch Otolaryngol Head Neck Surg 1994;120:852–5.

[58] Shikowitz MJ, Steinberg MB, Abramson AL. Hematoporphyrin derivative therapy of papillomas. Arch Otolaryngol Head Neck Surg 1986;112:42–6.

[59] Abramson AL, Hirschfield LS, Shikowitz MJ, et al. The pathologic effects of photodynamic therapy on the larynx. Arch Otolaryngol Head Neck Surg 1988;114:33–9.

[60] Abramson AL, Shikowitz MJ, Mullooly VM, et al. Clinical effects of photodynamic therapy on recurrent laryngeal papillomas. Arch Otolaryngol Head Neck Surg 1992;118:25–9.

[61] Shikowitz KJ, Abramson AL, Freeman K, et al. Efficacy of DHE photodynamic therapy for respiratory papillomatosis: immediate and long-term results. Laryngoscope 1998;107(7): 962–7.

[62] Shikowitz KJ, Abramson AL, Steinberg B, et al. Clinical trial of photodynamic therapy with meso-tetra (hydroxyphenyl) cholorin for respiratory papillomatosis. Arch Otolaryngol Head Neck Surg 2005;131:99–105.

[63] Goldstone SE, Palefsky JM, Winnitt MT, et al. Activity of HspE7, a novel immunotherapy, in patients with anogenital warts. Dis Colon Rectum 2002;45:502–7.

[64] Chu NR, Wu HB, Wu T, et al. Immunotherapy of a human papillomavirus (HPV) type 16 E7-expressing tumour by administration of fusion protein comprising Mycobacterium bovis bacilli Calmette-Guerin (BCG) hsp65 and HPV 16 E7. Clin Exp Immunol 2000;121: 216–25.

[65] Derkay CS, Smith RJH, McClay J, et al. HspE7 treatment of pediatric recurrent respiratory papillomatosis: final results of an open-label trial. Ann Otol Rhinol Laryngol 2005;114(9): 730–7.

[66] Armstrong LR, Derkay CS, Reeves WC. Initial results from the National Registry for juvenile-onset recurrent respiratory papillomatosis. Arch Otolaryngol Head Neck Surg 1999; 125:743–8.

[67] Lindeberg H, Elbrond O. Laryngeal papillomas: clinical aspects in a series of 231 patients. Clin Otolaryngol 1989;14:333–42.

[68] Cole RR, Myer CM, Cotton RT. Tracheotomy in children with respiratory papillomatosis. Head Neck 1989;111:226–30.

[69] Silverberg MJ, Thorsen P, Lindeberg H, et al. Clinical course of recurrent respiratory papillomatosis in Danish children. Arch Otolaryngol Head Neck Surg 2004;130:711–6.

[70] Gabbott M, Cossart YE, Kan A, et al. Human papillomavirus and host variables as predictors of clinical course in patients with juvenile-onset recurrent respiratory papillomatosis. J Clin Microbiol 1997;35(12):3098–103.

[71] Rimmel FL, Shoeimaker DL, Pou AM, et al. Pediatric papillomatosis: prognostic role for viral typing and cofactors. Laryngoscope 1997;107:915–8.

[72] Mounts P, Kashima H. Association of human papillomavirus subtype and clinical course in respiratory papillomatosis. Laryngoscope 1984;94:28–33.

[73] Gerein V, Rastorguev E, Gerein J, et al. Incidence, age at onset, and potential reasons of malignant transformation in recurrent respiratory papillomatosis patients: 20 years experience. Otolaryngol Head Neck Surg 2005;132:392–4.

[74] Ruparelia S, Unger ER, Nisenbaum R, et al. Predictors of remission in juvenile-onset recurrent respiratory papillomatosis. Arch Otolaryngol Head Neck Surg 2003;129:1275–8.

[75] Bishai D, Kahsima H, Shah K. The cost of juvenile-onset recurrent respiratory papillomatosis. Arch Otolaryngol Head Neck Surg 2000;126:935–9.

[76] Jacobson BH, Johnson A, Grywalski C, et al. The voice handicap index (VHI): development and validation. Am J Speech Lang Pathol 1997;6:66–70.

[77] Carding PN, Horsley IA. An evaluation study of voice therapy in non-organic dysphonia. Eur J Disord Commun 1992;27:137–58.
[78] Carding PN, Horsley IA, Docherty GJ. The effectiveness of voice therapy for patients with non-organic dysphonia. Clin Otolaryngol 1998;23:310–8.
[79] Hill DS, Akhtar S, Corroll A, et al. Quality of life issues in recurrent respiratory papillomatosis. Clin Otolaryngol 2000;25:153–60.
[80] Lindman JP, Gibbons MD, Morlier R, et al. Voice quality of prepubescent children with quiescent recurrent respiratory papillomatosis. Int J Pediatr Otolaryngol 2004;68:529–36.
[81] Snowden RT, Thompson J, Horwitz E, et al. The predictive value of serum interleukin in recurrent respiratory papillomatosis: a preliminary study. Laryngoscope 2001;111:404–8.
[82] Poetker DM, Sankler AD, Scott CL, et al. Survivin expression in juvenile-onset recurrent respiratory papillomatosis. Ann Otol Rhinol Laryngol 2002;111:957–61.
[83] Rahbar R, Vargas SO, Folkman J, et al. Role of vascular endothelial growth factor-A in recurrent respiratory papillomatosis. Ann Otol Rhinol Laryngol 2005;114:289–95.
[84] Buchinsky FJ, Derkay CS, Leal SM, et al. Multicenter initiative seeking critical genes in respiratory papillomatosis. Laryngoscope 2004;114(2):349–57.

ELSEVIER
SAUNDERS

Otolaryngol Clin N Am
39 (2006) 159–172

OTOLARYNGOLOGIC
CLINICS
OF NORTH AMERICA

Laser Applications in Laryngology:
Past, Present, and Future

Steven M. Zeitels, MD, FACS*,
James A. Burns, MD, FACS

*Center for Laryngeal Surgery and Voice Rehabilitation, Massachusetts General Hospital,
One Bowdoin Square, Boston, MA 02114, USA*

Endolaryngeal surgery has been a primary driver for the development of laryngology since its inception in the mid nineteenth century, and laser technology [1] has been a key element of that development over the past 30 years [2–5]. Endoscopic laryngeal surgery remained office-based despite the transition from indirect-mirror-guided interventions to direct-laryngoscopic (Kirstein 1895) procedures in the early twentieth century [6]. Kirstein [7,8] clearly envisioned the enhanced surgical precision provided by direct laryngoscopy and astutely foretold the changeover to direct endolaryngeal surgery. "Autoscopy is veritably a surgical method...I nevertheless believe that finally, in the course of years, autoscopy will be generally accepted as the standard method for endolaryngeal and endotracheal surgery" [8]. As is often the case, an advance in anesthesia (ie, topical cocaine) [9,10] allowed for surgical development. With the ability to administer effective local anesthesia with cocaine, Kirstein performed autoscopy (direct laryngoscopy) in his office with an assistant. Subsequently, Jackson [11] championed moving direct laryngoscopic surgery to the operating suite as illustrated in the first textbook of rigid endoscopy of the upper aerodigestive tract.

Throughout the twentieth century, seminal innovations such as the surgical microscope [12–15] and general endotracheal anesthesia greatly enhanced the precision and success of endolaryngeal surgery. This culminated in the introduction of the carbon dioxide (CO_2) laser to surgery in the 1970s by Polanyi [1], Jako [2], Strong [3,16], and Vaughan [5,17]. They coupled the CO_2 laser

The authors received the following instrumentation on loan: 585-nm pulsed-dye laser (Cynosure, Chelmsford, MA), 532-nm pulsed KTP (Laserscope), and the Thulium laser (LISA Laser Products OHG, Katlenburg-Lindau, Germany).

* Corresponding author.
E-mail address: zeitels.steven@mgh.harvard.edu (S.M. Zeitels).

doi:10.1016/j.otc.2005.10.001
oto.theclinics.com

to the surgical microscope, thereby creating a new means of precise hemostatic dissection. Clinically, the CO_2 laser is a fundamental tool for the endolaryngeal surgeon; however, its use has been limited to the operating room because the energy cannot be delivered through a fiber. Recently, the 585-nm pulsed-dye laser (PDL) [6,18–20] and the 532-nm potassium-titanyl-phosphate (KTP) laser [21–23] have become increasingly popular in endolaryngeal surgery. Unlike the CO_2 laser, both PDL and KTP lasers deliver energy through thin glass fibers. Therefore, the PDL and KTP lasers are well suited for use through the channel of a flexible laryngoscope in the office [6] as well as the speculum of a direct laryngoscope in the operating room. Most recently, a 2-μm continuous wave laser has been introduced, which retains some of the key cutting and ablative characteristics of the CO_2 laser, but it is delivered through 0.2- to 0.6-mm glass fibers.

It is common for laryngologic investigators and clinicians to use terms such as laser treatment, laser therapy, and laser management. This terminology should be abandoned because it is imprecise and can lead to confusion. Various lasers have dramatically different tissue interactions and associated surgical capabilities. In this sense, they represent a spectrum of tools that assist in achieving different outcomes, depending on the clinical problem. Although the CO_2 laser has been the primary laser used in laryngeal surgery for decades, today the laser most used in the present authors' practice are the fiber-based photoangiolytic lasers. Furthermore, it is inevitable that there will be further development of new laser technology as most surgical disciplines become increasingly minimally invasive and office-based.

Carbon dioxide laser

After introducing the CO_2 laser to laryngology and surgery, Jako, Strong, and Vaughan explored its use with various benign and malignant disorders, including carcinoma, stenosis, papilloma, nodules, polyps, cysts, and amyloidosis [24–26]. The seminal nature of their contributions is envisaged by the number of subsequent investigations by generations of surgeons in and outside laryngeal surgery. This continues today as developments in the CO_2 laser [27] enhance its function, primarily resulting in broader application in endoscopic surgical oncology. However, improvements in cold instruments and techniques along with the development of photoangiolytic lasers have caused most surgeons to abandon the CO_2 laser in the treatment of benign nonepithelial lesions of the phonatory mucosa.

It is worthwhile to review key considerations for using the CO_2 laser in laryngeal surgery, but the reader is cautioned that there is a wide spectrum of opinion on this issue. Therefore, the present authors provide a specific philosophy of management that is based on (1) known physiological principles of laryngeal function during phonation and deglutition; (2) laser-tissue interactions that have been well studied; and (3) 2 decades of experience with a majority of laryngeal pathologies.

The CO_2 laser functions primarily as a hemostatic scalpel when the beam is focused. When the beam is defocused, the CO_2 laser can also be used effectively to ablate and cytoreduce epithelial disease such as diffuse papillomatosis. Carbon dioxide lasers deliver nonionizing electromagnetic radiation that is well absorbed by water, which is ubiquitous in the laryngeal soft tissues. Operating at a wavelength 10.6 μm in the infrared region, the CO_2 laser causes thermal injury to soft tissue. For this reason, this laser is relatively contraindicated for the treatment of lesions of the vibratory membranes of the musculomembranous vocal folds. The heat that develops can result in fibrosis of the delicate superficial lamina propria (SLP), which is the primary oscillator responsible for voice production. The associated fibrosis diminishes mucosal pliability, which is the key determinate of voice quality if glottal closure is maintained [28]. Given that the geographic position of many vocal-fold lesions is on the medial phonatory surface, heat absorption and subsequent fibrosis are further exacerbated by unavoidable tangential dissection. Furthermore, optimal subepithelial resection [28–30] of common vocal-fold lesions such as nodules, polyps, and cysts is impossible with a CO_2 laser because attempted dissection at the epithelial basement membrane would result in vaporization of the epithelium. It is reasonable to use the CO_2 on the vibratory membranes when (1) there is no functional SLP present as may be encountered in patients who have had previous surgery; and (2) cancer has already invaded and replaced the SLP.

It should be remembered that Jako introduced both "cold" microlaryngeal hand instruments [12] (1962) as well as the CO_2 laser (1972) [2]. In addition to its hemostatic properties, the CO_2 laser was extremely valuable in microlaryngeal surgery because most surgeons could not perform delicate cold-instrument dissection from a distance under high magnification, especially with their nondominant hand (M.S. Strong, personal communication, 1994). Because the delivery system took the form of a joystick and a foot pedal, a majority of surgeons were able to perform precise bimanual surgery. However, the enhanced manual dexterity of the joystick is offset by the vaporization and ablation of varied amounts of the layered microstructure (epithelium and superficial lamina propria), primary tissues necessary for optimal vocal-fold vibration.

Jako correctly intended that the CO_2 laser should be used synergistically with cold instruments, not alternatively. Unfortunately, since he introduced both approaches, there have been divergent efforts by different investigators to convince colleagues that they should make a choice as to their preferred vocal-fold dissection method: cold-instrument or laser. Those who espouse that an exclusive choice is necessary, not based on soft-tissue interactions and physiologic principles of function, tend to be invested either by habit, previous academic work, or by other motivations. Unfortunately, clinically based investigations performed to elucidate the clinical effects of using a CO_2 laser for benign vocal-fold lesions inevitably suffer from a number of design flaws such as (1) cases were not been randomized; (2) small subject cohorts cases were not been stratified to account for differences in lesion type, size, and laryngoscopic exposure; (3) objective acoustic and aerodynamic measures were not obtained for conversation level and maximal range tasks; (4) those who assessed the results were not blinded to the treatment; (5) surgeons used different CO_2 lasers and had varied skill sets with different lasers and cold instrumentation; and (6) most importantly, the CO_2 laser resection was not compared with subepithelial resection, which is substantially more successful than cold-instrument amputation of most benign lesions (ie, nodules, polyps, and cysts) [28].

In summary, microspot CO_2 lasers are used optimally for epithelial lesions that require resection and whenever the preservation of superficial lamina propria is not necessary (ie, most supraglottic lesions), impossible (already lost from disease or prior surgery), or not appropriate (ie, when glottic cancer has invaded or replaced most of the SLP). The CO_2 laser is also valuable in treating selected posterior glottal disorders that require arytenoidectomy or dissection of subepithelial stenosis. The microspot CO_2 laser is ill suited to treat benign subepithelial masses of the phonatory vocal fold such as nodules, polyps, and cysts. These lesions are optimally resected by cold-instrument tangential dissection with maximal preservation of underlying SLP and complete preservation of overlying epithelium. Regardless of the dissection approach, it is valuable to use the subepithelial infusion technique [28,31–33], which is used to enhance the precise resection of these lesions.

Photoangiolytic 585-nm and 532-nm lasers

585-nm pulsed-dye laser

Anderson and colleagues [34–36] developed the concept of selective photothermolysis over 20 years ago for the treatment of dermatologic vascular malformations. This concept evolved into the 585-nm PDL because its wavelength is precisely selected to target an absorbance peak of oxyhemoglobin (approximately 571 nm) and to fully penetrate the intraluminal blood, thereby depositing heat uniformly into the vessel. The laser pulse width (0.5 ms) is precisely selected to contain the heat to the vessel without causing collateral damage to the extravascular soft tissue from heat conduction. After learning about vocal fold phonatory function, Anderson stated, "Treating vascular lesions in infants skin is similar to treating vocal folds, pliability must be maintained or restored." (R. Rox Anderson, personal communication, 1996)

Pilot studies were performed using the 585-nm pulsed-dye laser for laryngeal papillomatosis by Bower and colleagues [37] and McMillan and colleagues [38]. Shortly thereafter, Zeitels and Anderson initiated large-scale investigations [6,18,19] into the treatment of a spectrum of laryngeal lesions, so that over 300 procedures have been carried out. They created new treatment paradigms for mucosal dysplasia [19], papillomatosis [6,18,20], early glottic cancer [39], ectasias, varices, and hemorrhagic polyps [28]. Because these lesions are composed of aberrant or abundant microvasculature, a surgical angiolysis model of control is philosophically well suited. Similar to the dermatologic model, it was theorized that the microcirculation could be targeted to involute laryngeal lesions (dysplasia, cancer, papilloma, and varices) or facilitate cold-instrument resection (ectasias and polyps), while minimizing thermal trauma to the surrounding soft tissue, SLP, and epithelium. In theory, this would be ideal for maintaining the pliability of the vocal folds' layered microstructure (SLP and epithelium) and glottal sound production.

Early on, it became clear that the primary pathologies for which the PDL would provide the greatest advantage were papillomatosis and dysplasia. A PhotoGenica V 585-nm PDL (Cynosure Inc., Chelmsford, Ma), used primarily for cutaneous vascular lesions, was modified and used to photocoagulate the vocal-fold microvasculature (450-ms pulse width, 2.0 J/pulse max output, 2-Hz repetition rate, 0.6 mm fiber, approximately 1–2-mm spot size, 65–250 J/cm^2 fluence [energy delivery to the tissue]). The procedures were performed primarily through the Universal Modular Glottiscope (Endocraft LLC, Providence, RI) [40] or the Adjustable Bivalved Supraglottiscope (R. Wolf, Rosemont, IL) [41].

Initially, the PDL was used to enhance cold-instrument microflap epithelial resection without including any of the underlying SLP, the primary oscillator during vocal-fold vibration. However, it soon became clear that these lesions would involute without concurrent resection. Because the epithelium is not vaporized to expose the superficial lamina propria, bilateral treatment of disease was possible. Furthermore, if the epithelium was not completely removed during PDL irradiation, the internal surfaces of the anterior commisure could be treated simultaneously without fear of scarring, synechia, or webbing. Therefore, anterior commisure disease (internal aspect), which is usually treated with staged operations, can be treated simultaneously, thus minimizing the number of general anesthetic procedures with their attendant morbidity and cost. It is readily apparent that PDL treatment does offer relief of tumor burden without the long-term consequences of vocal fold scarring that results from repeated surgical procedures using the CO_2 laser or cold instruments.

The success with treating glottal keratosis with dysplasia by strict involution through photoangiolysis of the subepithelial microcirculation was somewhat unexpected. Understandably, erythroplastic lesions would be treated ideally with the PDL because of their vascularity. However, it was unclear how the PDL would enhance management of the substantially more common keratotic lesions. The present authors' prospective investigations revealed that the 585-nm pulsed-dye laser successfully involuted these lesions [19], and current experience reveals that 75% to 100% of the visible disease will involute, and the procedure can be repeated as necessary. Most commonly, this is now performed as an office-based procedure with topical anesthesia [6].

The PDL has been effective in treating papillomatosis and dysplasia without the associated clinically observed soft-tissue complications associated with the CO_2 laser (thermal damage, tissue necrosis, superficial lamina propria scarring, and anterior commisure web formation) [6,18,19]. The presumed mechanism of disease regression is the selective destruction of the subepithelial microvasculature and separation of the epithelium from the underlying SLP by denaturing the basement membrane zone-linking proteins [42]. This results in ischemia to the diseased mucosa, albeit not permanently. This microvascular "angiolysis" approach restricts survival and growth of neoplastic epithelium, while minimizing cytotoxicity to the delicate layered microstructure (SLP) of the vocal fold. Based on this experience, the present authors believe that pulsed angiolysis lasers are a platform technology that will likely serve as a driver for a variety of future innovations in the management of laryngeal diseases as well as other areas of the body in which superficial diseased mucosa is problematic (eg, Barrett's esophagus, dysplasia of the cervix, and granulation in the nose and ear).

Disadvantages of pulsed-dye laser treatments

Despite the assets of pulsed-dye laser treatment, there are shortcomings to these technologies. The laser is expensive and is not likely to exist in most surgical suites. From the present authors' investigations, it is apparent that PDL therapy is less efficient in the treatment of exophytic versus sessile lesions because of the superficial penetration (approximately 2 mm) of the laser energy. This may be an artifact of the relatively low power settings used in this study. The Photogenica V laser is capable of 5 J/pulse, and the typical power output in this study was generally 0.55 to 0.75 J/pulse. It is likely that exuberant exophytic lesions require an increase in power to reach the vasculature at the core of the papillomatous lesions.

Another disadvantage of PDL treatment is that it is difficult to accurately quantify the energy delivery and real-time tissue effects, despite the fact that this laser is unlikely to cause substantial soft-tissue injury to the vocal folds. Furthermore, given the extremely short pulse width (approximately 0.5 ms), it is not unusual for the vessel walls of the microcirculation to become breeched, resulting in extravasation of blood into the surrounding tissue. In the skin this is seen as purpura. In laryngeal lesions such as papillomatosis, the extravasated blood diverts the laser energy in the form of a heat sink, which diminishes the effectiveness of laser. The bleeding also diminishes visualization of the pathology, leading to diminished precision.

Lesions perpendicular to the axis of the straight cleaved fiber are optimal for effective irradiation. Medial-surfaced lesions requiring significant retraction of the vocal fold and the inner aspect of the anterior commisure would be better treated with a side-firing tip. A delivery system that could be set to several angles (30°, 45°, and 90°) would help to ensure proper application of energy to difficult areas such as the medial surfaces of the vocal folds or the subcordal anterior commisure region.

Office-based pulsed-dye laser treatment

Presently, a principle reason that the endolaryngeal treatment of glottal dysplasia and papilloma is performed primarily in the operating room is for the administration of general anesthesia. This approach allows for precise optimal management of the primary goals, which are diagnostic accuracy, regression of disease, and voice restoration and maintenance. However, there is an unavoidable morbidity associated with general anesthesia and a variety of costs associated with the preoperative evaluation and procedural intervention.

Consequently, a majority of patients with recurrent glottal dysplasia and papillomatosis are followed with known disease until the adverse effects of the lesions' growth justifies the morbidity and costs of the surgical intervention. All surgeons and patients acknowledge inherently the detractors associated with general anesthesia in microlaryngoscopic treatment because they are required to develop an individualized plan for repeated treatment. Essentially, readily observed disease is followed until one or a number of factors justify a decision to leave the watchful-waiting model to embark on surgical intervention. These factors include airway restriction, voice deterioration, and worrisome visual appearance on clinical laryngoscopy.

This current management approach in adult patients is based on pragmatic clinical factors that may not always align with optimal disease treatment. When these diseases occur in a more accessible region with less delicate function, such as the oral cavity or skin, they are often treated more frequently and by means of local anesthesia. There would be a lower threshold for intervention for laryngeal lesions if a safe and efficacious treatment modality existed that did not require general anesthesia. Given the success encountered with the 585-nm PDL in treating glottal papillomatosis [18] and dysplasia [19] with general anesthesia, the present authors redesigned the approach, using topical local anesthesia [6].

To date, the present authors' clinical office-based experience treating these lesions with the PDL exceeds 200 cases. The PhotoGenica V 585-nm PDL was engineered to accept a 0.6-mm core fiber used along with a Pentax model VNL-1530T flexible laryngoscope. Visual guidance was achieved by observing the PDL fiber through the distal working channel of the laryngoscope, which has a 2.0-mm internal diameter and a 5.1-mm outside diameter. Although the VNL-153OT still uses optical fibers for illumination, superior higher resolution imaging capability is provided through the placement of the charge-coupled device video chip in the distal end (examination tip) of the scope.

The initial prospective investigation of office-based procedures was performed on 51 patients in 82 cases of recurrent glottal papillomatosis

(30 patients) and dysplasia (52 patients) [6]. All individuals had previously undergone microlaryngoscopic management with histopathologic evaluation. Five cases could not be completed because of impaired exposure (2 patients), discomfort (3 patients). Of those patients who could be treated, there was $\geq 50\%$ disease involution in 68 of 77 (88%) cases and 25% to 50% disease regression in the remaining 9 of 77 (12%) patients. Patients' self-assessment of their voice revealed that 73 of 77 were improved or unchanged, 4 of 77 were slightly worse, and none was substantially worse. These data confirmed that diseased mucosa can normalize without resection or substantial loss of vocal function. The putative mechanisms, which vary based on the fluence (energy) delivered by the laser, are photoangiolysis of sublesional microcirculation, denaturing of epithelial basement membrane-linking proteins, and cellular destruction. This safe effective technique allowed the treatment of many patients (in a clinic setting), in which classical surgery-related morbidity would have often delayed intervention.

However, there is a surgical learning curve using the PDL because energy delivery to the tissue (fluence) is difficult to determine exactly. Therefore, it is suggested that a noncontact mode should be used until the surgeon is familiar with the laser. This reduces the primary potential morbidity, scarring of the superficial lamina propria, because the effective tissue penetration at this wavelength is approximately 2 mm. In a noncontact mode, the necessary level of manual precision is diminished with the PDL compared with effective microlaryngoscopic dissection with the CO_2 laser or cold instruments. One can envision the PDL fiber delivery of light similar in technique to air-brush shading of paint.

As stated earlier, quantifying the energy delivery of the PDL and the associated real-time tissue effects is difficult. This is the case regardless of anesthetic approach but is more pronounced without stereoscopic microlaryngoscopic visualization. These functional characteristics of the PDL contrast with the familiar properties of the carbon dioxide laser in which the mucosal surface is vaporized. In addition, the vocal fold is more difficult to treat in an awake patient with the flexible laryngoscope because the target tissue is moving. Finally, when using flexible fiber-optic laryngoscopes, there are unavoidable tangential vectors for visualization and laser delivery, which cannot be overcome by bimanual tissue retraction and facile fiber alignment. There are substantially greater degrees of freedom of fiber positioning using a malleable cannula through a rigid laryngoscope with general anesthesia.

Based on the shortcomings of the flexible laryngoscopic PDL treatment, the present authors believe that there are innovations achievable in the foreseeable future. A side-firing fiber tip would significantly enhance control over treating the medial vocalizing surface of the vocal fold. This would dramatically diminish the comparative advantage of bimanual dexterity with microlaryngoscopic surgery. Additionally, high-resolution (distal-chip camera) real-time stroboscopy would provide indirect assessment of acute edema of the SLP, which is an indirect metric for energy delivery. Presently, one could remove the distal chip flexible laryngoscope and assess by telescopic stroboscopy; however, this approach is cumbersome and time consuming, considering the window of opportunity before more local anesthesia is required. Alternatively, stroboscopic capability is available with other flexible fiber-optic laryngoscopes; however, the optical resolution is suboptimal as compared with the distal-chip technology.

Despite the fact that PDL treatment of diseased glottal epithelium by flexible laryngoscopy with local anesthesia was less efficacious than by microlaryngoscopy with general anesthesia, there are considerable advantages to the former. The reduced morbidity associated with local anesthesia in the clinic considerably facilitates the treatment of older patients, particularly those with substantial cardiovascular and pulmonary disease. This scenario is not uncommon in aging societies with a predilection for tobacco use. In the younger and working populations, there is less lifestyle disruption if general anesthesia is avoided in the operating room.

There are a number of limitations with the flexible laryngoscopic approach. A specimen for histopathologic analysis is not obtained routinely as part of the decision-making process for treatment. This is considered to be acceptable for a number of reasons. Most importantly, all patients have previously undergone microlaryngoscopic biopsies, and the indication to obtain further post-PDL intraoperative biopsies or treatment remained unchanged, based on laryngoscopic appearance during the office examination. Therefore, if the post-treatment clinic examination improved so that transparent normal-appearing epithelium was observed, a biopsy was unnecessary. However, if there was insufficient resolution or response to treatment after 3 to 4 weeks, the intraoperative option remained available. It is highly unlikely that there would be a clinically unrecognized new malignancy given the previous non-cancerous biopsy results and even less likely that a delay of several weeks would have a deleterious effect on long-term outcome.

Another disadvantage of the local anesthesia approach is that this treatment pathway may lead ultimately to more procedures. This is mainly because the threshold for intervention is decreased commensurate with the diminished morbidity associated with local anesthetic treatment. In addition, individual office-based operations are generally less effective compared with operative procedures under general anesthesia. The surgeon is understandably less aggressive using the PDL with local anesthesia because of reduced visual precision and the fact that the vocal folds are moving. Hopefully, with greater experience in this new treatment pathway, we will be able to more closely simulate the treatment capabilities that we achieve using general anesthesia.

Involution and treatment of early glottic carcinoma with pulsed-dye laser

Based on the success of treating involuting vocal-fold dysplasia with the 585-nm pulsed-dye laser (PDL), a correlative treatment strategy was initiated to involute or treat microinvasive early glottic cancer. This approach evolved as a consequence of Folkman's concepts of cancer growth resulting from tumor angiogenesis [43,44]. PDL treatment was carried out initially to involute limited areas of microinvasive vocal-fold carcinoma in a selected pilot group of six patients who presented with early bilateral glottic cancer in which staged endoscopic resection was planned. The vocal fold with a greater volume of cancer was treated conventionally and the contralateral side was treated with the PDL, without resecting the smaller volume of cancer.

It was believed that this approach did not pose a substantial risk to the patients because (1) the disease was of small volume; (2) early glottic cancer grows slowly and rarely metastasizes; (3) it is easy to follow patients closely during the postoperative healing period and to intervene immediately if clinically indicated; (4) the routine plan would have been to perform a microlaryngoscopic resection of the second vocal fold in a staged fashion to avoid airway stenosis; and (5) all conventional treatment options remained. Subsequently, PDL was used to treat a patient in whom disease recurred after two previous endolaryngeal resections. This is likely to be the first demonstration of using non-ionizing radiation without chemical enhancement to involute (without vaporization or resection) microinvasive vocal-fold cancer.

Despite treatment of bilateral disease, objective voice measures revealed overall improvements in postoperative vocal function as measured by aerodynamic efficiency, maximum phonatory ranges, and voice quality-related acoustic parameters. These results substantiated stroboscopic observations of postoperative improvements, which revealed normal epithelium and enhanced mucosal wave function of PDL-treated vocal folds.

The 585-nm pulsed-dye laser demonstrated the capacity to involute microinvasive vocal-fold cancer. This approach is conceptually attractive because it is repeatable and also enhances vocal function by improving mucosal pliability. These findings support the concept that the inhibition of neoplastic blood supply (antiangiogenesis and photoangiolysis) by means of nonionizing radiation results in tumor regression. These cases established the proof-of-concept that microinvasive cancer could be involuted by means of photoangiolysis and that mucosal function and pliability could be maintained or restored. No conclusions can be drawn about the long-term oncologic efficacy of this approach, but these observations warrant further investigation. It may be that at some point in the future, surgeons may adopt the approach of incremental treatment of cancer to diminish morbidity as espoused by radiation and medical oncology.

The yellow light emitted by the PDL does not penetrate deeply into soft tissues, and therefore the present authors are not suggesting that this specific technology should be transferred to other mucosal cancer models. Selective photothermolysis of the microvasculature extends approximately 2 to 3 mm deep in most soft tissues, depending on fluence. Therefore, in one or two treatments, the PDL would not be expected to adequately treat thicker and more deeply invasive tumors. The findings from this pilot group of patients does support the fact that further research into developing laser technology that is capable of selectively ablating intralesional or sublesional tumor vascularity is a laudable goal. In fact, the elements of this approach were identified by almost 40 years ago [45]. Kleinsasser described the aberrant microcirculation associated with microinvasive vocal fold carcinoma, whereas Jako had already commenced investigations into the use of laser technology. "Experiments using laser beams for destruction of discrete areas of vocal cords are presently being conducted" [45].

Pulsed potassium-titanyl-phosphate laser

The potassium-titanyl-phosphate (KTP) laser is a green light laser with a wavelength of 532 nm, which coincides with one of the absorbance peaks of oxyhemoglobin (approximately 541 nm). Similar to the PDL, the light from this laser can be delivered through a thin glass fiber. It has been used in a variety of scenarios to treat vascular lesions within the larynx; however, all previous work was carried out with a continuous-wave mode. The investigators have reported success with subglottic hemangiomas [22] as well as vocal-fold ectasias and varices [21]. Based on Anderson's concept of selective photothermolysis and experience with the 585-nm pulsed-dye laser, the present authors sought to determine whether a 532-nm pulsed KTP laser would provide a clinical advantage over the PDL. An experimental pulsed KTP laser was designed to deliver a 15-ms pulse width to provide enhanced photoangiolysis and diminish extravascular blood extravasation, which had been experienced with the PDL. The pulsed nature of this new KTP laser takes advantage of the fact that the energy delivery time is less than the thermal relaxation time of the tissue. Consequently, there is minimal collateral extravascular thermal soft tissue trauma compared with using the same laser in a continuous mode. The experience thus far has been very favorable in treating over 40 cases of papilloma and dysplasia, including use in the clinic and the operating room. There has been less blood extravasation into the surrounding tissue, and the cytology of overlying diseased (papilloma and dysplasia) epithelium has been virtually unaltered by the subepithelial photoangiolysis. This newly configured pulsed KTP laser shows great promise for laryngeal use and is currently under investigation.

Two-micron continuous wave laser

Recently, a 2-μm continuous wave laser was developed to simulate the cutting properties of the carbon dioxide laser. In a pilot study it has been reported to be efficacious for opening the tracheobronchial lumen for obstructing carcinoma [46]. The RevoLix laser (LISA Laser Products OHG, Katlenburg-Lindau, Germany) is a diode pumped solid state laser that has a thulium-doped yttrium-aluminum-garnet laser rod, which produces a continuous wave beam with a wavelength of 2013 nm. This wavelength has a target chromphore of water. Because it is a continuous wave laser, there are no high peak power pulses (eg, the holmium laser) that create a rapidly expanding and contracting steam bubble each time a laser pulse is absorbed by tissue.

There are a number of distinct advantages of the thulium 2-μm continuous wave laser, primarily because it can be delivered on a glass fiber. Similar to a CO_2 laser, efficient absorption of this laser's radiation by water facilitates its cutting and dissection characteristics. However, unlike a CO_2 laser, the energy is delivered by means of a fiber, which allows for tangential endoscopic dissection. The present authors have used this laser to perform a number of endoscopic partial laryngectomy procedures in both the glottis and the supraglottis. The most remarkable observation was that the procedure was never halted to stop bleeding from laser dissection during any case. Although preliminary observations suggest that there is increased thermal damage on the soft tissues at the margin of the cancerous section compared with the CO_2 laser, it does not seem excessive. These authors are currently conducting a study to evaluate this observation. Furthermore, tangential dissection is more effective with the thulium laser because of the angulation of the fiber delivery system. In contrast, the mirror-based delivery of CO_2 laser energy cannot be angulated substantially. The present authors have also used the thulium laser through the flexible laryngoscope to perform ablation of diffuse recurrent respiratory papillomatosis and lesions of the larynx, apart from the phonatory membranes, which would be susceptible to the heat from this laser. Based on the favorable experience thus far, this laser is being prospectively investigated to determine its optimal applications in laryngeal surgery.

Summary

Since their introduction in laryngology over 30 years ago, lasers have facilitated critically important innovations. These advances have accommodated well to our specialty, which has led in designing minimally invasive surgical approaches since mirror-guided interventions in the nineteenth century. Lasers discussed in this article will provide new platform technologies that will likely lead to the enhanced treatment of a number of benign and malignant laryngeal disorders. There is an expanding group of centers in which fiber-based technologies have already caused many procedures to be performed by means of local anesthesia in the clinic or office, especially for chronic diseases such as papillomatosis and dysplasia. This approach is likely to expand significantly because of diminished patient morbidity along with socioeconomic pressures of health-care delivery.

One of the substantial roadblocks to the dissemination of these clinical advancements is the cost required to install the laser technology in institutions and surgeons' offices. Furthermore, the critical development of these new lasers is limited by the relatively small number of patients with laryngeal disorders, which discourages industry from investing substantial research and development funding. To solve this problem, the present authors hope that laryngology will continue to serve as a model for high-performance minimally invasive surgery that can be translated to other mucosal diseases of the upper and lower aerodigestive tract, genitourinary organs, and the cervix. Broader use of these new lasers in other surgical disciplines should diminish costs for all surgeons and their associated institutions.

References

[1] Polanyi T, Bredermeier HC, Davis TW Jr. CO_2 laser for surgical research. Med Biol Eng Comput 1970;8:548–58.
[2] Jako GJ. Laser surgery of the vocal cords. Cope 1972;82:2204–15.
[3] Strong MS. Laser excision of carcinoma of the larynx. Laryngoscope 1975;85:1286–9.
[4] Strong MS, Vaughan CW, Cooperband SR, et al. Recurrent respiratory papillomatosis: management with the CO_2 laser. Ann Otol Rhinol Laryngol 1976;85:508–16.
[5] Vaughan CW. Transoral laryngeal surgery using the CO_2 laser: laboratory experiments and clinical experience. Laryngoscope 1978;88:1399–420.
[6] Zeitels SM, Franco RA, Dailey SH, et al. Office-based treatment of glottal dysplasia and papillomatosis with the 585-nm pulsed dye laser and local anesthesia. Ann Otol Rhinol Laryngol 2004;113(4):265–76.
[7] Kirstein A. Autoskopie des Larynx und der Trachea (Laryngoscopia directa, Euthyskopie, Besichtigung ohne Spiegel) [Autoscopy of the larynx and trachea (direct examination without mirror)]. Archiv fur Laryngologie und Rhinologie 1895;3:156–64.
[8] Kirstein A. [Autoscopy of the larynx and trachea (direct examination without mirror)]. Philadelphia: F.A. Davis Co., 1897.
[9] Jelinek E. Das Cocain als Anastheticum und Analgeticum fur den Pharynx und Larynx. Wien Med Wochenschr 1884;34:1334–7; 1364–7.
[10] Koller K. Ueber die Verwendung des Cocain zur Anasthesirung am Aug. Wien Med Wochenschr 1884;43:1276.
[11] Jackson C. Tracheo-bronchoscopy, esophagoscopy and gastroscopy. St. Louis (MO): The Laryngoscope Co; 1907.
[12] Jako GJ. Correspondence documents between Geza Jako and the Stuemar Instrument Company. 1962.
[13] Jako GJ. Microscopic laryngoscopy. Presented at the New England Otolaryngological Society. 1964.
[14] Kleinsasser O. Mikrochirurgie im Kehlkopf. Arch fur Ohren Nasen und Kehlkopfheilkunde 1964;183:428–33.
[15] Scalco AN, Shipman WF, Tabb HG. Microscopic suspension laryngoscopy. Ann Otol Rhinol Laryngol 1960;69:1134–8.
[16] Strong MS, Jako GJ. Laser surgery of the larynx: early clinical experience with continuous CO_2 laser. Ann Otol Rhinol Laryngol 1972;81:791–8.
[17] Vaughan CW, Strong MS, Jako GJ. Laryngeal carcinoma: transoral treatment using the CO_2 laser. Am J Surg 1978;136:490–3.
[18] Franco RA, Zeitels SM, Farinelli WA, et al. 585-NM pulsed dye laser treatment of glottal papillomatosis. Ann Otol Rhinol Laryngol 2002;111:486–92.
[19] Franco RA, Zeitels SM, Farinelli WA, et al. 585-nm pulsed dye laser treatment of glottal dysplasia. Ann Otol Rhinol Laryngol 2003;112(9 Pt 1):751–8.
[20] Zeitels SM. Papillomatosis. In: Linville M, editor. Atlas of phonomicrosurgery and other endolaryngeal procedures for benign and malignant disease. San Diego (CA): Singular; 2001. p. 119–31.
[21] Hsiung MW, Kang BH, Su WF, et al. Clearing microvascular lesions of the true vocal fold with the $KTP/532$ laser. Ann Otol Rhinol Laryngol 2003;112(6):534–9.

[22] Kacker A, April M, Ward RF. Use of potassium titanyl phosphate (KTP) laser in management of subglottic hemangiomas. Int J Pediatr Otorhinolaryngol 2001;59(1):15–21.

[23] Manolopoulos L, Stavroulaki P, Yiotakis J, et al. CO2 and KTP-532 laser cordectomy for bilateral vocal fold paralysis. J Laryngol Otol 1999;113(7):637–41.

[24] Strong MS, Healy GB, Vaughan CW, et al. Endoscopic management of laryngeal stenosis. Otolaryngol Clin North Am 1979;12(4):797–805.

[25] Strong MS, Jako GJ, Polanyi T, et al. Laser surgery in the aerodigestive tract. Am J Surg 1973;126(4):529–33.

[26] Strong MS, Jako GJ, Vaughan CW, et al. The use of CO_2 laser in otolaryngology: a progress report. Trans Sect Otolaryngol Am Acad Ophthalmol Otolaryngol 1976;82(5):595–602.

[27] Remacle M, Hassan F, Cohen D, et al. New computer-guided scanner for improving CO_2 laser-assisted microincision. Eur Arch Otorhinolaryngol 2005;262(2):113–9.

[28] Zeitels SM, Hillman RE, Desloge RB, et al. Phonomicrosurgery in singers and performing artists: treatment outcomes, management theories, & future directions. Ann Otol Rhinol Laryngol 2002;111(Suppl 190):S21–40.

[29] Hochman II, Zeitels SM. Phonomicrosurgical management of vocal fold polyps: the subepithelial microflap resection technique. J Voice 2000;14:112–8.

[30] Zeitels SM. Polyps. In: Linville M, editor. Atlas of phonomicrosurgery and other endolaryngeal procedures for benign and malignant disease. San Diego (CA): Singular; 2001. p. 37–56.

[31] Kass ES, Hillman RE, Zeitels SM. The submucosal infusion technique in phonomicrosurgery. Ann Otol Rhinol Laryngol 1996;105:341–7.

[32] Zeitels SM. Premalignant epithelium and microinvasive cancer of the vocal fold: The evolution of phonomicrosurgical management. Laryngoscope 1995;105(Suppl 67):S1–51.

[33] Zeitels SM. Nodules. In: Linville M, editor. Atlas of phonomicrosurgery and other endolaryngeal procedures for benign and malignant disease. San Diego (CA): Singular; 2001. p. 57–68.

[34] Anderson R, Parrish J. Selective photothermolysis: precise microsurgery by selective absorption of pulsed radiation. Science 1983;220:524–7.

[35] Anderson RR, Parrish JA. Microvasculature can be selectively damaged using lasers: a basic theory and experimental evidence in human skin. Lasers Surg Med 1981;1:263–76.

[36] Anderson RR, Jaenicke KF, Parrish JA. Mechanisms of selective vascular changes caused by dye lasers. Lasers Surg Med 1983;3:211–5.

[37] Bower CM, Flock S, Waner M. Flash pump dye laser treatment of laryngeal papillomas. Ann Otol Rhinol Laryngol 1998;107:1001–5.

[38] McMillan K, Shapshay SM, McGilligan JA. A 585-nanometer pulsed dye laser treatment of laryngeal papillomas: preliminary report. Laryngoscope 1998;108:968–72.

[39] Zeitels SM. 585nm Pulsed-dye laser treatment of glottal cancer: proof of concept and a possible harbinger of future treatment philosophy. Presented at the 84th annual meeting of the American Broncho-Esophagological Association. Phoenix, AZ. April 30–May 1, 2004.

[40] Zeitels SM. Universal modular laryngoscope/glottiscope system. Endocraft LLC, April 13, 1999. US patent 5 893 830. 1999.

[41] Zeitels SM. Adjustable supraglottiscope system. R. Wolf, March 3, 1992. US patent 5 092 314. 1992.

[42] Gray S, Pignatari SSN, Harding P. Morphologic ultrastructure of anchoring fibers in normal vocal fold basement membrane zone. J Voice 1994;8:48–52.

[43] Folkman J. Tumor angiogenesis: therapeutic implications. N Engl J Med 1971;285:1182–6.

[44] Folkman J. Angiogenesis. In: Braunwald ASFE, Kasper DL, Hauser SL, et al, editors. Harrison's textbook of internal medicine. Columbus (OH): McGraw Hill. 2001. p. 517–30.

[45] Jako GJ, Kleinsasser O. Endolaryngeal micro-diagnosis and microsurgery. Presented at the 120th annual meeting of the American Medical Association. New York, NY. 1966.

[46] Stanzel F, Raasch P, Haeussinger K. A new 2 micron laser in airway disobliteration: a feasibility and safety study. Presented at the 15th Annual Congress of the European Respiratory Society. Copenhagen, Denmark. September 17–21, 2005.

ELSEVIER
SAUNDERS

Otolaryngol Clin N Am
39 (2006) 173–189

OTOLARYNGOLOGIC
CLINICS
OF NORTH AMERICA

Endoscopic Treatment for Early Glottic Cancer: Indications and Oncologic Outcome

Giorgio Peretti, MD*, Cesare Piazza, MD,
Andrea Bolzoni, MD

*Department of Otolaryngology, University of Brescia,
Piazza Spedali Civili 1, Brescia 25123, Italy*

The term "early" laryngeal cancer has been used widely, but there is sometimes confusion as to its exact definition. As clearly defined by Ferlito and colleagues [1], early cancer is an invasive carcinoma confined to the lamina propria, not involving the adjacent muscles and cartilages but still capable of metastasis to the lymph nodes or distant sites. Strictly speaking, carcinoma in situ and deeply invasive carcinoma should be excluded from this definition of early cancer. Nevertheless, there is a general agreement in grouping Tis, T1, and T2 lesions together for diagnostic and therapeutic purposes. In this article, the broader definition of early glottic cancer will be used.

The natural progression of glottic cancer is influenced by the presence of well-known anatomical barriers such as the vocal ligament, conus elasticus, ventricular band, quadrangular membrane, and the cartilaginous framework, which delineates the visceral compartments of the larynx to which the neoplasm is usually confined until more advanced stages. Therefore, the pattern of growth and spread of these tumors are usually predictable, on the basis of their origin, localization, and adjacent anatomical structures [2–5].

The most frequent site of origin of glottic cancer is the free edge of the vocal cord, where it has a discrete tendency to remain confined to Reinke's space, superficially involving both the anterior commisure and the vocal process of the arytenoid. Deep extension is limited by the vocal ligament, which reduces the possibility of infiltration into the vocalis muscle. In

---

* Corresponding author.

E-mail address: g.peretti@tin.it (G. Peretti).

a cohort of 86 T1 tumors of the vocal cord, the present authors' group [6] found a 3.4% prevalence of superficial muscle infiltration on histologic evaluation. More advanced lesions involving the vocalis muscle reduce cord mobility and ultimately fix the entire hemilarynx. The clinical definition of such different features in vocal fold mobility is not always possible because of the lack of objective tools with which to measure the range of vocal cord or arytenoid motion. At any rate, indirect signs of tumor extension should be taken into account to distinguish between partial invasion of the vocal muscle (impaired mobility) and complete infiltration of the thyroarytenoid muscle and paraglottic space (vocal cord fixation), with possible involvement of the cricoarytenoid joint (hemilarynx fixation).

Superficial neoplastic extension to the anterior commisure at the glottic level rarely causes thyroid cartilage infiltration because of the presence of a solid barrier represented by Broyle's ligament. This anatomical structure, formed by the union of the thyroepiglottic ligament, the vocal ligaments, and the conus elasticus, is composed of dense fibroelastic tissue and has no glandular structures or blood or lymphatic vessels. On the other hand, tumors of the anterior commisure with supra- or subglottic extension have a propensity for spreading to the extralaryngeal tissues superiorly through the thyrohyoid membrane and inferiorly through the cricothyroid membrane. These areas are rich in glandular and vascular structures, which become denser in both the cranial and caudal directions [7–9].

Selection criteria for endoscopic treatment and instrumentation

One of the most rate-limiting factors for any endolaryngeal procedure is adequate exposure of the surgical field. Careful patient selection and the use of proper instrumentation are key factors in obtaining adequate exposure. Patient factors related to body habitus that may portend difficult exposure include cervical rigidity caused by arthrosis, short neck, micrognathia, macroglossia, and dental abnormalities (long teeth, prostheses, and malocclusion). These factors can be evaluated safely in a preoperative setting. A careful history should also be obtained regarding any previous radiation therapy or surgical treatment of the neck and spine that may have reduced the cervical extension, the opening of the mouth, or laryngeal suspension. Although the presence of such problems is not always an absolute contraindication to endoscopic procedures, preoperative counseling in these patients should always include different open-neck or nonsurgical options in the event that endoscopic visualization is inadequate.

The proper placement of the patient in the Boyce-Jackson position (ie, flexion of the neck on the chest and extension of the head on the neck at the occipitoatlantoid joint) is an essential prerequisite in optimizing exposure of the entire glottis, including the anterior commisure [10,11]. The selection of the most suitable laryngoscope often requires choosing among different shapes and dimensions. As a general rule, the ideal laryngoscope for exposure of the glottis and anterior commisure should be shaped according to the inverted V-shaped configuration of this region. The widest laryngoscope that can be intercalated safely between the anterior laryngeal structures and the anesthesia tube should be chosen. Working in the posterior part of the glottis during special steps of the surgical procedure requires repositioning the laryngoscope between the endotracheal tube and the interarytenoid region. Bimanual surgical procedures with the patient still in the Boyce-Jackson position are made possible by the use of an appropriate device that allows for true laryngeal suspension [12,13]. External manual or mechanical counterpressure of the larynx directed onto the cricoid and lower half of the thyroid cartilages helps substantially in obtaining adequate visualization of different portions of the larynx during the different steps of the procedure [14].

During any surgical procedure that uses laser devices, special care must be taken to avoid laser fires, including the use of anti-ignition endotracheal tubes with a double cuff and protection of the cuffs by wet sponges. Plume evacuators connected to the laryngoscope greatly improve visualization during laser use and play a role in protecting the surgical staff from biologic hazards. Antireflecting surgical instrumentation, adequate ocular protection, and protection of the patient and the operating room personnel are mandatory.

Preoperative and intraoperative diagnostic work-up

Appropriate phonomicrosurgical endoscopic management of early glottic cancer requires a meticulous evaluation of its superficial and deep extension (the so-called "invisible third" dimension) to minimize any excessive removal of surrounding healthy tissue. Indeed, the fine-tuning modulation of such a deep resection can have a significant impact on vocal outcome after endoscopic excision [15]. The present authors' diagnostic work-up begins with a preoperative endoscopic examination of the larynx by videolaryngostroboscopy (VLS) coupled with an evaluation using a 70° or 90° rigid telescope or flexible laryngoscope. Although VLS is associated with a high degree of intra- and interobserver variability because of its intrinsic subjectivity and the possibility of false-positive findings from adjacent inflammatory changes [16], it allows an initial evaluation of the lesion and its possible influence on the mucosal wave of the vocal cord. In fact, the maintenance of the mucosal wave is an indirect sign that the lesion is still located intraepithelially (up to carcinoma in situ), whereas a reduced or absent mucosal wave may indicate a lesion that has transgressed the basal membrane into the lamina propria (from microinvasive to frankly invasive carcinomas).

A more detailed, multiperspective endoscopic view of the larynx can be obtained subsequently by 0° and angled (30°, 70°, and 120°) rigid telescopes during suspension microlaryngoscopy [17,18]. In this way, zones of the endolarynx (anterior and posterior commisure, floor and roof of the ventricle, and subglottis), traditionally considered "hidden," can be visualized adequately (Fig. 1). By combining the use of angled telescopes with special probes or microinstrumentation to rotate and palpate the free edge of the true vocal cords, the false vocal cords can be lifted to inspect the ventricle, the arytenoids can be separated, and additional information can be collected.

In selected cases that are limited to the true vocal cord, a subepithelial saline infusion (SI) using the angled needle designed by Zeitels and Vaughan [19] allows for indirect confirmation of preoperative VLS findings. This provides further information about involvement of the lamina propria by the neoplastic growth. A complete hydrodissection of the mucoligamentous plane with consequent ballooning and lifting of the lesion from the underlying intermediate layer of the lamina propria suggests a purely intraepithelial

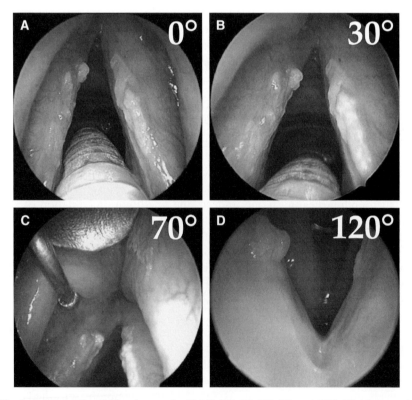

Fig. 1. Intraoperative rigid endoscopy by 0° (*A*), 30° (*B*), 70° (*C*), and 120° (*D*) telescopes in a patient who had erythroleukoplakia of both vocal cords. Note the exploration of the floor and bottom of the ventricle (*C*) by combination of an angled sucker and the 70° telescope. Subglottic extension of the lesions was ruled out by using the 120° endoscope.

extension of the neoplastic nests. Moreover, the artificial expansion of Reinke's space facilitates the subsequent removal of the lesion itself, serving as a heat sink to protect the vocal ligament from thermal damage from the laser. An incomplete or absent mucoligamentous hydrodissection after SI has the same implications of a reduced or absent mucosal wave on VLS and is associated with the likely transgression of the superficial layer of the lamina propria by neoplastic cells through the vocal ligament. The use of a SI in Reinke's space has drawbacks. The mucosa may balloon completely in cases of limited vocal ligament involvement by a few nests of neoplastic cells, yielding a false-negative impression of the extent of involvement. For this reason, the results of intraoperative SI should be always integrated with those of preoperative VLS. If the two tests give conflicting results, subepithelial or subligamental cordectomies should be tailored according to the more pessimistic scenario (ie, as if they were both positive for vocal ligament involvement). Applying such a simple diagnostic algorithm in a patient series from the authors' department, the combination of VLS and SI examinations resulted in a specificity, sensitivity, positive, negative predictive value, and accuracy of 89%, 100%, 88%, 100%, and 94%, respectively [20].

A number of ancillary tests have been advocated to intraoperatively define the macroscopic extension and nature of the erythroleukoplakia to be treated. The easiest and oldest technique was first introduced by Strong and coworkers [21], who described the use of supravital staining by 2% toluidine blue to precisely outline the superficial margins of the excisional biopsy (EB). This technique may be particularly useful in detecting multifocal patterns of cancerous growth. More sophisticated tools have been proposed by different authors [22–25] to evaluate the histology of lesions both in vivo and in situ. Contact endoscopy and autofluorescence provide the surgeon with the ability to understand the potentially malignant behavior of a glottic lesion before histologic examination is undertaken. Apart from concerns about cost effectiveness, contact endoscopy is limited in that only the superficial layers of the laryngeal epithelium can be visualized, and autofluorescence is limited by the masquerading effect of keratinization on the autofluorescent properties of the lesion. On the other hand, these techniques can be extremely useful from an iconographic point of view and may undergo further evolution as new stains and autofluorescent devices become available.

Recently, CT (with particular emphasis on the multislice technique) and MRI have played a definite role as imaging techniques for preoperative assessment, particularly in cases with anterior commisure involvement [26] and impairment of vocal cord mobility, to detect involvement of the paraglottic space [27,28]. The radiologic checklist for the endoscopic surgeon involved in the treatment of glottic tumors should include an assessment of the invasion of visceral spaces (with particular reference to submucosal supra- or subcommisural extension and posterolateral paraglottic space invasion with a transglottic pattern of growth) and laryngeal framework infiltration (at the level of the thyroid cartilage).

Classification of cordectomies

One of the most significant advances in the treatment of glottic cancer is the ability to perform endoscopic laser-assisted partial cordectomies, instead of the standard total cordectomy by traditional open-neck approaches. This technique makes the precise endoscopic modulation of the superficial and deep extent of resection possible, tailored to the individual neoplastic pattern of spread. Minimizing healthy tissue removal has become the cornerstone of the so-called "phonomicrosurgical" approach to vocal cord cancer [15]. To standardize common surgical language and make it possible to compare oncologic and functional outcome from different institutions, the European Laryngological Society published a consensus paper with a classification that includes five types of endoscopic cordectomies (Fig. 2) [29].

Type I or subepithelial cordectomy is the excision of the epithelium through the superficial layer of the lamina propria or Reinke's space. In the present authors' practice, this procedure is indicated whenever a glottic lesion presents with a normal mucosal wave at preoperative VLS and intraoperative complete mucoligamentous hydrodissection after SI, indicating an intraepithelial precancerous or neoplastic lesion up to carcinoma in situ. Type II or subligamental cordectomy is the removal of the intermediate and deep layers of lamina propria (which together form the vocal ligament), including the very superficial fibers of the adjacent vocal muscle. The present authors perform this resection in all cases of suspected invasion of the vocal ligament by microinvasive or invasive carcinomas not reaching the anterior commisure as evaluated by VLS (reduced or absent mucosal wave) and SI (incomplete or absent mucosal ballooning). Type III or transmuscular cordectomy is the removal of the medial part of the thyroarytenoid muscle for lesions previously sampled for biopsy elsewhere or inadequately excised without correct orientation and evaluation of the surgical margins. In the present authors' opinion, a second (complementary) procedure is indicated in these cases, in which there may be equivocal evidence of close or positive margins with or without the postoperative appearance of persistent disease at endoscopy. Because of the reduced accuracy of our diagnostic work-up in distinguishing between scar tissue, postsurgical inflammation, and residual disease, a deeper resection is mandatory in such cases to get clear margins. Type IV or total cordectomy is the compartmental resection of the entire vocal cord (including the fat-containing space lateral to the thyroarytenoid muscle) through a subperichondral plane along the thyroid lamina. The present authors use this technique in the presence of indirect signs of vocal muscle infiltration as shown by reduced vocal cord mobility during preoperative laryngoscopic examination, radiologic evidence of the involvement of

I	**Subephitelial cordectomy**: limited to the superficial layer of the lamina propria	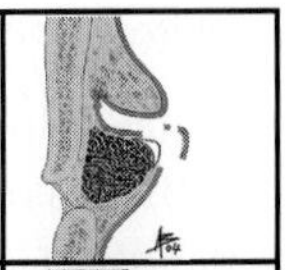
II	**Subligamental cordectomy**: limited to the mucosa, Reinke's space, the vocal ligament, and the very superficial part of the vocal muscle	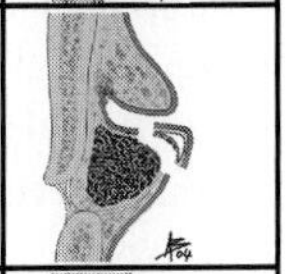
III	**Transmuscular cordectomy**: limited to the medial portion of the vocal muscle	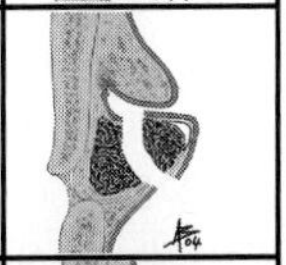
IV	**Total cordectomy**: involving the entire vocal cord together with the inner perichondrium	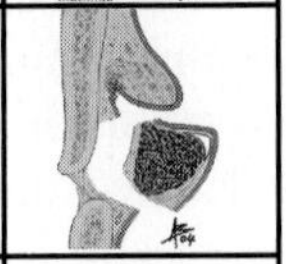
Va	**Extended cordectomy (a)**: extended to the contralateral vocal cord	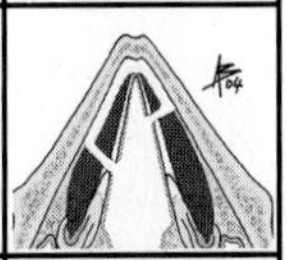
Vb	**Extended cordectomy (b)**: extended to the arytenoid cartilage	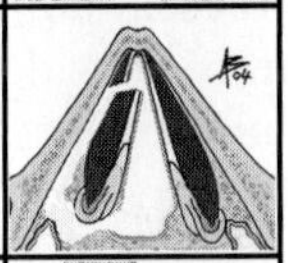
Vc	**Extended cordectomy (c)**: extended to the supraglottic region	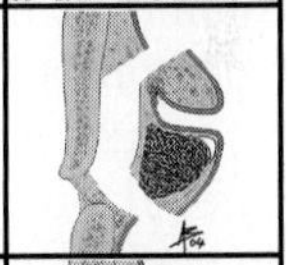
Vd	**Extended cordectomy (d)**: extended to the subglottic region	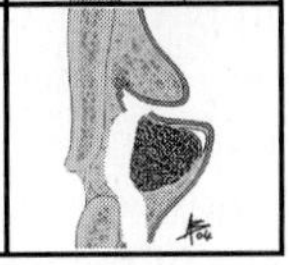

Fig. 2. Classification of endoscopic cordectomies by the European Laryngological Society [29].

the paraglottic space, and intraoperative stiffness on palpation. Type V or extended cordectomy is any kind of excision involving the whole or part of one vocal fold, with involvement of adjacent subsites. In detail, Remacle and coworkers [29] further subclassified extended cordectomies into four groups according to the subsite resected: type Va for contralateral vocal cord; type Vb for arytenoid; type Vc for ventricle and false fold; and type Vd for subglottis. In these lesions, a precise three-dimensional evaluation of the extent of surgical resection requires the integration between clinical-endoscopic tools with radiologic imaging, which allows the visualization of visceral spaces and cartilaginous framework involvement by neoplastic disease.

Excisional biopsy approach for Tis–T1a lesions

The EB concept in the management of early laryngeal cancer was first introduced by Blakeslee and colleagues [30] as the "en bloc" removal of the entire lesion, with a rim of surrounding healthy tissue. In this way, precise histopathologic diagnosis of the whole specimen and definitive therapeutic excision of the neoplasm are obtained in a single procedure, as long as clear surgical margins have been ensured. The performance of an EB without previous information about the nature of the lesion to be treated endoscopically can be difficult even for the skilled head and neck surgeon, who is accustomed to planning treatment only after intraoperative staging and histopathologic diagnosis. Such a change of mindset is made possible by the recent, previously described diagnostic advances that reduce the false-positive rate to a minimum. Indeed, the precise phonomicrosurgical modulation of the deep extension of tissue removal is fine-tuned based on the diagnostic work-up, detailed in the present report. In dealing with precancerous or frankly neoplastic lesions of the vocal cords, overtreatment is obviously preferable to undertreatment, even though the optimal compromise between adequate oncologic resection margins and vocal outcome should always remain one of the main treatment goals [6].

In the present authors' opinion, performing EB by type I and II cordectomies can be considered an ideal first-line treatment option in patients who have not undergone a biopsy and are affected by glottic erythroleukoplakia consistent with a diagnosis of Tis limited to one vocal cord and T1a without anterior commisure involvement (Fig. 3) [31]. This holds true not only from an oncologic point of view but also for functional outcomes and cost-effectiveness ratio concerns when the endoscopic approach is compared with both traditional open-neck techniques and radiation therapy [32–34]. By contrast, in patients who have undergone previous random biopsies, "mucosal stripping," or incomplete endoscopic excision (with close or positive surgical margins), a disruption of the normal multilayered vocal cord structure does not allow one to distinguish between iatrogenic alterations and neoplastic tissue of the vocal cord. In such a situation, minimization of resection of the deeper tissue margins is therefore not possible and a cordectomy (type III) is usually recommended as definitive treatment [6,20].

Compartmental approach for T1b–T2 lesions

For the management of more advanced glottic tumors, endoscopic surgery does not represent the treatment of choice but is one of several possible therapeutic tools to be chosen on the basis of patient- and tumor-related variables. The advantages of endoscopic techniques include limited morbidity in terms of the reduced need for a tracheotomy and a nasogastric feeding tube, a short hospitalization time with reduced financial and societal costs, respect of the laryngeal framework integrity, and no preclusion of further

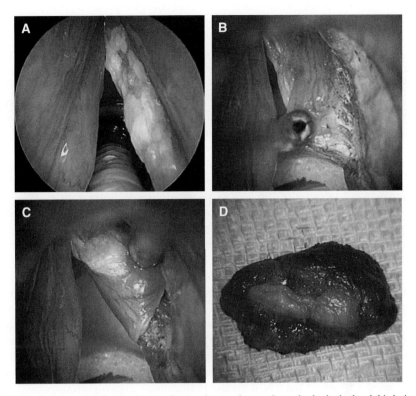

Fig. 3. Intraoperative rigid endoscopy by 0° telescope in a patient who had a leukoplakic lesion limited to the right vocal cord (*A*). A subligamental cordectomy (type II) was performed because of impaired mucosal wave at VLS and incomplete mucoligamentous hydrodissection with SI of Reinke's space. Note the superior incision line with exposure of the vocal muscle (*B*) and the demarcation of the posteroinferior margin of the EB (*C*). The leukoplakic lesion was therefore removed en bloc within macroscopically healthy tissues (*D*).

complementary or salvage treatments. More traditional open surgical alternatives as well as other emerging treatment protocols (eg, concomitant chemoradiation and radiation therapy or neoadjuvant chemotherapy followed by surgery) should always be considered during preoperative patient counseling. In the management of these lesions, the EB concept loses its advantages, and endoscopic procedures must be considered as compartmental resections following criteria similar to those observed during organ preservation surgery. Not only is a previous biopsy therefore mandatory but even en bloc removal is not considered an essential prerequisite. In fact, the piecemeal technique has been advocated strongly by a number of authors [35–40] as a useful tool in precisely evaluating the deep extension of the tumor. This technique takes advantage of the fact that different types of tissues are characterized by different interaction properties when cut through with the laser. Moreover, such an approach is recommended for practical reasons when lesions are so large that they are not amenable to complete and three-dimensional visualization through the laryngoscope.

Anterior commisure involvement at the level of the glottis does not represent a limit to endoscopic treatment as long as supra- or subcommisural extensions can be excluded safely by accurate pre- and intraoperative evaluation with proper imaging and endoscopy. When these superficial or deep infiltrations are present or suspected, intraoperative infrapetiolar exploration as described by Zeitels [41] should be performed. This maneuver aims to exclude any pre-epiglottic space invasion or inner perichondral infiltration of the thyroid cartilage. Subglottic extension of the tumor more than 1 cm caudal to the anterior commisure is a contraindication to endoscopic management because of the lack of proper tangential exposure.

Tumors involving the lateral supra- or subglottic regions are easily controlled when superficially spreading to the false cords and ventricle or to the mucosal lining of the cricoid cartilage. Deeper extension to the vocalis muscle does not have a negative impact on endoscopic local control if the fat-containing space medial to the thyroid lamina is spared. Clinically suspected or evident paraglottic space neoplastic involvement presents a different problem. Tucker and colleagues [42–43] originally defined the paraglottic space as a laryngeal compartment composed of connective tissue, limited anterolaterally by the thyroid cartilage, inferomedially by the conus elasticus, superomedially by the ventricle and quadrangular membrane, and dorsally by the piriform sinus [42,43]. Other authors [44–48], in agreement with the latest version of the TNM system [49], define the paraglottic space at the glottic level as the purely fat-containing, areolar tissue-filled space lateral to the thyroarytenoid muscle. Because of the narrow dimensions of this space at the glottic level, the detection of its early involvement in vocal cord cancer can present a challenge even for the experienced radiologist [27,28]. The paraglottic space can be involved by glottic neoplasms, passing either through the vocal muscle or through the ventricle and false vocal cord or at the level of the subglottis underneath the conus elasticus. Hence, the extralaryngeal extension can involve the posterior cricothyroid membrane and the adjacent soft tissues. Tumors arising primarily in the ventricle that progress directly through its floor into the paraglottic space and then in a craniocaudal direction (becoming transglottic) are less common. When neoplasms gain access to the paraglottic compartment, there are no further barriers to the transglottic spread tumor to adjacent laryngeal subsites and extralaryngeal soft tissues. In the present authors' experience, such aggressive behavior is associated frequently with the impairment of vocal cord mobility because of the involvement of the posterolateral paraglottic space. In such cases, endoscopic vertical partial laryngectomy with arytenoidectomy is necessary. Lesser procedures should be considered inadequate because of the high risk of persistent disease in the thyroarytenoid space [48].

A second-look microlaryngoscopic evaluation at the end of the healing process (30–60 days after the first endoscopic procedure) plays a definite role in the therapeutic approach to T1b and T2 lesions. On the basis of histologic evaluation of the previous specimen, specifically oriented re-excision can be performed in this setting to areas suspected for persistent disease.

Oncologic outcome

Close follow-up, including VLS examination bimonthly in the first year and with decreasing frequency in subsequent years, is mandatory whenever a phonomicrosurgical approach is performed for Tis and T1 vocal-fold lesions. Close follow-up allows for the early detection of alterations in the superficial healing process of the surgical bed, which are suggestive of persistent or recurrent disease. In the present authors' experience, approximately 14% of Tis and T1 lesions needed re-excision; one third for positive deep margin of resection and the remainder for postoperative endoscopic suspicion of persistent disease within the first 6 months of follow-up. However, in these cases, the second surgical specimen turned out to have residual foci of carcinoma in only 33% of cases, or 4.5% of the entire cohort of our patients [50].

From an oncologic standpoint, during the last 2 decades, the endoscopic resection of Tis and T1 glottic cancer has been shown to be a sound technique by a number of authors, with results comparable to radiation therapy and open-neck surgery [35–38,51–58]. An ultimate local control rate of 90% with laser alone and a laryngeal preservation rate of 94.4% have been reported by the authors' group [50]. These results are comparable to those of the most recent series in which ultimate local control rates with the endoscopic approach range between 77% and 100%, and laryngeal preservation rates range between 90% and 100% (Table 1) [59–62]. Excellent ultimate local control with laser alone is also seen when the endoscopic approach is used as salvage treatment in cases of recurrent cancer, particularly with superficial or multifocal patterns of spread [63]. The high laryngeal preservation rate can be maintained by shifting to salvage supracricoid laryngectomy in cases of submucosal recurrence in the visceral spaces and by shifting to radiation therapy in cases of multifocal superficial spreading disease without affecting the success rate in terms of local control and still preserving appreciable laryngeal function. Moreover, no increase in the postoperative complication rate has been observed in laryngeal conservation surgery after endoscopic failure, in contrast with that observed after radiation therapy [64].

The T2 category, even in the latest version of the TNM classification system [49], includes lesions that are extremely heterogeneous in terms of local extension and prognosis. In these situations, endoscopic treatment should be considered as a therapeutic option, to be decided on the basis of different patient and tumor variables. Apart from the obvious patient related factors (gender, professional activity, general status, and previous therapeutic attempts), the characteristics of the tumor (size, sites and subsites involved,

Table 1
Review of the most recent literature concerning series of patients affected by T1 glottic cancer treated with endoscopic surgery

Study	Number of patients	Local control (5 years) (%)	Laryngeal preservation (5 years) (%)
Spector et al [57] 1992	55 T1a	77	90
	6 T1b		
Moreau [59] 2000	26 Tis	100	100
	62 T1a		
	24 T1b		
Eckel et al [60] 2001	161	86.3	91.7
Peretti et al [50] 2001	13 Tis	92	94.4
	75 T1	90	
Gallo et al [61] 2002	12 Tis	100	100
	117 T1a	94	
	22 T1b	91	
Steiner et al [62] 2005	333 T1a	89.3	97.6

Abbreviations: Tis, carcinoma in situ; T1a, tumor involving one vocal cord; T1b, tumor involving both vocal cords with or without extension to the anterior commissure.

superficial and deep extension, and positive lymph nodes) must be regarded as fundamental in influencing the success rate after endoscopic resection. In fact, good oncologic outcomes (ranging from 79%–100% for local control with laser alone) have been observed in patients with T2 neoplasms with superficial extension to the supra- or subglottis (lateral portion) or with involvement of the vocalis muscle compartment but without invasion of the fat tissue medial to the thyroid lamina (Giorgio Peretti, MD, unpublished observations, 2005). This subset of T2 lesions should therefore be considered the most suitable for endoscopic treatment.

In contrast, in the case of anterior commisure tumors extending to the supra- or subglottic regions, local control with laser alone decreased to 68%, which is still comparable to results obtained after radiation therapy [65–70] or after open frontolateral laryngectomy [71–73] but significantly worse than those reported after supracricoid laryngectomy, especially when combined with neoadjuvant chemotherapy [74–77]. Laryngeal preservation rates after endoscopic surgery for T2 glottic cancer are approximately 90% in virtually every series of the most recent literature and are therefore comparable to those achieved with subtotal laryngectomy (Table 2) [78–80].

The present authors' results in dealing with lesions preoperatively staged as cT2 but postoperatively upstaged to pT3 for histologic evidence of deep infiltration at the level of the posterolateral paraglottic space (according to the UICC AJCC TNM Classification System, 6th edition [49]) have been completely disappointing [48]. This is therefore, at least in the present authors' experience, to be regarded as a relative contraindication for an endoscopic approach alone in favor of multimodality protocols such as supracricoid laryngectomy with neoadjuvant chemotherapy, laser surgery

Table 2
Review of the most recent literature concerning series of patients affected by T2 glottic cancer treated with endoscopic surgery

Study	Number of patients	Local control (5 years) (%)	Laryngeal preservation (5 years) (%)	Comments
Eckel [60] 2001	91	82.9	89.3	37% of recurrence were AC+
Steiner et al [78] 2004	75 (T2a)	79 (AC+) 74 (AC−)	93 (AC+) 97 (AC−)	60% of recurrence had subglottic extension and 30% required total laryngectomy
Steiner et al [79] 2005	212 (T2a–b)	84 (T2a) 74 (T2b)	95 (T2a) 85 (T2b)	—
Motta et al [80] 2005	236	61 (unilateral) 55 (bilateral)	82.5	—
Peretti et al (unpublished series, June 2005)	67	82	94	—

Abbreviations: T2a, tumor with normal vocal cord mobility; T2b, tumor with impaired vocal cord mobility; AC, anterior commisure; +, involved by the tumor; −, not involved by the tumor.

followed by radiation therapy, and concomitant chemoradiation therapy organ preservation regimens. To improve success rates in these challenging cases, other authors have proposed various types of extended resections resembling endoscopic frontolateral laryngectomies with or without arytenoidectomy [40,81]. Even with these larger lesions, an endoscopic approach should remain a fundamental part of the management to precisely stage the lesion. Endoscopic partial resection of the tumor allows one to clearly evaluate its deep extension and subsequently complete the treatment by a further endoscopic procedure or with more conventional therapeutic approaches.

Summary

The present authors' treatment approach for the comprehensive management of early glottic cancer (Tis–T2) can be categorized into two basic therapeutic scenarios. Tis and T1a lesions of the midcord are treated preferably by an EB, which, after appropriate pre- and intraoperative diagnostic workup, including at least VLS, SI into the Reinke's space, and rigid endoscopy, allows the achievement, in a single procedure, of a precise diagnosis and definitive treatment of the lesion. Postoperative voice quality has been shown to be comparable to that of controls. Moreover, this approach is associated with minimal morbidity, short hospitalization time, and a high cost-effectiveness ratio. On the other hand, T1b and T2 tumors deserve special attention because comparable oncologic outcomes can be achieved with other surgical and nonsurgical therapeutic modalities. Therefore, the appropriate preoperative counseling, including other voice-sparing options (eg, radiation or chemoradiation therapy), should be always discussed with the patient. Great caution should be also observed with T2 lesions in which there is impaired vocal cord mobility because of the possibility of invasion through the vocal muscle into the paraglottic space (T3). In such cases, frustrating results have been obtained in the present authors' series by endoscopic surgery alone, and further complementary treatment modalities should always be considered.

References

[1] Ferlito A, Carbone A, DeSanto LW, et al. "Early" cancer of the larynx: the concept as defined by clinician, pathologist, and biologist. Ann Otol Rhinol Laryngol 1996;105:245–50.
[2] Russ JE, Sullivan C, Gallager HS, et al. Conservation surgery of the larynx: a reappraisal based on whole organ study. Am J Surg 1979;138:588–96.
[3] Kirchner JA, Carter D. Intralaryngeal barriers to the spread of cancer. Acta Otolaryngol 1987;103:503–13.
[4] Beitler JJ, Mahadevia PS, Silver CE, et al. New barriers to ventricular invasion in paraglottic laryngeal cancer. Cancer 1993;73:2648–52.
[5] Buckley JG, MacLennan K. Cancer spread in the larynx: a pathologic basis for conservation surgery. Head Neck 2000;22:265–74.
[6] Peretti G, Piazza C, Balzanelli C, et al. Vocal outcome after endoscopic cordectomies for Tis and T1 glottic carcinoma. Ann Otol Rhinol Laryngol 2003;112:174–9.
[7] Kirchner JA. Two hundred laryngeal cancers: patterns of growth and spread as seen in serial section. Laryngoscope 1977;87:474–82.
[8] Hirano M, Kurita S, Matsuoka H, et al. Vocal fold fixation in laryngeal carcinomas. Acta Otolaryngol 1991;111:449–54.
[9] Laccourreye O, Salzer SJ, Brasnu D, et al. Glottic carcinoma with a fixed true vocal cord: outcomes after neoadjuvant chemotherapy and supracricoid partial laryngectomy with cricohyoidoepiglottopexy. Otolaryngol Head Neck Surg 1996;114:400–6.
[10] Boyce JW. Duties of the second assistant in endoscopy per os. In: Jackson C, editor. Tracheobronchoscopy, esophagoscopy and gastroscopy. St. Louis (MO): The Laryngoscope Co; 1907. p. 145–7.
[11] Jackson C. Position of the patient for peroral endoscopy. In: Jackson C, editor. Peroral endoscopy and laryngeal surgery. St. Louis (MO): The Laryngoscope Co; 1915. p. 77–8.
[12] Grundfast KM, Vaughan CW, Strong MS, et al. Suspension microlaryngoscopy in the Boyce position with a new suspension gallows. Ann Otol Rhinol Laryngol 1978;87:560–6.
[13] Zeitels SM, Burns JE, Dailey SH. Suspension laryngoscopy revisited. Ann Otol Rhinol Laryngol 2004;113:16–22.
[14] Zeitels SM, Vaughan CW. "External counterpressure" and "internal distention" for optimal laryngoscopic exposure of the anterior glottal commisure. Ann Otol Rhinol Laryngol 1994;103:669–75.
[15] Zeitels SM. Premalignant epithelium and microinvasive cancer of the vocal fold: the evolution of phonomicrosurgical management. Laryngoscope 1995;105(Suppl 3):S1–51.
[16] Colden D, Zeitels SM, Hillman RE, et al. Stroboscopic assessment of vocal fold keratosis and glottic cancer. Ann Otol Rhinol Laryngol 2001;110:293–8.

[17] Andrea M, Dias O. Newer techniques of laryngeal assessment. In: Cummings CW, Fredrickson JM, Harker LA, et al, editors. Otolaryngology head and neck surgery. 3rd edition. St. Louis (MO): Mosby; 1998. p. 1967–78.

[18] Andrea M, Dias O. Rigid and contact endoscopy of the larynx. In: Ferlito A, editor. Diseases of the larynx. Edinburgh: Churchill Livingstone; 2000. p. 101–11.

[19] Zeitels SM, Vaughan CW. A submucosal vocal fold infusion needle. Otolaryngol Head Neck Surg 1991;105:478–9.

[20] Peretti G, Piazza C, Berlucchi M, et al. Pre- and intraoperative assessment of mid-cord erythroleukoplakias: a prospective study on 52 patients. Eur Arch Otorhinolaryngol 2003;260: 525–8.

[21] Strong MS, Vaughan CW, Incze J. Toluidine blue in diagnosis of cancer of the larynx. Arch Otolaryngol Head Neck Surg 1970;91:515–9.

[22] Andrea M, Dias O, Santos A. Contact endoscopy during microlaryngeal surgery: a new technique for endoscopic examination of the larynx. Ann Otol Rhinol Laryngol 1995; 104:333–9.

[23] Fryen A, Glanz H, Lohmann W, et al. Significance of autofluorescence for the optical demarcation of field cancerisation in the upper aerodigestive tract. Acta Otolaryngol 1997;117: 316–9.

[24] Malzahn K, Dreyer T, Glanz H, et al. Autofluorescence endoscopy in the diagnosis of early laryngeal cancer and its precursor lesions. Laryngoscope 2002;112:488–93.

[25] Arens C, Glanz H, Dreyer T, et al. Compact endoscopy of the larynx. Ann Otol Rhinol Laryngol 2003;112:113–9.

[26] Barbosa MM, Araújo VJF, Boasquevisque E, et al. Anterior vocal commisure invasion in laryngeal carcinoma diagnosis. Laryngoscope 2005;115:724–30.

[27] Murakami R, Furusawa M, Baba Y, et al. Dynamic helical CT of T1 and T2 glottic carcinomas: predictive value for local control with radiation therapy. AJNR Am J Neuroradiol 2000;21:1320–6.

[28] Murakami R, Nishimura R, Baba Y, et al. Prognostic factors of glottic carcinomas treated with radiation therapy: value of the adjacent sign on radiological examinations in the sixth edition of the UICC TNM staging system. Int J Radiat Oncol Biol Phys 2005;61:471–5.

[29] Remacle M, Eckel HE, Antonelli AR, et al. Endoscopic cordectomy, a proposal for a classification by the Working Committee, European Laryngological Society. Eur Arch Otorhinolaryngol 2000;257:227–31.

[30] Blakeslee D, Vaughan CW, Shapshay SM, et al. Excisional biopsy in the selective management of T1 glottic cancer: a three-year follow-up study. Laryngoscope 1984;94:488–94.

[31] Peretti G, Cappiello J, Nicolai P, et al. Endoscopic laser excisional biopsy for selected glottic carcinomas. Laryngoscope 1994;104:1276–9.

[32] Cragle SP, Brandenburg JH. Laser cordectomy or radiotherapy: cure rates, communication, and cost. Otolaryngol Head Neck Surg 1993;108:648–54.

[33] Myers EN, Wagner RL, Johnson JT. Microlaryngoscopic surgery for T1 glottic lesions: a cost-effective option. Ann Otol Rhinol Laryngol 1994;103:28–30.

[34] Brandenburg JH. Laser cordotomy versus radiotherapy: an objective cost analysis. Ann Otol Rhinol Laryngol 2001;110:312–8.

[35] Steiner W. Experience in endoscopic laser surgery of malignant tumours of the upper aerodigestive tract. Adv Otolaryngol 1988;39:135–44.

[36] Thumfart WF, Eckel HE. Endolaryngeal laser surgery in the treatment of laryngeal cancers: the current Cologne concept. HNO 1990;38:174–8.

[37] Eckel H, Thumfart WF. Laser surgery for the treatment of larynx carcinomas: indications, techniques, and preliminary results. Ann Otol Rhinol Laryngol 1992;101:113–8.

[38] Steiner W. Results of curative laser microsurgery of laryngeal carcinomas. Am J Otolaryngol 1993;14:116–21.

[39] Rudert HH, Werner JA. Endoscopic resections of glottic and supraglottic carcinomas with the CO2 laser. Eur Arch Otorhinolaryngol 1995;252:146–8.

[40] Steiner W, Ambrosch P. Endoscopic laser surgery of the upper aerodigestive tract: with special emphasis on cancer surgery. Stuttgart: Thieme; 2001.

[41] Zeitels SM. Infrapetiole exploration of the supraglottis for exposure of the anterior glottal commisure. J Voice 1998;12:117–22.

[42] Tucker GF, Smith HR. A histological demonstration of the development of laryngeal connective tissue compartments. Trans Am Acad Ophthalmol Otolaryngol 1962;66:308–18.

[43] Tucker GF. Some clinical inferences from the study of serial laryngeal sections. Laryngoscope 1963;73:728–48.

[44] Maguire A, Dayal VS. Supraglottic anatomy: the pre- or the peri-epiglottic space? Can J Otolaryngol 1974;3:432–45.

[45] Sato K, Kurita S, Hirano M. Location of the preepiglottic space and its relationship to the paraglottic space. Ann Otol Rhinol Laryngol 1993;102:930–4.

[46] Reidenbach MM. The paraglottic space and transglottic cancer: anatomical considerations. Clin Anat 1996;9:244–51.

[47] Reidenbach MM. Borders and topographic relationships of the paraglottic space. Eur Arch Otorhinolaryngol 1997;254:193–5.

[48] Peretti G, Piazza C, Mensi MC, et al. Endoscopic treatment of cT2 glottic carcinoma: prognostic impact of different pT subcategories. Ann Otol Rhinol Laryngol 2005;114:579–86.

[49] Union Internationale Contre le Cancer. TNM classification of malignant tumours. 6th edition. New York: Wiley-Liss; 2002.

[50] Peretti G, Nicolai P, Piazza C, et al. Oncological results of endoscopic resections of Tis and T1 glottic carcinomas by carbon dioxide laser. Ann Otol Rhinol Laryngol 2001; 110:820–6.

[51] Ossoff RH, Sisson GA, Shapshay SM. Endoscopic management of selected early vocal cord carcinoma. Ann Otol Rhinol Laryngol 1985;94:560–4.

[52] Wetmore SJ, Key JM, Suen JY. Laser therapy for T1 glottic carcinoma of the larynx. Arch Otolaryngol Head Neck Surg 1986;112:853–5.

[53] McGuirt WF, Koufman JA. Endoscopic laser surgery: an alternative in laryngeal cancer treatment. Arch Otolaryngol Head Neck Surg 1987;113:501–5.

[54] Wolfensberger M, Dort JC. Endoscopic laser surgery for early glottic carcinoma: a clinical and experimental study. Laryngoscope 1990;100:1100–5.

[55] Davis RK, Kelly SM, Parkin JL, et al. Selective management of early glottic cancer. Laryngoscope 1990;100:1306–9.

[56] Zeitels SM. Phonomicrosurgical treatment of early glottic cancer and carcinoma in situ. Am J Surg 1996;172:704–9.

[57] Spector JG, Sessions DG, Chao KS, et al. Stage I (T1N0M0) squamous cell carcinoma of the laryngeal glottis: therapeutic results and voice preservation. Head Neck 1999;21:707–17.

[58] Peretti G, Nicolai P, Redaelli De Zinis LO, et al. Endoscopic CO2 laser excision for Tis, T1, and T2 glottic carcinomas: cure rates and prognostic factors. Otolaryngol Head Neck Surg 2000;123:124–31.

[59] Moreau PR. Treatment of laryngeal carcinomas by laser endoscopic microsurgery. Laryngoscope 2000;110:1000–6.

[60] Eckel HE. Local recurrence following transoral laser surgery for early glottic carcinoma: frequency, management and outcome. Ann Otol Rhinol Laryngol 2001;110:7–15.

[61] Gallo A, de Vincentiis M, Manciocco V, et al. CO2 laser cordectomy for early-stage glottic carcinoma: a long-term follow-up of 156 cases. Laryngoscope 2002;112:370–4.

[62] Steiner W, Ambrosch P, Palme CE, et al. Laser microsurgical resection of T1a glottic carcinoma: results of 333 cases. Presented at the 126th Annual Meeting of the American Laryngological Association. Boca Raton, FL, May 13–14, 2005 [abstract].

[63] Peretti G, Piazza C, Bolzoni A, et al. Analysis of recurrence in 322 Tis, T1, or T2 glottic carcinomas treated by carbon dioxide laser. Ann Otol Rhinol Laryngol 2004;113:853–8.

[64] Spriano G, Pellini R, Romano G, et al. Supracricoid partial laryngectomy as salvage surgery after radiation failure. Head Neck 2002;24:759–65.

[65] Mendenhall WM, Amdur RJ, Morris CG, et al. T1–T2N0 squamous cell carcinoma of the glottic larynx treated with radiation therapy. J Clin Oncol 2001;19:4029–36.

[66] Jørgensen K, Godballe C, Hansen O, et al. Cancer of the larynx: treatment results after primary radiotherapy with salvage surgery in a series of 1005 patients. Acta Oncol 2002;41: 69–76.

[67] Johansen LV, Grau C, Overgaard J. Glottic carcinoma: patterns of failure and salvage treatment after curative radiotherapy in 861 consecutive patients. Radiother Oncol 2002;63: 257–67.

[68] Johansen LV, Grau C, Overgaard J. Laryngeal carcinoma: multivariate analysis of prognostic factors in 1252 consecutive patients treated with primary radiotherapy. Acta Oncol 2003; 42:771–8.

[69] Garden AS, Forster K, Wong P-F, et al. Results of radiotherapy for T2N0 glottic carcinoma: does the "2" stand for twice-daily treatment? Int J Radiat Oncol Biol Phys 2003;55:322–8.

[70] Colasanto JM, Haffty BG, Wilson LD. Evaluation of local recurrence and second malignancy in patients with T1 and T2 squamous cell carcinoma of the larynx. Cancer J 2004; 10:61–6.

[71] Laccourreye O, Weinstein G, Brasnu D, et al. Vertical partial laryngectomy: a critical analysis of local recurrence. Ann Otol Rhinol Laryngol 1991;30:357–62.

[72] Laccourreye O, Gutierrez-Fonseca R, Garcia D, et al. Local recurrence after vertical partial laryngectomy, a conservative modality of treatment for patients with stage I–II squamous cell carcinoma of the glottis. Cancer 1999;85:2549–56.

[73] Laccourreye O, Laccourreye L, Garcia D, et al. Vertical partial laryngectomy versus supracricoid partial laryngectomy for selected carcinomas of the true vocal cord classified as T2N0. Ann Otol Rhinol Laryngol 2000;109:965–71.

[74] Laccourreye O, Muscatello L, Laccourreye L, et al. Supracricoid partial laryngectomy with cricohyoidoepiglottopexy for "early" glottic carcinoma classified as T1–T2N0 invading the anterior commisure. Am J Otolaryngol 1997;18:385–90.

[75] Chevalier D, Laccourreye O, Brasnu D, et al. Cricohyoidoepiglottopexy for glottic carcinoma with fixation or impaired motion of the true vocal cord: 5-year oncologic results with 112 patients. Ann Otol Rhinol Laryngol 1997;106:364–9.

[76] Laccourreye O, Diaz EM Jr, Bassot V, et al. A multimodal strategy for the treatment of patients with T2 invasive squamous cell carcinoma of the glottis. Cancer 1999;85:40–6.

[77] Laccourreye O, Bassot V, Brasnu D, et al. Chemotherapy combined with conservation surgery in the treatment of early larynx cancer. Curr Opin Oncol 1999;11:200–3.

[78] Steiner W, Ambrosch P, Rodel RM, et al. Impact of anterior commisure involvement on local control of early glottic carcinoma treated by laser microresection. Laryngoscope 2004; 114:1485–91.

[79] Steiner W, Martin A, Ambrosch P, et al. Laser microsurgical treatment of pT2/3N0 carcinoma of the glottis: results of 301 cases. Presented at the 85th Annual meeting of the American Broncho-Esophagological Association. Boca Raton, FL, May 13–14, 2005 [abstract].

[80] Motta G, Esposito E, Motta S, et al. CO2 laser surgery in the treatment of glottic cancer. Head Neck 2005;27:566–74.

[81] Davis RK, Hadley K, Smith ME. Endoscopic vertical partial laryngectomy. Laryngoscope 2004;114:236–40.

ELSEVIER
SAUNDERS

Otolaryngol Clin N Am
39 (2006) 191–204

OTOLARYNGOLOGIC
CLINICS
OF NORTH AMERICA

Reconstruction of Glottic Defects after Endoscopic Cordectomy: Voice Outcome

Marc Remacle, MD, PhD*, Georges Lawson, MD,
Dominique Morsomme, Speech Th,
Jacques Jamart, MD

University Hospital of Louvain at Mont-Godinne, Therasse Avenue 1, 5530 Yvoir, Belgium

Endoscopic cordectomy is a recognized treatment for T1 and selected T2 glottic carcinoma [1–4]. Oncologic effectiveness has been demonstrated repeatedly with identical survival rates for radiotherapy and surgery (cause-specific survival rate $\geq$ 90%) [5–8]. If the local control is ultimately similar after surgery and radiotherapy, the functional disadvantages after surgery are moderate and clearly are counterbalanced by a significant decrease in long-term laryngeal preservation rate after radiotherapy (90.1% after radiotherapy versus 97.4% after surgery) [5]. Results of various studies that compared voice outcome after surgery or radiotherapy are controversial; voice quality is reported to be equivalent [6,7,9] or better after radiotherapy [8,10–12].

Although laryngeal cancer has an impact on patients' lifestyles, they seldom relate this to vocal dysfunction [3,13,14]. Whereas evaluation of preoperative and postoperative objective results showed significant voice improvement after types I and II cordectomies (European Laryngological Society [ELS] classification) [15], the postoperative vocal outcome was not significantly different from the preoperative pattern after types III, IV, and V cordectomies [16]. Once the body layer of the vocal fold is injured, vocal quality decreases significantly. Even if there is no linear correlation with the amount of tissue removed [17], a significant glottic gap may persist, which in some cases, leads to poor voice quality. The development of thick, and sometimes partially stenosing, synechiae at the anterior commissure also is a major factor that results in poor vocal outcome after extended cordectomy [18].

---

* Corresponding author.
E-mail address: remacle@orlo.ucl.ac.be (M. Remacle).

0030-6665/06/$ - see front matter © 2005 Elsevier Inc. All rights reserved.
doi:10.1016/j.otc.2005.10.010   *oto.theclinics.com*

Indications and techniques

One hundred and forty-five patients were operated on by endoscopic approach for glottic carcinoma in our department between 1995 and 2004. There were 115 men (79%) and 31 women (21%), with a mean age of 58 (± 14) years. The median follow-up was 42 months.

There were 29 cases of carcinoma in situ (20%), 70 cases of T1a lesions (48%), 22 cases of T1b lesions (15%), 14 cases of T2 lesions (10%), and 10 cases of T3–T4 lesions (7%). Forty-six subligamental cordectomies (type II), 38 transmuscular cordectomies (type III), 15 total cordectomies (type IV), and 46 extended cordectomies (type V) (cordectomy type according to ELS classification) were performed [19].

Postoperative speech therapy was recommended to all the patients. Among them, 10 patients (6.9% of all of the cordectomies and 16.4% of the total and extended cordectomies) considered their voice to be insufficient, and were offered surgery for voice rehabilitation. This included 8 men and 2 women with a mean age of 55 years (range: 19–70 years).

Six of the men had a significant glottic gap, and four patients (two men and two women) had anterior synechiae. Four of them had undergone a total cordectomy and six had undergone an extended cordectomy. A minimum 6-month period of recovery after cordectomy was observed before proceeding with reconstructive surgery. This time period was chosen to allow adequate healing, to verify the absence of early recurrence, and to evaluate the voice rehabilitation that was achieved by voice therapy.

Medialization thyroplasty was performed for glottic gaps, and transoral placement of a laryngeal keel after laser-assisted section was performed for anterior synechiae.

The voice assessment tools that were used in this study included the voice handicap index (VHI) self-assessment questionnaire [20]; Grade (G) of the perceptual GRBAS scale [21]; maximum phonation time (MPT; normal range: 20–25 seconds); phonation quotient (PQ; the quotient obtained by dividing the vital capacity by the MPT [normal range: 150–250 mL/s]; estimated subglottic pressure (normal value 6.1 hPa) [22]; and stroboscopy for qualitative assessment of glottic closure.

Medialization thyroplasty was performed under general anesthesia using a laryngeal mask airway (The Laryngeal Mask Company, Henley-on-Thames, United Kingdom), under fiberoptic laryngoscopic guidance [23]. The laryngeal mask airway consists of a tube attached to a silicone and polyvinyl chloride membrane. The membrane takes the exact shape of the upper laryngeal circumference upon which it is placed in the same manner as a cap on a bottle. The membrane encloses the larynx (Fig. 1).

The joint that connects the laryngeal mask to the ventilation tube is angled, and contains a small valve through which a fiberoptic laryngoscope can be passed. To assess surgical progress or completion of the thyroplasty, the fiberoptic laryngoscope is connected to a camera, and lowered into the

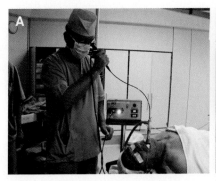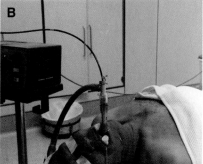

Fig. 1. Installation for fiberscopy through the laryngeal mask.

larynx above the glottic plane. Without hampering the patient's ventilation, the operator is able to verify the appropriate position of the vocal fold inside a perfectly free glottic plane (Fig. 2).

Two types of implants have been used: the Vocom hydroxyapatite implant (Smith-Nephew, Memphis, Tennessee) from Cummings and Flint [24] and the Montgomery implant [25]. The hydroxyapatite implant is used if the dissection cannot be performed sufficiently along the vocal cord level to permit use of the Montgomery implant.

The landmarks that are used for establishing the thyroid cartilage window were determined according to the particular technique of each of the implants. The cartilage window is left intact to minimize the risk of tearing the fibrous tissue of the vocal cord bed during dissection and positioning of the implant. The dissection, between the inner wall of the thyroid cartilage and the fibrous tissue around the window, requires meticulous care and must continue in close contact with the cartilage when the inner perichondrium is not identified. This elevation of the fibrous tissue must cover a large enough area to ensure that the implant is put in place without fibrous tissue resistance and consequent tearing. This dissection is lengthier and more laborious than is the dissection that is required for vocal cord paralysis.

Care must be taken to medialize the scar tissue as close as possible to the laryngeal midline; however, the authors do not believe that medialization to the degree attained for paralysis is feasible. Before closure, the authors cover the window with fibrin glue (Immuno, Vienna, Austria) and place a small suction drain that remains in place for 24 hours.

Laser-assisted section of anterior synechiae and placement of laryngeal keel was performed transorally under subglottic jet-ventilation, according to the technique that was proposed by Lichtenberger and Toohill [26]. The section was performed through the middle of the synechia, and care was taken to extend the section up to the thyroid cartilage anterior angle. In the last 4 years, the authors also have used mitomycin-C, in

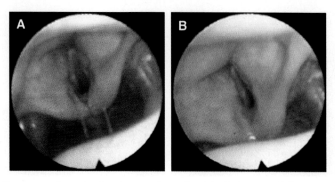

Fig. 2. Fiberscopy through the laryngeal mask. (*A*) Before medialization. (*B*) After medialization.

a concentration of 2 mg/mL, which is applied locally for 2 minutes after completion of the section. The keel was handmade with a 0.2-mm thick sheet of silastic (Fig. 3). The sheet was folded and glued with a medical adhesive for silicone (Dow Corning, Midland, Michigan) on the flexible sheath of a pediatric catheter. The size of the keel was altered to fit the dimensions of the synechia, and a nonresorbable suture (00) was passed through the sheath. Under rigid telescope control, the Lichtenberger needle-carrier [27] (Wolf, Knittlingen, Germany) was used to pass the suture from inside to outside. One end of the suture was passed under the anterior commissure, through the cricothyroid ligament, and the second end was passed above the anterior commissure, through the petiole of the epiglottis and the thyroid cartilage (Fig. 4). If the thyroid cartilage was too ossified at this level, the needle was passed at a level that was several millimeters more superior.

Under telescope control, the keel was placed carefully between the two vocal cords at the level of the anterior commissure. The keel must be in close contact with the thyroid cartilage to minimize any recurrence of synechiae. The suture was knotted tightly on a silastic or cotton pad placed on the neck. Patients were awakened in the operating room.

After 4 weeks, the keel was removed under general anesthesia. A new application of mitomycin-C also was put on the edges of the vocal cords at that time (Fig. 5). Patients were given oral antibiotics and nebulized steroids for 5 to 6 days.

These patients also were started on a proton pump inhibitor and antitussive medication, and the correct position of the keel was checked every week by fiberoptic laryngoscopy. Dressing on the pad and local care once per week were recommended to avoid any superinfection of the skin.

Food intake was resumed on the evening of the operation and the patients were discharged on the following day. Restrictions on voice use and on physical activities were recommended strongly after surgery for anterior synechiae.

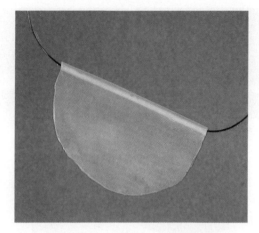

Fig. 3. Handmade sheet-silastic keel.

Results

The authors did not observe any preoperative or immediate postoperative complications in the group that underwent medialization thyroplasty or the anterior glottic synechia group. All patients were awakened in the operating room, and were returned to the ward after a short stay in the recovery room. No patient exhibited stridor or dyspnea and none required intubation. Fits of coughing could be observed for a few hours after surgery in patients who had undergone keel placement. This problem was solved with nebulized lidocaine and antitussive medication.

A hydroxyapatite implant was used for four of the patients who underwent medialization thyroplasty and a Montgomery implant was used for the other two patients. One woman underwent a medialization thyroplasty as a second-stage procedure after undergoing lysis of anterior glottic synechiae and keel placement. This patient received a hydroxyapatite implant because the fibrosis at the glottic level precluded the use a Montgomery implant.

One skin superinfection was observed after 3 weeks around the cotton pad in the anterior glottic synechia group. The patient was given antibiotics, and the keel was removed immediately. This patient healed properly without recurrence of the synechia. No keel dislocation was observed. Granulomas were observed around the puncture sites of the suture in the larynx but were too small to warrant resection or laser vaporization.

The vocal cords were not healed fully when the keel was taken out. Healing generally was observed after 6 weeks. One patient presented a partial recurrence of the synechia of 3 to 4 mm, but no other recurrence was observed.

One hydroxyapatite implant extrusion was observed after 8 months. The patient returned to the department after coughing up the implant, and complaining of sudden deterioration of his voice. The wound was allowed to

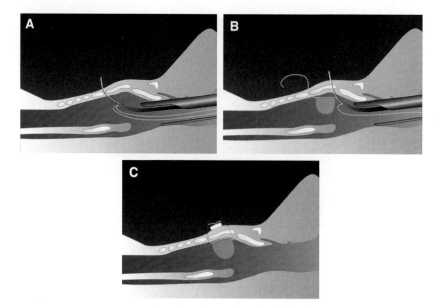

Fig. 4. Transoral keel placement according to Lichtenberger.

heal for 4 weeks, and a Montgomery implant was placed. The voice quality returned to its previous level. It has been 23 months since the replacement of the stent.

Comparison between the individual or median preoperative and postoperative values showed a significant improvement, mainly for the self-evaluation scores of the VHI, G, and the MPT (Tables 1 and 2). Improvement was much less significant for the PQ and for the estimated subglottic pressure. Stroboscopy showed improved or complete glottic closure, but typically it was irregular. Ventricular dysphonia usually persisted after medialization thyroplasty, which made observation of the glottis difficult. Persistent vibratory asymmetry and vocal stiffness also were observed.

Discussion

Endoscopic cordectomy and quality of life

Statistical evaluation of preoperative and postoperative results show that the voice can be affected significantly after total or extended endoscopic cordectomy [16,28].

Although staged resections can be performed in cases of bilateral keratosis, Reinke's edema, or papillomatosis to prevent anterior glottic synechiae, resection of cancer that involves the anterior commissure is a one-stage surgery [29].

Although laryngeal cancer has an impact on patient lifestyle, patients seldom relate this to vocal dysfunction [13], and influence of voice on

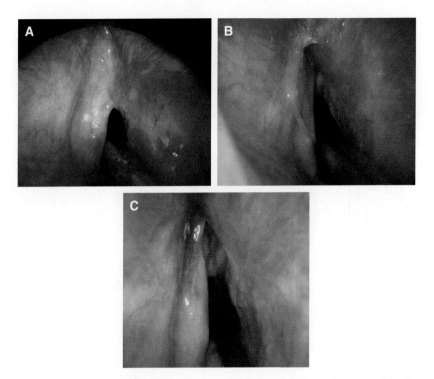

Fig. 5. Endoscopic view. (*A*) Anterior glottic synechia after extender cordectomy of the right vocal cord. (*B*) Sheet-silastic keel in place. (*C*) Aspect of the anterior commissure 4 weeks later, immediately after the keel was pulled out of the larynx.

the quality of life seems to be minor [3]. This also was observed in our series of 10 patients with only 6.9% of all the cordectomy patients and 16.4% of total and extended cordectomy patients considering their voice as inadequate.

From this point of view, self-report symptom questionnaires are convenient and consistent tools for assessing the voice outcome following endoscopic cordectomy. For instance, early vocal fatigue and increased effort to speak easily can be assessed this way. VHI was used for our study, but other questionnaires are available [30,31].

Objective voice assessment after endoscopic cordectomy

Vocal cord vibration is unstable after endoscopic cordectomy, and renders some digitized voice analyses variable, depending on the software and algorithms that are used. This may explain why the study by Bertino and colleagues [32], which compared voice quality after cordectomy with or without reconstruction, using only acoustic analysis, did not show any difference between the two groups. On the contrary, Zeitels and colleagues

Table 1
Breakdown of the cases and voice assessment

Surgery	Sex	Age (year)	VHI		G(rade)		MPT (s)		PQ (mL/s)		Subglottic pressure (hPa)		Glottic closure after surgery
			preop	postop	preop	postop	preop	postop	preop	postop	preop	postop	
Medialization thyroplasty	Male	67	52	42	3	3	5	10	486	254	17	25	Improved irregular ventricular dysphonia
	Male	47	67	47	3	2	2	16	235	153	15.2	28	Improved irregular ventricular dysphonia
	Male	70	55	25	2	1	5	7	625	491	26.7	15.9	Improved irregular ventricular dysphonia
	Male	51	66	10	3	2	9	10	407	535	21	21	Improved irregular ventricular dysphonia
	Male	62	62	15	3	1	9	13	367	284	7.6	14.2	Improved irregular ventricular dysphonia
	Male	67	88	24	3	1	1	7.4	1354	189	31.4	21.1	Improved irregular ventricular dysphonia
Surgery for glottic anterior synechia	Male	57	65	22	3	2	10	14	320	242	25	18	Complete irregular
	Male	56	82	75	2	2	6	7	641	428	13	14	Improved irregular ventricular dysphonia
Surgery for anterior synechia and medialization thyroplasty	Female	19	74	41	3	2	6	11	682	358	23	15	Complete irregular
	Female	52	56	42	2	2	6	16	658	228	9.8	8.9	Completed regular

Abbreviations: postop, postoperative value; preop, preoperative value.

Table 2
Voice assessment. Median values

Value	VHI preop	VHI postop	G preop	G postop	MPT (s) preop	MPT (s) postop	PQ (mL/s) preop	PQ (mL/s) postop	Subglottic pressure (hPa) preop	Subglottic pressure (hPa) postop
Median	65.5	33	3	2	6	10.5	555.5	269	19	16.95
Minimum	52	10	2	1	1	7	235	153	7.6	8.9
Maximum	88	75	3	3	10	16	1354	535	31.4	28
P	<.001		.002		.003		.04		<0.5	

Abbreviations: G, Grade; postop, postoperative value; preop, preoperative value.

[18] demonstrated positive results after glottic reconstruction following cordectomy, which also was based on digitized acoustic measurements.

Scales for perceptual evaluation [17,21] and basic aerodynamic measurements (MPT, PQ) remain valuable [28]. Studies that included these tools [17,28,33] showed improvement after reconstruction. Sittel and colleagues [33], for example, used a dysphonia index that ranged from 0 (normal) to 3 (aphonia), which includes objective parameters as well as expert voice ratings and patient's perception.

In our study, results were significantly better with VHI, G(rade) from the GRBAS scale, MPT, and PQ than with the estimated subglottic pressure that was measured with the workstation EVA (Evaluation vocale assistée, SQ-LAB, Aix-en Provence, France) [22].

Speech therapy

According to Sittel and colleagues [17], there is no evidence of significant benefit from speech therapy after cordectomy, but we propose it empirically to prevent the development of ineffective supraglottic hyperkinetic dysfunction, at least in cases of type I or type II cordectomy.

As Moore [34] pointed out many years ago, speech therapy often is recommended when possible. Therapy that is applicable to voice following partial laryngectomy combines five areas: strengthening glottic closure and loudness of the voice; improving the efficiency of breath expenditure; increasing the articulatory skill and intelligibility of speech; recognizing and compensating for hearing loss; and aiding the patient to reduce detrimental environmental influences and to adjust to his environmental requirements.

6-Month interval

We recommend a 6-month interval after cordectomy before engaging in further surgery that is aimed at voice improvement. This allows the vocal cord to heal fully and to form a fibrous neo-cord that, by itself, can provide a satisfactory functional outcome. The 6-month interval also permits the diagnosis of early recurrence. Furthermore, medialization thyroplasty does not conceal possible late recurrence; in fact, the implant forces the entire fibrous block inward toward the laryngeal lumen.

Injection laryngoplasty

Injection laryngoplasty [35] is futile after total or extended cordectomy, because the tight scar tissue does not lend itself to augmentation. Collagen or fat augmentation are indicated only for limited scarring (eg, after surgical, iatrogenic injury after excision of vocal cord lesions).

Medialization thyroplasty according to Tucker

The use of a superior rim of thyroid cartilage that was advocated recently by Sittel and colleagues [33] for medialization thyroplasty already was proposed by Tucker [36], but a slow resorption can be expected [37]. According to this technique, elevation of the inner perichondrium and the fibrotic tissue from the upper margin of the thyroid cartilage downward to a point below the level of the vocal cord is easier than through the classic thyroplasty window; however, it may restrict the size of the implant.

Medialization laryngoplasty with Gore-Tex according to Zeitels and colleagues

Zeitels and colleagues [38] reported a prospective study on 142 patients who underwent 152 Gore-Tex medialization laryngoplasties. The study included 14 cancer reconstructions. Endoscopic removal was necessary for one case because of persistent granulation. According to Zeitels and colleagues, Gore-Tex is especially useful for medialization of complex anatomic soft tissue defects (eg, those that result from cancer resection), with superior ease in handling, placement, and in vivo adjustability.

General anesthesia and laryngeal mask

It is accepted commonly that thyroplasty should be performed under local anesthesia to assess the vocal result immediately, and directly provide the technical modifications that are required to improve this result. In certain instances, however, local anesthesia is awkward for the patient and complicates surgery (eg, anxious patient, nonstandard anatomic configuration).

Moreover, for certain operations, such as for sulcus vergeture or presbyphonia, the gain in phonation intensity or duration cannot be estimated by subjective auditory appreciation under operating room conditions. In those instances, the authors perform thyroplasty under general anesthesia. The use of laryngeal mask airway and fiberoptic laryngoscopy allow excellent control of the medialization [39,40].

Because elevating the fibrous tissue from the inner surface of the thyroid cartilage is a lengthy and laborious step, the authors prefer general anesthesia for medialization thyroplasty following endoscopic cordectomy. This step is critical. Care must be taken to avoid any tear toward the lumen, with consequent risk of implant extrusion. This elevation must cover a sufficiently large area to ensure easy placement of the implant [23].

Implants

The Montgomery implant [25] is the authors' preferred implant because of its suppleness, ease of handling, and rounded edges that protect the fibrous tissue from erosion and tear. It cannot always be used if there is extended scar at the vocal cord level. In those instances, hand-made or preshaped implants [24], with axes perpendicular to the vocal cord, are advisable. In this regard, Gore-Tex as proposed by Zeitels and colleagues [38], is useful.

Flaps and laryngofissure

More extended reconstruction by open neck approaches have been proposed in cases of glottic gap, including bipedicled strap muscle transposition [41], bilateral omohyoid muscle flaps [42], vestibular fold flap [32,43], and composite myo-mucosal reconstruction [44]. These approaches require major dissection of the thyroid cartilage or laryngofissure [32,42–44], without significantly better voice results.

Mitomycin C

Topical application of mitomycin C reduces the rate of stenosis after surgical lysis [45–47], which makes the use of a keel unnecessary for selected cases [48]. A concentration of 0.4 mg/mL usually is proposed with durations of application ranging from 4 [47] to 5 minutes [46]. Two-minute duration of application has proved to be insufficient [49]. The authors use a concentration of 2 mg/mL for 2 minutes or longer (P.R. Monnier, personal communication, 1999).

Keel placement

Transoral keel placement is favored by several investigators [26,50–52], and makes laryngofissure unnecessary [53]. The transoral approach was described first with the passage of the suture from outside to inside [51,52]. The synechia is lysed using microsurgical technique or with laser. Following this, two 16-gauge needles are driven through the anterior neck skin in the midline so that the more inferior of the two passes just below the lower border of the thyroid cartilage; the more superior one passes through the thyroid notch precisely in the midline.

A fine wire suture is passed through each of these, and is grasped endoscopically by the surgeon. The wires are fixed to a Teflon keel. The keel is placed into the anterior commissure while an assistant gently pulls on the wires from the outside. The wires are fixed on the skin.

The authors consider the Lichtenberger [27] technique to be superior; it allows easier placement from inside to outside with the needle-carrier under rigid telescope control.

Summary

Medialization thyroplasty for correction of glottic gap, keel placement after laser-assisted section, and topical application of mitomycin-C for anterior glottic synechiae are effective procedures for voice restoration after endoscopic cordectomy. Only a minority of patients (16.4% of the authors' patients after total or extended cordectomies) request this voice restoration. In this regard, self-evaluation questionnaires (eg, VHI) probably are the most useful tools, along with stroboscopy, for voice assessment.

Careful elevation of the fibrous tissue from the inner surface of the thyroid cartilage is a tedious and lengthy step, but is critical in successful medialization after cordectomy; therefore, general anesthesia is preferable.

Transoral keel placement is still advisable in cases of thick synechiae. The Lichtenberger technique has been a major advancement to the transoral approach, and is the preferred technique of the authors.

References

[1] Casiano RR, Cooper JD, Lundy DS, et al. Laser cordectomy for T1 glottic carcinoma: a 10-year experience and videostroboscopic findings. Otolaryngol Head Neck Surg 1991; 104(6):831–7.
[2] Damm M, Sittel C, Streppel M, et al. Transoral CO_2 laser for surgical management of glottic carcinoma in situ. Laryngoscope 2000;110(7):1215–21.
[3] Lopez LA, Nunez BF, Llorente Pendas JL, et al. [Laser cordectomy: oncologic outcome and functional results] Acta Otorrinolaringol Esp 2004;55(1):34–40.
[4] Eckel HE, Thumfart W, Jungehulsing M, et al. Transoral laser surgery for early glottic carcinoma. Eur Arch Otorhinolaryngol 2000;257(4):221–6.
[5] Bron LP, Soldati D, Zouhair A, et al. Treatment of early stage squamous-cell carcinoma of the glottic larynx: endoscopic surgery or cricohyoidoepiglottopexy versus radiotherapy. Head Neck 2001;23(10):823–9.
[6] Cragle SP, Brandenburg JH. Laser cordectomy or radiotherapy: cure rates, communication, and cost. Otolaryngol Head Neck Surg 1993;108(6):648–54.
[7] Delsupehe KG, Zink I, Lejaegere M, et al. Voice quality after narrow-margin laser cordectomy compared with laryngeal irradiation. Otolaryngol Head Neck Surg 1999;121(5): 528–33.
[8] Jones AS, Fish B, Fenton JE, et al. The treatment of early laryngeal cancers (T1–T2 N0): surgery or irradiation? Head Neck 2004;26(2):127–35.
[9] Morris MR, Canonico D, Blank C. A critical review of radiotherapy in the management of T1 glottic carcinoma. Am J Otolaryngol 1994;15(4):276–80.
[10] Elner A, Fex S. Carbon dioxide laser as primary treatment of glottic T1S and T1A tumours. Acta Otolaryngol Suppl 1988;449:135–9.
[11] Dickens WJ, Cassisi NJ, Million RR, et al. Treatment of early vocal cord carcinoma: a comparison of apples and apples. Laryngoscope 1983;93(2):216–9.
[12] Krengli M, Policarpo M, Manfredda I, et al. Voice quality after treatment for T1a glottic carcinoma–radiotherapy versus laser cordectomy. Acta Oncol 2004;43(3):284–9.

[13] Schuller DE, Trudeau M, Bistline J, et al. Evaluation of voice by patients and close relatives following different laryngeal cancer treatments. J Surg Oncol 1990;44(1):10–4.

[14] Keilmann A, Bergler W, Artzt M, et al. Vocal function following laser and conventional surgery of small malignant vocal fold tumours. J Laryngol Otol 1996;110(12):1138–41.

[15] Remacle M, Eckel HE, Antonelli A, et al. Endoscopic cordectomy. A proposal for a classification by the Working Committee, European Laryngological Society. Eur Arch Otorhinolaryngol 2000;257(4):227–31.

[16] Peretti G, Piazza C, Balzanelli C, et al. Preoperative and postoperative voice in Tis-T1 glottic cancer treated by endoscopic cordectomy: an additional issue for patient counseling. Ann Otol Rhinol Laryngol 2003;112(9 Pt 1):759–63.

[17] Sittel C, Eckel HE, Eschenburg C. Phonatory results after laser surgery for glottic carcinoma. Otolaryngol Head Neck Surg 1998;119(4):418–24.

[18] Zeitels SM, Hillman RE, Franco RA, et al. Voice and treatment outcome from phonosurgical management of early glottic cancer. Ann Otol Rhinol Laryngol Suppl 2002;190:3–20.

[19] Dufour X, Lawson G, Trussart C, et al. Chirurgie partielle endoscopique des cancers glottiques T1B,T2, T3. Indication et résultats [abstract]. Revue Soc Fr ORL 2004;84:80 [in French].

[20] Benninger MS, Ahuja AS, Gardner G, et al. Assessing outcomes for dysphonic patients. J Voice 1998;12(4):540–50.

[21] Yamaguchi H, Shrivastav R, Andrews ML, et al. A comparison of voice quality ratings made by Japanese and American listeners using the GRBAS scale. Folia Phoniatr Logop 2003; 55(3):147–57.

[22] Giovanni A, Heim C, Demolin D, et al. Estimated subglottic pressure in normal and dysphonic subjects. Ann Otol Rhinol Laryngol 2000;109(5):500–4.

[23] Remacle M, Lawson G, Mayne A. Use of a laryngeal mask during medialization laryngoplasty. Rev Laryngol Otol Rhinol (Bord) 2003;124(5):335–8.

[24] Cummings CW, Purcell LL, Flint PW. Hydroxylapatite laryngeal implants for medialization. Preliminary report. Ann Otol Rhinol Laryngol 1993;102(11):843–51.

[25] Montgomery WW, Montgomery SK. Montgomery thyroplasty implant system. Ann Otol Rhinol Laryngol Suppl 1997;170:1–16.

[26] Lichtenberger G, Toohill RJ. New keel fixing technique for endoscopic repair of anterior commissure webs. Laryngoscope 1994;104(6 Pt 1):771–4.

[27] Lichtenberger G. Endo-extralaryngeal needle carrier instrument. Laryngoscope 1983; 93(10):1348–50.

[28] Remacle M, Lawson G, Hedayat A, et al. Medialization framework surgery for voice improvement after endoscopic cordectomy. Eur Arch Otorhinolaryngol 2001;258:267–71.

[29] Desloge RB, Zeitels SM. Endolaryngeal microsurgery at the anterior glottal commissure: controversies and observations. Ann Otol Rhinol Laryngol 2000;109(4):385–92.

[30] Rosen CA, Lee AS, Osborne J, et al. Development and validation of the voice handicap index-10. Laryngoscope 2004;114(9):1549–56.

[31] Wilson JA, Webb A, Carding PN, et al. The Voice Symptom Scale (VoiSS) and the Vocal Handicap Index (VHI): a comparison of structure and content. Clin Otolaryngol Allied Sci 2004;29(2):169–74.

[32] Bertino G, Bellomo A, Ferrero FE, et al. Acoustic analysis of voice quality with or without false vocal fold displacement after cordectomy. J Voice 2001;15(1):131–40.

[33] Sittel C, Friedrich G, Zorowka P, et al. Surgical voice rehabilitation after laser surgery for glottic carcinoma. Ann Otol Rhinol Laryngol 2002;111(6):493–9.

[34] Moore GP. Voice problems following limited surgical excision. Laryngoscope 1975;85(4): 619–25.

[35] Ford CN, Bless DM. Selected problems treated by vocal fold injection of collagen. Am J Otolaryngol 1993;14(4):257–61.

[36] Tucker HM. Management of the patient with an incompetent larynx. Am J Otolaryngol 1979;1(1):47–56.

[37] Guay ME, Miller FR, Bauer TW, et al. Vocal fold medialization using autologous cartilage in a canine model: a preliminary study. Laryngoscope 1995;105(10):1049–52.

[38] Zeitels SM, Mauri M, Dailey SH. Medialization laryngoplasty with Gore-Tex for voice restoration secondary to glottal incompetence: indications and observations. Ann Otol Rhinol Laryngol 2003;112(2):180–4.

[39] Grundler S, Stacey MR. Thyroplasty under general anesthesia using a laryngeal mask airway and fibreoptic bronchoscope. Can J Anaesth 1999;46(5 Pt 1):460–3.

[40] Razzaq I, Wooldridge W. A series of thyroplasty cases under general anaesthesia. Br J Anaesth 2000;85(4):547–9.

[41] Su CY, Chuang HC, Tsai SS, et al. Bipedicled strap muscle transposition for vocal fold deficit after laser cordectomy in early glottic cancer patients. Laryngoscope 2005;115(3): 528–33.

[42] Calcaterra TC. Bilateral omohyoid muscle flap reconstruction for anterior commissure cancer. Laryngoscope 1987;97(7 Pt 1):810–3.

[43] Martins Mamede RC, Ricz HM, Guiar-Ricz LN, et al. Vestibular fold flap for post-cordectomy laryngeal reconstruction. Otolaryngol Head Neck Surg 2005;132(3):478–83.

[44] Milutinovic Z. Composite myo-mucosal reconstruction of the vocal fold. Eur Arch Otorhinolaryngol 1995;252(2):119–22.

[45] Spector JE, Werkhaven JA, Spector NC, et al. Prevention of anterior glottic restenosis in a canine model with topical mitomycin-C. Ann Otol Rhinol Laryngol 2001;110(11): 1007–10.

[46] Roh JL, Yoon YH. Prevention of anterior glottic stenosis after transoral microresection of glottic lesions involving the anterior commissure with mitomycin C. Laryngoscope 2005; 115(6):1055–9.

[47] de Mones E, Lagarde F, Hans S, et al. [Mitomycin C: prevention and treatment of anterior glottic synechia] Ann Otolaryngol Chir Cervicofac 2004;121(4):229–34.

[48] Unal M. The successful management of congenital laryngeal web with endoscopic lysis and topical mitomycin-C. Int J Pediatr Otorhinolaryngol 2004;68(2):231–5.

[49] Hartnick CJ, Hartley BE, Lacy PD, et al. Topical mitomycin application after laryngotracheal reconstruction: a randomized, double-blind, placebo-controlled trial. Arch Otolaryngol Head Neck Surg 2001;127(10):1260–4.

[50] Casiano RR, Lundy DS. Outpatient transoral laser vaporization of anterior glottic webs and keel placement: risks of airway compromise. J Voice 1998;12(4):536–9.

[51] Dedo HH. Endoscopic Teflon keel for anterior glottic web. Ann Otol Rhinol Laryngol 1979; 88(4 Pt 1):467–73.

[52] Tucker HM. Laryngeal webs—management of specific lesions. Surgery for phonatory disorders. New York: Churchill Livingstone; 1981.

[53] Montgomery WW, Montgomery SK. Manual for use of Montgomery laryngeal, tracheal, and esophageal prostheses: update 1990. Ann Otol Rhinol Laryngol Suppl 1990;150:2–28.

ELSEVIER
SAUNDERS

Otolaryngol Clin N Am
39 (2006) 205–221

OTOLARYNGOLOGIC
CLINICS
OF NORTH AMERICA

Eosinophilic Esophagitis: Its Role in Aerodigestive Tract Disorders

Dana M. Thompson, MD[a],*,
Amindra S. Arora, MBBChir[b],
Yvonne Romero, MD[b], Eileen H. Dauer, MD[c]

[a]Division of Pediatric Otolaryngology, Department of Otorhinolaryngology,
Mayo Clinic College of Medicine, 200 First Street, SW, Rochester, MN 55905, USA
[b]Department of Gastroenterology, Mayo Clinic College of Medicine, 200 First Street,
SW, Rochester, MN 55905, USA
[c]Department of Otolaryngology-Head and Neck Surgery,
Malcolm Grow Medical Center, 1050 West Perimeter Road,
Andrews Air Force Base, MD 20762, USA

Eosinophilic esophagitis (EE) is a chronic inflammatory disorder of the esophagus that is rapidly emerging as a distinct clinical disease entity of importance. It is characterized by an isolated, dense eosinophilic epithelial infiltration of the esophagus with unusual structural alterations that are often overlooked by radiologists and endoscopists. The disease affects patients of all ages, but traditionally, it is appreciated mainly in the pediatric literature. The presenting symptoms are usually gastrointestinal in nature. Epigastric pain, chest pain, dysphagia, and food impaction are common in adults and children. Vomiting, regurgitation, feeding disorders, and failure to thrive are additional findings in children with EE. Recent reports highlight the upper airway and respiratory symptoms of rhinitis, sinusitis, pneumonia, wheezing, globus, hoarseness, dysphonia, and cough in children [1,2]. Additionally, EE has been attributed as a causative factor in airway findings of subglottic stenosis and chronic laryngeal edema refractory to traditional reflux therapy in a case report of a child [3]. With the crossover of upper airway symptoms and findings along with the expanding role of otolaryngologist in the treatment and management of esophageal disorders and dysphagia, it is important for otolaryngologist to recognize and appropriately treat or refer patients who have EE for further management.

* Corresponding author.
E-mail address: thompson.danam@mayo.edu (D.M. Thompson).

0030-6665/06/$ - see front matter © 2005 Elsevier Inc. All rights reserved.
doi:10.1016/j.otc.2005.10.002
oto.theclinics.com

Eosinophilic disease involving the esophagus was first described by Dobbins and colleagues in 1977 [4]. The report describes an adult patient with asthma, hay fever, and severe dysphagia. Endoscopic biopsies demonstrated eosinophilic infiltration of the small bowel and esophagus and, for the first time, established involvement of the esophagus in eosinophilic gastroenteritis. The clinicopathologic entity now known as isolated "eosinophilic esophagitis" was described in the 1978 by Landres and colleagues [5], when they reported a patient with severe dysphagia who demonstrated marked eosinophilia in esophageal biopsies obtained during open myotomy. This patient had no evidence of systemic or other gastrointestinal disease.

Although many symptoms of EE overlap with those of reflux disease, even the earliest literature describes a distinct clinicopathologic entity, with unique radiographic, endoscopic, and histopathologic findings [5–8]. After these scattered reports in the 1980s, descriptions the clinical entity EE were virtually absent until the mid 1990s. In 1993, Attwood and colleagues [9] described a fairly unique group of patients who had high concentrations of intraepithelial eosinophils and significant dysphagia. Histopathologic analysis of biopsy specimens taken from these dysphagic patients showed a more pronounced eosinophilic infiltration compared with a similar group of patients who had gastroesophageal reflux disease (GERD). The authors concluded that, although low-grade eosinophilia is sometimes associated with GERD (averaging 3.3 eosinophils per high power field), high-grade intraepithelial eosinophilic infiltrates seem to represent a distinct disease process [9]. Since then, the number of reported adult and child patients who have EE has steadily increased. The exact reason for the escalating epidemiology and reported prevalence of EE is poorly understood, but there are some plausible explanations for this trend.

Before 1995, the presence of eosinophils in the esophagus was associated routinely with GERD symptoms and reflux esophagitis; therefore, patients who had this finding were assumed to have pathologic GERD. Because the symptoms can be similar to those seen in GERD patients, these patients were treated accordingly, with acid suppression or fundoplication. Since then, numerous authors have examined the clinical characteristics of small groups of patients who have a symptom complex similar to GERD, who do not respond to standard antireflux therapies (including fundoplication) [2,10–12]. It was not until these patients experienced a mild or no response did clinicians begin to realize that the eosinophilic infiltrate represented a separate disease entity that required different therapy. Reports of pediatric EE suggest that the prevalence of the disease in those with refractory reflux symptoms is high, with two recent reports demonstrating EE as the cause of reflux-like symptoms in 68% to 94% of children who were unresponsive to proton pump inhibitor therapy [13,14]. Through these reports, the clinical features and prevalence of EE have become gradually more defined in the pediatric population. However, the prevalence in adults has not been as well studied. Increased physician awareness of the disease may contribute to a perceived escalating prevalence. Other reports suggest that there is an environmental component to this disease [15,16] that may be contributing to the increased incidence (discussed below).

Cause and pathophysiology of eosinophilic esophagitis

Knowledge of the cause and pathophysiology of EE is evolving and has yet to be clearly defined. Eosinophils may function as an effector or a modulator in this inflammatory reaction. There is evidence to support EE as an allergic disease, a disease of immune dysregulation, a result of severe acid reflux disease, or a combination of any of the three. Most authors agree that EE appears to be driven by a combination of allergic and immunologic responses. The inflammatory pattern seems to involve an initial injury followed by an eosinophilic response, in which these eosinophils are activated in situ in the esophagus [17].

Eosinophils are tissue-dwelling cells with a tissue-to-blood ratio of 100–300:1. Whereas the majority of human eosinophils reside in the gastrointestinal tract, very few eosinophils are found in the normal esophagus [18], and some investigators would argue that no eosinophils should exist in the esophagus [16,19]. Thus, the marked infiltration of eosinophils into the esophagus clearly suggests a role for eosinophils in the pathogenesis of EE. Eosinophils are important effector cells in epithelial inflammation at the interface between the external and internal milieu, such as skin (eg, atopic dermatitis) and lung (eg, bronchial asthma) [20]. The esophagus is another epithelial interface between the external and internal milieu where foreign antigens, including allergens and pathogens, enter and reside. The route of entry and initial sensitization of the antigen may occur in the form of swallowed food, aeroallergens, pathogens, and secretions from the upper and lower airways. In response to the antigen or pathogen, eosinophils cause epithelial injury through release of a diverse array of mediators, such as cytotoxic granule proteins, reactive oxygen intermediates, lipid mediators, and cytokines [20]. The antigens that mount this eosinophilic response include food [13,21–24], aeroallergens [15,16,19,25], and possibly fungi [15,16,19,25]. The current data suggest both IgE-mediated (extrinsic and allergic) and non-IgE-mediated (intrinsic and nonallergic) immune responses against ingested antigens are operative in EE.

Food allergy is clearly associated with EE in children; its role in adults remains yet to be determined. Whether the mounted response is IgE- or non-IgE-mediated is debatable. Food hypersensitivity in the form of a type IV (cell-mediated) reaction, rather than a type I reaction (IgE-mediated), has been offered and supported as the cause of the eosinophilic response. Liacouras and colleagues [22,23] support this mechanism based on their experience with patients who have EE, whose skin prick and radio-allergosorbent (RAST) test results are negative for allergies (both IgE-dependent). Liacouras also postulates that with type IV food hypersensitivity, the symptoms occur within hours to days after ingestion of the causative food and that mast-cell activation is probably related [22,23]. This author (Liacouras) has found that skin patch testing to food antigens (non-IgE-dependent) often shows a delayed reaction (type IV reaction). This finding may help increase the identification of potential food allergies in the cause of EE and aid in treatment. In contrast, an atopic predisposition, increased IgE levels, and a positive response to skin prick and RAST testing of food antigens, reported by many authors, suggest that an IgE-mediated mechanism is present [1,2,12,14,21,24]. These findings, combined, suggest that both IgE-mediated and non-IgE-mediated mechanisms have a role in the pathogenesis of food antigen-induced EE. Because not all patients who have EE have demonstrated food allergy, some authors [15,16] argue that food allergy is not the full cause of EE but may be a specific variant or trigger.

Environmental aeroallergens have been implicated as a possible contributor. EE patients commonly report a symptom exacerbation during pollen season [15,16], with the normalization of symptoms and esophageal histology in the off-peak season [15]. The portal of entry of the antigen into the esophagus is unknown. It is possible that the antigen is swallowed as a result of the passive ingestion of aeroallergens deposited in the oronasal cavity. Another possibility is that there is a direct connection between pulmonary and tracheal antigens and the esophagus. This theory is based on experiments carried out in an animal model showing that the repeated delivery of specific allergens or the T_H2 cytokine interleukin (IL)-13 to the lung of mice induces experimental EE [25]. The proposed immunopathogenesis of aeroallergen antigens in EE are the roles of IL-5 and eotaxin (a prototypic eosinophil-directed cytokine and a chemokine) [16,20] in the induction of epithelial inflammation and eosinophilic response. This has been studied extensively in mouse models by Mishra and associates [25,26]. They have shown a central role for IL-5 in trafficking eosinophils into the esophagus in both the pulmonary sensitization model [25] and the intestinal challenge model [26]. Abolishing IL-5 resulted in the complete disappearance of esophageal eosinophils, although abolishing eotaxin resulted in significant but partial decrease in esophageal eosinophils [25]. Most recently, these authors have shown in mice that the intratracheal administration of IL-13 but not IL-4 induces eosinophilic infiltration in the esophagus, which depends on IL-5 and partially on eotaxin [27]. These findings suggest that esophageal eosinophilic inflammation is linked mechanistically with pulmonary inflammation [16]. For the otolaryngologic patient population, the next step would be to evaluate if it is linked with laryngeal inflammation or chronic rhinosinusitis.

In contrast to animal models, the number of immunologic studies on patients who have EE has been sparse. The esophagus shows an increased infiltration of $CD3^+$ [14,28] and $CD8^+$ T cells [14], $CD1a^+$ dendritic cells [14], and mast cells [28]. Straumann and colleagues [28] have shown augmented expression of IL-5 in cells infiltrating the epithelial cell layer in EE, whereas differences in eotaxin and RANTES (regulated on activation normal T cell expressed and secreted) expression were slight to minimal. The marked expression of eotaxin in eosinophils themselves in the esophagus is described in a single case report [29]. Functionally, polyclonal, nonspecific stimulation of peripheral blood mononuclear cells with phytohemagglutinin did not result in augmented IL-5 production or attenuated interferon-γ production [28]. Although these data provide some insights, a detailed immunologic study on EE in clinical settings is urgently required.

Gastroesophageal reflux disease and eosinophilic esophagitis

The contribution of reflux disease to EE is not well understood. If the reflux of gastric contents into the tubular esophagus is a significant contributing factor, it is likely that acid exposure causes damage to the epithelium that mounts an eosinophilic response in the healing process. This theory is challenged because not all patients who have biopsy-proven GERD have an eosinophilic infiltrate. Additionally, although the treatment of acid reflux disease may improve some of the symptoms of EE, it does not change the histology [23]. Ambulatory pH level data on patients who have EE have been reported as normal; however, a summary of raw data and criteria for "normal" have not been available [12,30] for a critical review. The results of a recent study that presented the raw ambulatory pH level data from pediatric patients who had EE were interpreted by the authors as negative for GERD [11]. However if these same data were interpreted using Koufman and colleagues' [31] criteria for laryngopharyngeal reflux, the data would be interpreted as positive for GERD in the setting of an airway disease. A recent summary of 71 pediatric patients who had EE and mixed airway and esophageal symptoms reported abnormal pH data on 41% of those tested [1]. Rothenberg [16] and colleagues [19] propose that there is an intermediate group of patients who have a moderate number of eosinophils seen on biopsy results who have both GERD and an allergic or atopic disease. It is likely that GERD and EE can coexist in the same patient, but in this setting, it is less likely that the disease is primary eosinophilic esophagitis and will be refractory to treatment directed only toward reflux disease. Until placebo-controlled prospective studies evaluating acid exposure, pH data, impedance data (to detect the role of gastric contents, not just acid), EE, and responses to treatment are available, the contribution of GERD as a cause of EE remains inconclusive.

Clinical presentation

EE occurs in adults and children, but the majority of the patients reported in the literature are children. The clinical features of EE differ slightly between children and adults. In adults and children, EE is seen more

commonly in males who present with GERD symptoms that are refractory
to standard reflux therapies and dysphagia, with or without food impaction.
Other common features include peripheral blood eosinophilia and increased
IgE levels.

Typical symptoms in children include vomiting, regurgitation, epigastric
pain, and poor eating [2,14,32]. Young children may demonstrate food refusal and failure, whereas adolescents experience dysphagia. Less common
symptoms include growth failure and failure to thrive, hematemesis, and
water brash [32]. Any child who presents with food impaction that requires
endoscopic extraction should be evaluated for the possibility of EE. Most
children who have EE have atopic conditions, including asthma, atopic
dermatitis, and food allergy. The most common food allergies are milk,
peanuts, and soy. An atopic predisposition is seen more commonly in children than in adults, but this finding may be the result of more widespread
allergy testing in children for other reasons. Further studies evaluating adult
and allergic disease in the setting of EE are needed.

In contrast to symptoms demonstrated in children with EE, adults present more commonly with solid food dysphagia that is often accompanied by
solid food impaction. Many cases require endoscopic dilation of strictured
segments and may even be misdiagnosed with a Schatzki's ring. The dysphagia is usually longstanding in duration, can date back to childhood [33,34],
and often is not associated with significant weight loss. These adults often
compensate for their dysphagia by eating slowly. As more gastroenterolo-
gists have become aware of the adult presentation and presence of EE,
more information about adult forms of the disease are available. Many of
these adults have a history of unexplained eosinophilic inflammation of
the esophageal mucosa. A study by Croese and colleagues [35] has reported
that symptoms of adult EE were present for an average of 54 months, with
a maximum of 15 years, before diagnosis. The diagnosis was delayed for an
average of 7 years because the sentinel features were overlooked during initial endoscopy, and biopsies were not taken. Almost 60% of the patients in
their series had esophageal strictures that were treated by esophageal dilation, which consistently relieved symptoms. Repeat dilations were often required. Esophageal tears were present almost uniformly after dilation, but
no perforations were reported. Similar to pediatric patients, the allergy history, peripheral eosinophilia, and elevated IgE levels were present in these
patients [35].

The link between EE and upper airway symptoms in children was first
highlighted by Orenstein and colleagues [2], who noted that 62% of patients
who had EE also had wheezing, pneumonia, sinusitis, or congestion. The
first description of EE in the otorhinolaryngology literature [3] is the case
of a 2-year-old girl who presented with stridor, choking, vomiting, and subglottic stenosis refractory to surgery. When antireflux therapy failed to prevent a recurrence of her symptoms, she was treated for EE with oral
corticosteroids, and she improved dramatically and was successfully

decannulated [3]. Additional upper airway and laryngeal symptoms of recurrent cough, choking episodes, hoarseness and globus sensation, and apnea and stridor have been reported in children who had EE [1]. Upper airway symptoms are highlighted below in an adult and pediatric case.

Male gender, atopic predisposition, blood eosinophilia, elevated IgE, and positive skin prick or RAST seem to be useful initial clues in suspecting EE, particularly in the setting of GERD symptoms refractory to standard antireflux therapy. The absence of IgE-related features (negative RAST or skin prick testing) does not exclude the possibility of EE because non-IgE-mediated EE does exist, as discussed above.

Diagnosis

Endoscopy with biopsy is required to identify eosinophilic esophagitis. The endoscopic features of EE may be quite subtle or very obvious. Several reports have commented on findings of subtle esophageal mucosal granularity, adherent white exudate, concentric rings, (the "trachealization" effect of the esophagus) (Fig. 1), vertical linear furrowing, a "crepe-paper" appearance (also seen in lichen planus of the esophagus), and low esophageal strictures (Fig. 2) [1,2,12,36–40]. These findings can be found throughout the esophagus or in a more focal part of the esophagus. A small-caliber "stenotic" esophagus has been described in EE, and in adults, what was once known as "congenital esophageal stenosis" has now come to be recognized as EE in many cases [37]. Vasilopoulos and colleagues [40] reported on five male patients who had dysphagia and a small-caliber esophagus, four of whom were later found to have evidence of EE on histology. In this group of patients, dilation relieved the symptoms. This study suggested that the clue to the

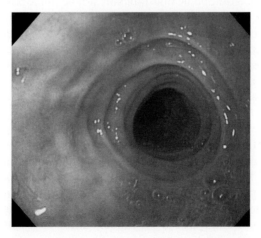

Fig. 1. Concentric rings, also known as the "trachealization" effect, seen the esophagus of a patient who has EE.

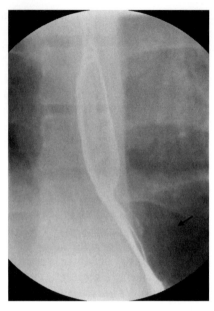

Fig. 2. Contrast esophagram demonstrating a lower esophageal stricture caused by EE.

diagnosis was in reinspecting the esophagus after dilation and finding the mucosal tears. The presence of mucosal tears has been described in several other studies. Indeed, some endoscopists have suggested that EE should be characterized by a fragile esophageal mucosa or the so-called crepe-paper mucosa [35,40]. However, one must remember that the finding of crepe-paper esophagus is also seen in lichen planus involvement of the esophagus.

In selecting the site for esophageal biopsies, the endoscopist should be mindful that the eosinophilic infiltrate may not be homogenous. Some areas of the esophagus may demonstrate abnormalities whereas others do not. Visual abnormalities are not always present in EE because dense eosinophilic infiltrates have been reported in visually normal esophageal examinations [1,23]. Because of these inconsistencies between the gross appearance of the esophagus and abnormal histology, multiple biopsies from different levels of the esophagus (distal, mid, and proximal) are necessary to increase diagnostic yield. Nevertheless, in the visually abnormal esophagus, biopsies directed to areas of plaque, granularities, ring formation and furrowing likely provide the greatest diagnostic yield [1].

Currently, an endoscopic biopsy with histologic evaluation is required to diagnose EE. The nonspecific findings of epithelial inflammation include basal zone hyperplasia, and increased papillary size is seen in both EE and GERD. Because of the presence of the low-grade eosinophilic infiltration that can be seen in GERD [41], investigators have sought to establish a quantitative cut-off value for eosinophilic infiltration, to differentiate EE from GERD. Most studies agree that EE can be diagnosed if the eosinophil infiltration is ≥20 eosinophils/high power field (HPF) (magnification ×400), as seen in Fig. 3 [2,22,32,34,41,42]. However, typical EE symptoms and endoscopic findings have been seen in patients who have ≤15 eosinophils/HPF [1,23]. Ruchelli and colleagues [43] found that a cut-off value of ≥7 eosinophils/HPF provides 85% accuracy for diagnosing EE and 86% predictive value for failure with conventional antireflux and promotility therapy. The number of eosinophils per high power field for the determination of pathologic EE is still evolving.

The clinician must have an increased index of suspicion, knowledge of the clinical presentation, and the corroboration of other laboratory data to suspect EE, to avoid overlooking the diagnosis. Ancillary tests such as allergy testing, peripheral blood eosinophil counts, and IgE levels may also assist in the diagnosis, but their precise value is not fully defined. It is possible that the correlation of positive ancillary tests will prove especially helpful in cases in which the eosinophil count is ≤15 eosinophils/HPF in cases of suspected EE [1].

Treatment

The treatment of EE continues to evolve and is widely debated. Current therapies are directed at eliminating or abating the eosinophilic response. Because several studies have shown convincingly that food allergy is a common cause of EE in children, diets in which the causative antigen has been eliminated have been advocated and used successfully [13,21]. Markowitz and colleagues [13] treated pediatric patients using an elemental diet with an amino acid-based formula. They were able to demonstrate a decrease in eosinophils from 33 to 1 eosinophil/HPF. The practicality of this approach is difficult because this formula is not palatable; therefore, many patients require an administration of the formula through a nasogastric tube

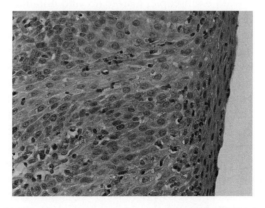

Fig. 3. Esophageal biopsy demonstrating ≥20 eosinophils/HPF (H&E stain, original magnification ×400).

[23]. The role of food elimination as a form of treatment has not been studied extensively in adults.

Medical treatment seems to be a more practical approach to the treatment of the symptoms of EE. Options include the use of systemic corticosteroids, topically ingested steroids, a leukotriene receptor antagonist, and anti-IL-5. Topically ingested steroids appear to be the most effective treatment with the least potential for side effects [14,23,34,44,45]. The protocol at the authors' institutions is to teach the patient a "bad inhaler technique" using a fluticasone inhaler. Fluticasone is prescribed at a dose of 220 µg per puff, four puffs twice per day, after breakfast and the evening meal (total dosage of 1760 µg/d) for 6 weeks. The patient is instructed to not use the spacer device of the inhaler to maximize the drug delivery to the esophagus. After shaking the inhaler, the patient is instructed to take a deep breath and, at the point of maximum held inspiration, to depress the inhaler and swallow the aerosol with each puff. To decrease problems with transient dry mouth and deposition of steroid in the mouth (potentially leading to candidiasis), the patient is instructed to rinse the mouth with water and spit. In patients in whom candidiasis or thrush does occur, nystatin, 100,000 units per 5 mL daily, swish and swallow, is prescribed for 5 days. After using their fluticasone spray, patients are instructed to avoid food or drink for 3 hours after dispensing [34,44]. This swallow technique with the inhaler is difficult to teach to small children. The delivery of nasal fluticasone (110–220 µg per dose) mixed in chocolate syrup has been found to be equally successful (Dana M. Thompson, MD, unpublished data) in the toddler patient group. Symptoms generally improve within days to a few weeks after treatment. Treatment responses have been excellent, showing some reversal of endoscopic findings and symptom improvement. Post-treatment histologic evaluation has demonstrated a reduction in the number of eosinophils as well as other markers of eosinophilic inflammation (CD3$^+$ and CD8$^+$ lymphocytes) [14,46]. The current data suggest that patients treated with swallowed fluticasone have improved endoscopic, histologic, and immunologic parameters associated with EE [14,46].

Oral corticosteroids have also proven effective for the treatment of EE [47,48], with a recently published post-treatment reduction in eosinophil count from 34 to 1.5 eosinophils/HPF [48]. However, the potential for serious side effects makes systemic steroids a less desirable option for first-line therapy and is probably best reserved for relapses or resistant cases.

Montelukast (montelukast sodium, Singulair, Merck), a leukotriene receptor antagonist, has also been used in the treatment of EE [49–51]. Leukotrienes are released predominantly by eosinophils, basophils, and mast cells and are involved in eosinophil attraction and migration. The clinical effects of leukotrienes include smooth muscle constriction, airway edema, mucous hypersecretion, and reduction of ciliary motility [52]. Montelukast works by selectively inhibiting the eosinophil leukotriene D4 receptor. Its primary use has been in the treatment of asthma [53]. The proposed theory behind using this drug for symptomatic treatment of EE is that it selectively blocks the D4 receptor of the cysteinyl leukotriene present on the eosinophils. By blocking this receptor, montelukast theoretically reduces the inflammatory action of the eosinophil. Although this treatment does not result in a reduction in the number of eosinophils present, their action is nullified [49,50,52]. The study by Attwood and colleagues [49] reported the use of this drug in eight patients treated with 10-100 mg per day. Initially, seven of eight patients demonstrated a complete subjective improvement in dysphagia. The patients were placed subsequently on a maintenance does of 20 to 40 mg per day. Six of the eight patients reported a recurrence of symptoms within 3 weeks of stopping the medication. No biopsies were performed after the medication was taken, therefore the degree of esophageal eosinophilia on medication or after treatment is unknown.

The monoclonal antibody anti-IL-5 may play a role in the treatment of patients who have severe EE. IL-5 is a strong eosinophilic activator and is involved in regulating the production and recruitment of eosinophils. Anti-IL-5 therapy (mepolizumab) has recently gained attention as a potential treatment for severe refractory cases of EE. A recent pilot study of 6 weeks of intravenous anti-IL-5 administration for hypereosinophilic syndromes, which included one patient who had EE, has shown efficacy with no serious adverse effects and the benefit of glucocorticoid-sparing effects [54]. Additional studies with larger patient populations will be needed to substantiate these results. Regardless of which medical therapy is used for the treatment of EE, the disease appears to be a chronic condition in which initial clinical improvement and reduction of the esophageal eosinophilia are shown, but on withdrawal of these medications, symptoms [1,23] and abnormal histology may recur [1,23]. Symptom-free intervals after withdrawal from medications appear to be patient-dependent.

Endoscopy with dilation can be an important adjunctive treatment for EE patients, particularly in adults who have a history of food impaction. The risk of esophageal mucosal rents from dilation is high and can be quite frightening. Fortunately, actual esophageal perforations occurring after dilatations in this setting have rarely been reported. Adult patients will often require repeated dilations to maintain symptom-free periods [33,35]. It is very possible that adults have developed strictures caused by damage from long-standing eosinophilic disease that went unrecognized. The role of early identification of EE and treatment in adult patients may prevent stricture formation and thus the need for dilation. Prospective studies will be required to answer this question.

Prognosis

Straumann and colleagues [33] have recently reported the natural history of 30 adult patients who had EE. During the mean follow-up of 7.2 years, dysphagia persisted in 29 patients (97%). Eosinophilic inflammation was confined to the esophagus and did not progress into the stomach or duodenum. EE did not show a malignancy potential for cancer or hypereosinophilic syndrome during the follow-up. Quality of life indicators showed that socioprofessional activities were moderately impacted in a minority of these EE patients (3%), whereas 50% of the patients indicated only a mild impact. Although these data suggest that EE is likely controllable and nondisabling, it should be emphasized that 71% (15/21) of adult EE patients [34,55] and 24% (5/21) of pediatric EE patients [11] do experience serious food impaction, requiring endoscopic intervention for the removal of a food bolus.

Further insights into the natural history of EE may be extrapolated from other allergic disorders, such as atopic dermatitis and bronchial asthma. Patients who develop these diseases during early childhood often outgrow them as they mature. Other patients continue to struggle with these problems into adulthood. Thus, limited data exist for the natural history of EE, and the long-term prognosis for pediatric EE patients is therefore uncertain. Additionally, it is not uncommon for patients to have both asthma and EE, and steroid treatment for asthma is common practice; therefore, it is not know how many patients who have asthma also have inadvertent, partially treated EE.

Case examples

Case 1

A 29 year old man presented with a 3 month history of mild dysphonia, globus sensation and 9 month history of dysphagia progressing to food impaction. As a professional musician and singer, his concerns prompted an otolaryngologic consultation for further evaluation. His past medical history was significant for biopsy proven and treated GERD. He had an additional contributing history of asthma, atopy, cat allergy and seasonal rhinitis. Incidentally, this episode occurred at the height of pollen season. During the previous 8 years, he had undergone three esophagogastroduodenoscopic (EGD) examinations with dilation for a presumed Schatzki's ring. He noted immediate improvement of dysphagia and food impaction. Videostrobolaryngoscopy demonstrated bilateral vocal fold nodules and mild posterior glottic edematous changes without erythema. A contrast esophagram was unremarkable. The EGD was reported as visually normal. Dilation was undertaken, but biopsies were not obtained by the examining endoscopist because of the visually normal appearance of the esophageal mucosal lining. Food impaction and dysphagia symptoms resolved. Thirteen months later, at age 30, the patient presented to the emergency department with symptomatic food impaction requiring urgent EGD, with removal of an impacted bolus and dilation of the esophagus. This episode likewise occurred at the height of pollen season. Biopsies were not obtained. GERD was assumed to be responsible for his symptoms, prompting the initiation of proton pump inhibitor (PPI) therapy. Laryngoscopy 3 months after the initiation of PPI therapy showed persistent vocal-fold nodules and mild posterior glottic edematous changes. He had persistent globus sensation despite PPI therapy and dilation of the esophagus. Given his asthma and atopic history along with food impaction, a diagnosis of EE was entertained. The patient was referred for EGD with an express request for biopsies. The examination was visually normal; however, distal, mid, and proximal esophageal biopsies demonstrated 41 eosinophils/HPF. He was treated with a 6-week course of oral fluticasone and continued PPI therapy. Three-month and 9-month post therapy laryngoscopic examinations showed a resolution of the vocal-fold nodules. The patient also reported symptomatic resolution of globus, dysphonia, and dysphagia.

This case illustrates the importance of correlating the clinical history of atopy, asthma, food impaction, and the failure to improve with reflux medications to recognize that EE is part of the clinical spectrum. Another clue to the diagnosis in this patient is the exacerbation of his symptoms with the peaking of pollen season, to which he was allergic. This case also illustrates that globus, dysphonia, and perhaps vocal-fold nodule formation may be part of the airway clinical spectrum of EE. It was not until EE was recognized and treated did the vocal fold nodules disappear in this professional singer. This patient's history of seasonal rhinitis, atopy, and asthma also supports the possibility of the respiratory tract (sinonasal or tracheal-bronchial) as the portal of entry of the antigen responsible for his EE.

Case 2

A 33-month-old boy presented with a history of 12 episodes of "recurrent croup" requiring emergency department evaluation and management. There was no seasonal variation to the croup episodes. The symptoms responded to racemic epinephrine and intravenous dexamethasone. His medical history was significant for a 28-month period of recurrent emesis and regurgitation for which he was treated first with ranitidine, starting at 8 months of age. Because there was no improvement, lansoprazole was added at 18 months of age. Although his condition improved overall after the addition of lansoprazole, he continued to have trouble with regurgitation. His parents also noted a brassy quality to his voice. He was described as a picky eater and was at the 16th percentile for weight. The result of RAST testing for food allergies was negative. Because of the recurrent nature of his breathing symptoms, voice quality, and persistent emesis, he was taken to the operating room for microlaryngoscopy, rigid bronchoscopy, and esophagoscopy. Microlaryngoscopy demonstrated bilateral vocal cord nodules and laryngeal edematous changes. Bronchoscopy showed a grade I subglottic stenosis, mild mucosal edematous changes, and cobble-stoning effect. Esophagoscopy showed mild mucosal edema and furrowing effect. Esophageal biopsies taken from the distal and mid esophagus demonstrated 40 eosinophils/HPF. The child was treated with oral fluticasone mixed in chocolate syrup for 6 weeks. Repeat endoscopy with biopsy, performed 8 weeks after treatment, showed no evidence of subglottic stenosis and a resolution of the esophageal eosinophilia. By 3 months after fluticasone treatment, the vocal nodules had disappeared, and the symptom of emesis had resolved. At 1 year after the diagnosis and treatment of EE, he has had two episodes of croup, no further regurgitation or emesis, and no recurrence of vocal-fold nodules, and he is now at the 56th percentile for weight.

This case is also illustrates the need for providers to have a high index of suspicion to accurately diagnose EE. This child's persistent symptoms of emesis and food refusal despite maximum medical reflux therapy provided the clue that EE was a strong possibility. This case, like the first, highlights that upper airway manifestations are part of the spectrum of EE and respond to EE treatment. The subglottic inflammation present in this case was likely responsible for the recurrent nature of the croup-like illnesses. Interestingly, the number of these episodes decreased dramatically after the identification and treatment of EE. It may be that EE is a precursor or a contributing factor to the formation of subglottic stenosis in high-risk patients.

Summary

Eosinophilic esophagitis is a unique clinicopathologic entity that has slowly gained attention over the past decade but has not been well recognized in the field of otolaryngology. The precise cause of the disease is unknown but is likely associated with food and environmental allergic antigens. Both IgE-mediated and non-IgE-mediated mechanisms are involved in the pathophysiology of the disease. Otolaryngologists should be familiar with the presentation because many patients experience concomitant pharyngolaryngeal and airway symptoms. As the otolaryngologist's role in the evaluation and management of esophageal disease continues to expand, it will be imperative to consider EE as a potential diagnosis among young children with feeding disorders and adolescents and adults with dysphagia. Esophagoscopy with biopsies of the proximal, mid, and distal esophagus are essential in diagnosing EE. Food allergy testing (RAST or skin prick or patch) may be helpful in identifying possible causative agents that should be restricted or eliminated. Peripheral eosinophil counts and IgE, although frequently elevated, are less specific for the disease. Swallowed or inhaled corticosteroids have been shown to be effective and well tolerated, but other options exist for refractory cases.

References

[1] Dauer EH, Freese DK, El-Youssef M, et al. Charateristics of eosiniphilic esophagitis in children. Ann Otol Rhinol Laryngol 2005;114:827–33.

[2] Orenstein SR, Shalaby TM, Di Lorenzo C, et al. The spectrum of pediatric eosinophilic esophagitis beyond infancy: a clinical series of 30 children. Am J Gastroenterol 2000;95: 1422–30 [erratum appears in Am J Gastroenterol 2001;96(7):2290].

[3] Hartnick C, Liu J, Cotton R, et al. Subglottic stenosis complicated by allergic esophagitis: case report. Ann Otol Rhinol Laryngol 2002;111:57–60.

[4] Dobbins J, Sheahan D, Behar J. Eosinophilic gastroenteritis with esophageal involvement. Gastroenterology 1977;72:1312–6.

[5] Landres R, Kuster G, Strum W. Eosinophilic esophagitis in a patient with vigorous achalasia. Gastroenterology 1978;74:1298–301.

[6] Lee RG. Marked eosinophilia in esophageal mucosal biopsies. Am J Surg Pathol 1985;9: 475–9.

[7] Picus D, Frank PH. Eosinophilic esophagitis. AJR Am J Roentgenol 1981;136:1001–3.

[8] Feczko PJ, Halpert RD, Zonca M. Radiographic abnormalities in eosinophilic esophagitis. Gastrointest Radiol 1985;10:321–4.

[9] Attwood S, Smyrk T, Demeester T, et al. Esophageal eosinophilia with dysphagia: a distinct clinicopathologic syndrome. Dig Dis Sci 1993;38:109–16.

[10] Liacouras CA. Failed Nissen fundoplication in two patients who had persistent vomiting and eosinophilic esophagitis. J Pediatr Surg 1997;32:1504–6.

[11] Cheung KM, Oliver MR, Cameron DJ, et al. Esophageal eosinophilia in children with dysphagia. J Pediatr Gastroenterol Nutr 2003;37:498–503.

[12] Fox VL, Nurko S, Furuta GT. Eosinophilic esophagitis: it's not just kid's stuff. Gastrointest Endosc 2002;56:260–70.

[13] Markowitz JE, Spergel JM, Ruchelli E, et al. Elemental diet is an effective treatment for eosinophilic esophagitis in children and adolescents. Am J Gastroenterol 2003;98: 777–82.

[14] Teitelbaum JE, Fox VL, Twarog FJ, et al. Eosinophilic esophagitis in children: immunopathological analysis and response to fluticasone propionate. Gastroenterology 2002;122: 1216–25.

[15] Fogg MI, Ruchelli E, Spergel JM. Pollen and eosinophilic esophagitis. J Allergy Clin Immunol 2003;112:796–7.

[16] Rothenberg ME. Eosinophilic gastrointestinal disorders (EGID). J Allergy Clin Immunol 2004;113:11–28.

[17] Justinich CJ, Ricci A Jr, Kalafus DA, et al. Activated eosinophils in esophagitis in children: a transmission electron microscopic study. J Pediatr Gastroenterol Nutr 1997;25:194–8.

[18] Kato M, Kephart GM, Talley NJ, et al. Eosinophil infiltration and degranulation in normal human tissue. Anat Rec 1998;252:418–25.

[19] Rothenberg ME, Mishra A, Collins MH, et al. Pathogenesis and clinical features of eosinophilic esophagitis. J Allergy Clin Immunol 2001;108:891–4.

[20] Gleich GJ, Adolphson CR, Leiferman KM. The biology of the eosinophilic leukocyte. Annu Rev Med 1993;44:85–101.

[21] Kelly KJ, Lazenby AJ, Rowe PC, et al. Eosinophilic esophagitis attributed to gastroesophageal reflux: improvement with an amino acid-based formula. Gastroenterology 1995;109: 1503–12.

[22] Liacouras CA. Eosinophilic esophagitis in children and adults. J Pediatr Gastroenterol Nutr 2003;37(Suppl 1):S23–8.

[23] Liacouras CA, Ruchelli E. Eosinophilic esophagitis. Curr Opin Pediatr 2004;16:560–6.

[24] Spergel JM, Beausoleil JL, Mascarenhas M, et al. The use of skin prick tests and patch tests to identify causative foods in eosinophilic esophagitis. J Allergy Clin Immunol 2002;109: 363–8.

[25] Mishra A, Hogan SP, Brandt EB, et al. An etiological role for aeroallergens and eosinophils in experimental esophagitis. J Clin Invest 2001;107:83–90.

[26] Mishra A, Hogan SP, Brandt EB, Rothenberg ME. IL-5 promotes eosinophil trafficking to the esophagus. J Immunol 2002;168:2464–9.

[27] Mishra A, Rothenberg ME. Intratracheal IL-13 induces eosinophilic esophagitis by an IL-5, eotaxin-1, and STAT6-dependent mechanism. Gastroenterology 2003;125:1419–27.

[28] Straumann A, Bauer M, Fischer B, et al. Idiopathic eosinophilic esophagitis is associated with a T(H)2-type allergic inflammatory response. J Allergy Clin Immunol 2001;108: 954–61.

[29] Fujiwara H, Morita A, Kobayashi H, et al. Infiltrating eosinophils and eotaxin: their association with idiopathic eosinophilic esophagitis. Ann Allergy Asthma Immunol 2002;89: 429–32.

[30] Munitiz V, Martinez de Haro LF, Ortiz A, et al. Primary eosinophilic esophagitis. Dis Esophagus 2003;16:165–8.

[31] Koufman JA, Aviv JE, Casiano RR, et al. Laryngopharyngeal reflux: position statement of the committee on speech, voice, and swallowing disorders of the American Academy of Otolaryngology-Head and Neck Surgery [review article]. Otolaryngol Head Neck Surg 2002; 127:32–5.

[32] Markowitz JE, Liacouras CA. Eosinophilic esophagitis. Gastroenterol Clin North Am 2003; 32:949–66.

[33] Straumann A, Spichtin HP, Grize L, et al. Natural history of primary eosinophilic esophagitis: a follow-up of 30 adult patients for up to 11.5 years. Gastroenterology 2003;125: 1660–9.

[34] Arora AS, Perrault J, Smyrk TC. Topical corticosteroid treatment of dysphagia due to eosinophilic esophagitis in adults. Mayo Clin Proc 2003;78:830–5.

[35] Croese J, Fairley SK, Masson JW, et al. Clinical and endoscopic features of eosinophilic esophagitis in adults. Gastrointest Endosc 2003;58:516–22.

[36] Furuta GT. Clinicopathologic features of esophagitis in children. Gastrointest Endosc Clin N Am 2001;11:683–715.

[37] Langdon DE. "Congenital" esophageal stenosis, corrugated ringed esophagus, and eosinophilic esophagitis. Am J Gastroenterol 2000;95:2123–4.

[38] Gupta SK, Fitzgerald JF, Chong SK, et al. Vertical lines in distal esophageal mucosa (VLEM): a true endoscopic manifestation of esophagitis in children? Gastrointest Endosc 1997;45:485–9.

[39] Siafakas CG, Ryan CK, Brown MR, et al. Multiple esophageal rings: an association with eosinophilic esophagitis: case report and review of the literature. Am J Gastroenterol 2000;95:1572–5.

[40] Vasilopoulos S, Murphy P, Auerbach A, et al. The small-caliber esophagus: an unappreciated cause of dysphagia for solids in patients with eosinophilic esophagitis. Gastrointest Endosc 2002;55:99–106.

[41] Ahmad M, Soetikno RM, Ahmed A. The differential diagnosis of eosinophilic esophagitis. J Clin Gastroenterol 2000;30:242–4.

[42] Walsh SV, Antonioli DA, Goldman H, et al. Allergic esophagitis in children: a clinicopathological entity. Am J Surg Pathol 1999;23:390–6.

[43] Ruchelli E, Wenner W, Voytek T, et al. Severity of esophageal eosinophilia predicts response to conventional gastroesophageal reflux therapy. Pediatr Dev Pathol 1999;2:15–8.

[44] Faubion WA Jr, Perrault J, Burgart LJ, et al. Treatment of eosinophilic esophagitis with inhaled corticosteroids. J Pediatr Gastroenterol Nutr 1998;27:90–3.

[45] Noel RJ, Putnam PE, Collins MH, et al. Clinical and immunopathologic effects of swallowed fluticasone for eosinophilic esophagitis. Clin Gastroenterol Hepatol 2004;2:568–75.

[46] Noel RJ, Putnam PE, Rothenberg ME. Eosinophilic esophagitis. N Engl J Med 2004;351: 940–1.

[47] Zein NN, Perrault J, Freese DK, et al. Idiopathic eosinophilic esophagitis in children: a distinct syndrome. Gastroenterology 1996;110:A305.

[48] Liacouras CA, Wenner WJ, Brown K, et al. Primary eosinophilic esophagitis in children: successful treatment with oral corticosteroids. J Pediatr Gastroenterol Nutr 1998;26:380–5.

[49] Attwood SE, Lewis CJ, Bronder CS, et al. Eosinophilic oesophagitis: a novel treatment using Montelukast. Gut 2003;52:181–5.
[50] Schwartz DA, Pardi DS, Murray JA. Use of montelukast as steroid-sparing agent for recurrent eosinophilic gastroenteritis. Dig Dis Sci 2001;46:1787–90.
[51] Neustrom MR, Friesen C. Treatment of eosinophilic gastroenteritis with montelukast [letter]. J Allergy Clin Immunol 1999;104(2 Pt 1):506.
[52] Samuelsson B. Leukotrienes: mediators of immediate hypersensitivity reaction and inflammation. Science 1983;220:568–75.
[53] Sampson A, Holgate S. Leukotriene modifiers in the treatment of Asthma. BJM 1998;316: 1257–8.
[54] Garrett JK, Jameson SC, Thomson B, et al. Anti-interleukin-5 (mepolizumab) therapy for hypereosinophilic syndromes. J Allergy Clin Immunol 2004;113:115–9.
[55] Arora AS, Yamazaki K. Eosinophilic esophagitis: asthma of the esophagus? Clin Gastroenterol Hepatol 2004;2:523–30.

ELSEVIER
SAUNDERS

Otolaryngol Clin N Am
39 (2006) 223–227

OTOLARYNGOLOGIC
CLINICS
OF NORTH AMERICA

Index

Note: Page numbers of article titles are in **boldface** type.

A

Acellular dermis, for injection laryngoplasty, 47

Adam's apple, reduction of, 80, 81

Adductor laryngeal breathing dystonia, 87–88, 101

Aeroallergens, environmental, eosinophilic esophagitis and, 208

Airway, upper, symptoms of eosinophilic esophagitis in, 210–211

Alloderm implant, in injection laryngoplasty, 47, 120
in sulcus vocalis, 34–35

Anesthesia, for medialization thyroplasty, 61–62
for office-based laryngeal procedures, 113–116
general, for endoscopic cordectomy for glottic carcinoma, 200–201

Ansa cervicalis nerves, and selective adductor denervation reinnervation surgery, 105

Arytenoid adduction, 58, 63–65
cricoarytenoid area exposure in, 65–66
cricoarytenoid joint identification in, 66
edema in, 66
future intubation and, 66–67
recurrent laryngeal nerve and, 66
surgical landmarks for, 63, 64
suturing in, 64–65

B

Biopsy, and laryngoscopy, office-based, 131–132

Botulinum toxin, cautions in use of, 95
in laryngeal dystonia, 93–98
injection techniques for use of, 96–97
mechanism of action of, 94–95
outcomes in use of, 97–98
resistance to, 95

side effects of, 94–95
structure and preparation of, 93–94
types of, 93

Bovine collagen, for injection laryngoplasty, 45

Brush biopsy, of larynx, in-office, 128–131

C

Carbon dioxide laser, for ablation of laryngeal papilloma, 141–142
in laryngology, 160–162

Child(ren), management of laryngeal papilloma in, **135–158**

Chondrolaryngoplasty, 80, 81

Cidofovir, in laryngeal papilloma, 144–146
injection of, for papilloma management, 124–125
equipment for, 125
indications for, 124
sites for, 125

Cold excision, of laryngeal papilloma, 141–142

Collagen, autologous, for injection laryngoplasty, 46–47
bovine, for injection laryngoplasty, 45
injection of, in sulcus vocalis, 33

Cordectomy(ies), endoscopic, in glottic carcinoma, and quality of life, 196–197
classification of, 178–179
indications for, 192
results of, 195–196
six-month evaluation following, 199–200
speech therapy following, 199
techniques for, 192–194
voice assessment following, 192, 197–199
reconstruction of glottic defects after, **191–204**

Corticosteroids, oral, in eosinophilic esophagitis, 214

Cricothyroid approximation, 70–71
to elevate vocal pitch, 80–82

Cricothyroid subluxation, 71–72

Cymetra, in injection laryngoplasty, 47

D

Dysphonia, laryngeal surgery in. See
Laryngeal framework surgery.
paralytic, approximation laryngeal
framework surgery in, versus
injection augmentation, 68–69
spasmodic, adductor, classification of,
101
selective adductor
denervation
reinnervation surgery
in, 102–103
treatment with laryngeal
adductor
reinnervation surgery,
101–109
voice breaks in, 102

Dystonia, adductor laryngeal breathing,
87–88, 101
laryngeal. See also *Dysphonia,
spasmodic.*
botulinum toxin in, 93–98
clinical classification of, 91–92
dystonias associated with, 88
etiology of, 88–89
evaluation of, 89–91
hyperfunction of laryngeal
muscles in, 87–88
synonyms for, 87
treatment options in, 92–93

E

Endolarynx, in surgical position, 19, 20
surgery of, 159

Endoscopic cordectomy. See
Cordectomy(ies), endoscopic.

Endoscopy, for treatment of early glottic
carcinoma, **173–189**
with biopsy, in eosinophilic
esophagitis, 211–213
with dilation, in eosinophilic
esophagitis, 215

Eosinophilic esophagitis. See *Esophagitis,
eosinophilic.*

Esophagitis, eosinophilic, and upper airway
symptoms, 210–211
case examples of, 216–218
cause and pathophysiology of,
207–209

clinical presentation of, 209–211
diagnosis of, 211–213
endoscopy with biopsy in,
211–213
environmental aeroallergens and,
208
food allergy and, 207–208
gastroesophageal reflux disease
and, 206, 209
prognosis in, 215–216
role in aerodigestive tract
disorders, **205–221**
symptoms of, 205, 206
treatment of, 213–215

F

Fascia, for injection laryngoplasty, 47

Fascia implant (superficial or deep), in
sulcus vocalis, 36

Fat, for injection laryngoplasty, 47–48

Fat implant (superficial lamina propria), in
sulcus vocalis, 36

Fat injection, deep, in sulcus vocalis, 35–36

Fiberscopy, through laryngeal mask airway,
192–193, 194

Fibroblast growth factor, for injection
laryngoplasty, 48

Food allergy, eosinophilic esophagitis and,
207–208

G

Gastroesophageal reflux disease, and
eosinophilic esophagitis, 206, 209

Glottic carcinoma, early, endoscopic
treatment for, **173–189**
classification of
cordectomies for,
178–179
instrumentation for,
174–175
preoperative and
intraoperative
work-up for, 175–178
selection criteria for, 174
endoscopic treatment of,
oncologic outcome of,
183–185
involution and treatment of, with
pulsed-dye laser, 167–169
T1b-T2 lesions, endoscopic
treatment of,
compartmental approach
for, 180–183

Changing Your Address?

Make sure your subscription changes too! When you notify us of your new address, you can help make our job easier by including an exact copy of your Clinics label number with your old address (see illustration below.) This number identifies you to our computer system and will speed the processing of your address change. Please be sure this label number accompanies your old address and your corrected address—you can send an old Clinics label with your number on it or just copy it exactly and send it to the address listed below.

We appreciate your help in our attempt to give you continuous coverage. Thank you.

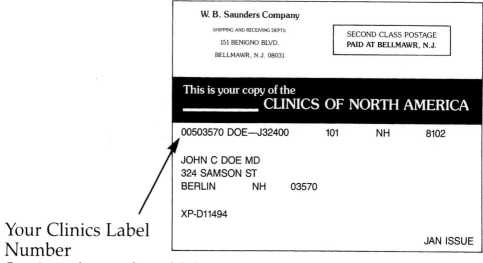

Your Clinics Label Number
Copy it exactly or send your label along with your address to:
W.B. Saunders Company, Customer Service
Orlando, FL 32887-4800
Call Toll Free 1-800-654-2452

Please allow four to six weeks for delivery of new subscriptions and for processing address changes.